THE 1983 YEAR BOOKS

The YEAR BOOK series provides in condensed form the essence of the best of the recent international medical literature. The material is selected by distinguished editors who critically review more than 500,000 journal articles each year.

Anesthesia: *Drs. Kirby, Miller, Ostheimer, Saidman, and Stoelting.*

Cancer: *Drs. Clark, Cumley, and Hickey.*

Cardiology: *Drs. Harvey, Kirkendall, Kirklin, Nadas, Resnekov, and Sonnenblick.*

Critical Care Medicine: *Dr. Rogers.*

Dentistry: *Drs. Cohen, Beaudreau, Hendler, Johnson, Moyers, Robinson, and Silverman.*

Dermatology: *Drs. Sober and Fitzpatrick.*

Diagnostic Radiology: *Drs. Bragg, Keats, Kieffer, Kirkpatrick, Koehler, Sorenson, and White.*

Drug Therapy: *Drs. Hollister and Lasagna.*

Emergency Medicine: *Dr. Wagner.*

Endocrinology: *Drs. Schwartz and Ryan.*

Family Practice: *Dr. Rakel.*

Medicine: *Drs. Rogers, Des Prez, Cline, Braunwald, Greenberger, Bondy, Epstein, and Malawista.*

Neurology and Neurosurgery: *Drs. De Jong, Sugar, and Currier.*

Nuclear Medicine: *Drs. Hoffer, Gottschalk, and Zaret.*

Obstetrics and Gynecology: *Drs. Pitkin and Zlatnik.*

Ophthalmology: *Dr. Ernest.*

Orthopedics: *Dr. Coventry.*

Otolaryngology: *Drs. Strong and Paparella.*

Pathology and Clinical Pathology: *Dr. Brinkhous.*

Pediatrics: *Drs. Oski and Stockman.*

Plastic and Reconstructive Surgery: *Drs. McCoy, Brauer, Haynes, Hoehn, Miller, and Whitaker.*

Psychiatry and Applied Mental Health: *Drs. Freedman, Kolb, Lourie, Meltzer, Nemiah, and Weiner.*

Sports Medicine: *Drs. Krakauer, Shephard and Torg, Col. Anderson, and Mr. George.*

Surgery: *Drs. Schwartz, Najarian, Peacock, Shires, Silen, and Spencer.*

Urology: *Drs. Gillenwater and Howards.*

TOPICS IN ADOLESCENT MEDICINE

A Year Book Special Edition

Topics in Adolescent Medicine

A Year Book Special Edition

Edited by

ROBERT B. SHEARIN, M.D.

*Director, Children and Youth Ambulatory Service,
and Division of Adolescent Medicine;
Associate Professor of Pediatrics,
Department of Pediatrics,
Georgetown University Medical Center,
Washington, D.C.*

YEAR BOOK MEDICAL PUBLISHERS
CHICAGO • LONDON

Printed in U.S.A.

Library of Congress Catalog Card Number: 83–060526

International Standard Book Number: 0–8151–7675–9

Table of Contents

Acknowledgments

The abstracts included in this book were selected from volumes published in the 1982 and 1983 YEAR BOOK Series. Authors of editorial comments which accompany individual abstracts are identified by their initials. The following list is a key to the YEAR BOOK sources used.

A.S.N.—Alexander S. Nadas, M.D.—CARDIOLOGY
C.E.D.—Charles E. Driscoll, M.D.—FAMILY PRACTICE
D.E.R.—David E. Rogers, M.D.—MEDICINE
D.F.R.—Dale F. Redig, D.D.S.—DENTISTRY (1982)
D.K.W.—David K. Wagner, M.D.—EMERGENCY MEDICINE
E.B.—Eugene Braunwald, M.D.—MEDICINE
F.H.E.—Franklin H. Epstein, M.D.—MEDICINE
————H.A. Peterson, M.D.—ORTHOPEDICS (1982)
H.B.G.R.—Hamilton B.G. Robinson, D.D.S., M.S., Sc.D.(Hon.)—DENTISTRY
————Howard J. Weinstein, M.D.—PEDIATRICS (1982)
H.W.—Herbert Weiner, M.D.—PSYCHIATRY AND APPLIED MENTAL HEALTH
H.Y.M.—Herbert Y. Meltzer, M.D.—PSYCHIATRY AND APPLIED MENTAL HEALTH
J.A.S.—James A. Stockman, III, M.D.—PEDIATRICS
J.C.N.—John C. Nemiah, M.D.—PSYCHIATRY AND APPLIED MENTAL HEALTH
————Jackson E. Fowler, Jr., M.D.—UROLOGY (1982)
J.S.T.—Joseph S. Torg, M.D.—SPORTS MEDICINE
L.C.L.—Louis C. Lasagna, M.D.—DRUG THERAPY
L.E.H.—Leo E. Hollister, M.D.—DRUG THERAPY
L.J.K.—Lewis J. Krakauer, M.D., F.A.C.P.—SPORTS MEDICINE
M.B.C.—Mark B. Coventry, M.D., M.S.—ORTHOPEDICS
M.J.C.—Martin J. Cline, M.D.—MEDICINE
M.L.H.—Merle L. Hale, B.A., D.D.S., M.S.—DENTISTRY (1982)
N.J.G.—Norton J. Greenberger, M.D.—MEDICINE
O.S.—Oscar Sugar, M.D.—NEUROLOGY AND NEUROSURGERY
P.G.C.—Phillip G. Couchman, M.D.—FAMILY PRACTICE
————R.A. Klassen, M.D.—ORTHOPEDICS (1982)
R.D.C.—Robert D. Currier, M.D.—NEUROLOGY AND NEUROSURGERY
R.E.M.—Robert E. Moyers, D.D.S., Ph.D.—DENTISTRY
R.E.R.—Robert E. Rakel, M.D.—FAMILY PRACTICE
————R.H. Fitzgerald, Jr., M.D.—ORTHOPEDICS (1982)
R.J.S.—Roy J. Shephard, M.D., Ph.D.—SPORTS MEDICINE
R.L.C.—Randolph Lee Clark, B.S., M.D., M.Sc. (Surgery), D.Sc. (Hon.)—CANCER
R.L.D.—Richard L. Dobson, M.D.—DERMATOLOGY (1982)
R.M.P.—Roy M. Pitkin, M.D.—OBSTETRICS AND GYNECOLOGY
R.N.D.J.—Russell N. De Jong, M.D.—NEUROLOGY AND NEUROSURGERY

R.O.B.—Raymond O. Brauer, M.D.—PLASTIC AND RECONSTRUCTIVE SURGERY

R.S.L.—Reginald S. Lourie, M.D.—PSYCHIATRY AND APPLIED MENTAL HEALTH

R.W.A.—Richard W. Altreuter, M.D.—EMERGENCY MEDICINE

S.J.D.—Steven J. Davidson, M.D.—EMERGENCY MEDICINE

S.S.H.—Stuart S. Howards, M.D.—UROLOGY

T.B.S.—Theodore B. Schwartz, M.D.—ENDOCRINOLOGY

W.G.R.—Will G. Ryan, M.D.—ENDOCRINOLOGY

W.P.H.—W. Proctor Harvey, M.D.—CARDIOLOGY

Journals Represented

Acta Dermato-Venereologica (Stockholm)
Acta Odontologica Scandinavica
American Family Physician
American Heart Journal
American Journal of Cardiology
American Journal of Diseases of Children
American Journal of Epidemiology
American Journal of Medicine
American Journal of Obstetrics and Gynecology
American Journal of Orthodontics
American Journal of Psychiatry
American Journal of Roentgenology
American Journal of Sports Medicine
Annals of Allergy
Annals of Emergency Medicine
Annals of Internal Medicine
Annals of Plastic Surgery
Annals of Rheumatic Diseases
Archives of Dermatological Research
Archives of Dermatology
Archives of Disease in Childhood
Archives of General Psychiatry
Archives of Internal Medicine
Archives of Neurology
Archives of Otolaryngology
Archives of Surgery
Arthritis and Rheumatism
Athletic Training
Biological Psychiatry
Blood
British Journal of Dermatology
British Journal Obstetrics and Gynaecology
British Journal of Psychiatry
British Medical Journal
Canadian Journal of Psychiatry
Cancer
Cancer Treatment Reports
Chemotherapy
Chest
Chirurg
Circulation
Clinical Endocrinology
Clinical and Experimental Dermatology
Clinical Pediatrics (Philadelphia)
Clinical Pharmacology and Therapeutics

Clinical Science
Comprehensive Psychiatry
Cutis
Dermatologica
Developmental Medicine and Child Neurology
European Journal of Orthodontics
European Journal of Respiratory Diseases
Fertility and Sterility
Foot and Ankle
Gastroenterology
Hospital Practice
International Journal of Andrology
International Journal of Dermatology
International Journal of Radiation Oncology, Biology, Physics
Journal of Adolescent Health Care
Journal of Allergy & Clinical Immunology
Journal of the American Academy of Child Psychiatry
Journal of the American Academy of Dermatology
Journal of the American Dental Association
Journal of the American Medical Association
Journal of Bone and Joint Surgery (American volume)
Journal of Bone and Joint Surgery (British volume)
Journal of Child Psychology and Psychiatry
Journal of Clinical Endocrinology & Metabolism
Journal of Dermatology (Tokyo)
Journal of Family Practice
Journal of the Medical Society of New Jersey
Journal of the National Cancer Institute
Journal of Nervous and Mental Disease
Journal of Neurosurgery
Journal of Oral and Maxillofacial Surgery
Journal of Sports Medicine and Physical Fitness
Journal of Trauma
Journal of Urology
Lancet
Mayo Clinic Proceedings
Medical Aspects of Human Sexuality
Medical Journal of Australia
Nature
Neurology (New York)
New England Journal of Medicine
Obstetrics and Gynecology
Oral Surgery, Oral Medicine, Oral Pathology
Pediatrics
Physician and Sportsmedicine
Postgraduate Medicine
Psychological Medicine
Psychosomatic Medicine
Scandinavian Journal of Clinical and Laboratory Investigation
Scandinavian Journal of Urology and Nephrology
Science
Seminars in Perinatology
Southern Medical Journal
Urology

Introduction

The strength of this Year Book Special Edition lies in the fact that it brings together under one cover diverse and expert opinion and summaries of major articles from all disciplines that address the health of adolescents and young adults. Its purpose is to offer the clinician a review and quick reference to the major problems which confront him on a daily basis. With the exception of two articles in the General Topics section which are new selections from the *Journal of Adolescent Health Care,* the articles in this book were chosen from the approximately 8,000 articles selected by the 94 YEAR BOOK Editors for inclusion in the current editions of the 24 medical specialty and dentistry YEAR BOOKS.

I have organized the book into fifteen sections covering major topics which impact on adolescent health care. In each section, my general comments provide an overview. These are followed by the YEAR BOOK abstracts, most of which are accompanied by comments from experts in the particular field. At the end of each section, a list of other key articles gleaned from the YEAR BOOKS is offered.

The number of articles dealing with adolescents and young adults has grown in recent years as more health care professionals administer to this age group. Within the YEAR BOOK series, adolescents as a group are distinguished in only two volumes, the YEAR BOOK OF PEDIATRICS and the YEAR BOOK OF PSYCHIATRY, but adolescent patients are included in most if not all of the others. They may represent the age extremes of children or adults in a study of a specific disease, or a paper may discuss a problem characteristic of adolescence, for example acne. As I reviewed the YEAR BOOKS, I was pleasantly surprised at the wealth of material available.

It is hoped this small volume will prove useful to students, teachers, and practitioners who work with adolescents.—R. B. SHEARIN

General Topics

"When I was fourteen I was amazed at how ignorant my father was, but when I reached the age of twenty-one I was surprised how much he had learned in seven years."—WILL ROGERS

Adolescent health care also has matured since 1968 and today, health care professionals are offering treatment programs, conducting research, and making observations that benefit this once forgotten age group. The articles in this section demonstrate the variety of areas of adolescent medicine that are being studied. This general section includes many broad topics as well as those articles which do not seem to fit into a specific section. Of general concern are two articles which point out the need for improving the health care environment in order to improve compliance in the adolescent. Even though the article by Neinstein deals with psychiatric care and the one by Kellam et al. deals with general health care, the principles offered are similar: The first recommends that health care facilities analyze factors in their own environment which may influence the appointment keeping of the adolescent, while the second suggests that the presence of peer leaders in the environment in which the adolescent is seen will improve compliance and appointment-keeping behavior.

The article on mothers of adolescent mothers offers insight for the health care professional working with a pregnant adolescent and her offspring. The mother-daughter relationship here becomes an extremely important concept. In this situation, addition of the infant to the family is not clearly detrimental and may improve the relationship between the mother of an adolescent mother and her daughter.

Another interesting article is the one on vomiting and parotid enlargement. Parotid enlargement in an adolescent patient may be a clinical sign of persistent or recurrent vomiting and the only presenting feature of bulimia or anorexia nervosa. This is a clinical pearl to add to our armamentarium for early diagnosis of bulimia or anorexia nervosa in adolescents.

Today the number of teenagers receiving tetracycline for acne is astronomical. Most health care professionals assume that there are no side effects from the use of this antibiotic. The article on tetracycline-induced esophageal ulcers indicates the contrary.

Lowering Broken Appointment Rates at a Teenage Health Center. Broken and cancelled appointments are a frustrating problem in all clinics and health care centers. Lawrence S. Neinstein (Univ. of Southern California School of Medicine, Los Angeles) under-

J. Adolesc. Health Care 3:110–113, 1982.

took a prospective study at an adolescent health center in Los Angeles, a multidisciplinary clinic for subjects aged 12–21 years, in order to elucidate the behavior of adolescents who miss appointments, and to evaluate a new triage system aimed at discouraging families with no intention of coming from making appointments. All new patient appointments over a 3-month period were recorded, and chief complaints stratified to well-adolescent care, noncosmetic problems, and cosmetic problems such as obesity. Under the triage system introduced a year later, an appointment was arranged only after the return of a form requesting identifying and medical information.

The results from the first group of adolescents are given in Table 1. About 40% of initial appointments were broken. Overall, teenagers seen for well-adolescent care had a higher no-show rate than those with noncosmetic complaints; those with cosmetic problems all showed up. When funding source was analyzed in regard to waiting time to appointment, no significant difference in scheduling appointments was found between public-funded and privately funded adolescents, although publicly funded patients had a higher no-show rate overall. The two triage methods—scheduling appointments based on telephone interviews (I) versus use of a two-page form (II)—are compared in Table 2. The 2 groups were similar in age and sex, distance from the center, source of funding, and type of chief complaint. The no-show rate was significantly lower for method II. The waiting time to appointments declined from 40 to 8 days with this method.

This study demonstrated a decrease in the rate of broken appoint-

TABLE 1.—COMPARISON OF SHOW VERSUS NO-SHOW ADOLESCENTS WITH APPOINTMENT (METHOD I).

	Shows 59.2%	No shows 39.8%
Total group (138)	(n = 83)	(n = 55)
Sex		
Female	53.7%	46.4%
Male	46.3%	53.7%
Age (mean ± SD)	14.5 ± 1.8	14.4 ± 1.6
Grade	9.2 ± 1.8	8.9 ± 1.6
Days to appointment	37.1 ± 20.5	44.1 ± 19.9
Distance to center (miles)	7.5 ± 4.3	7.3 ± 3.5
Funding		
Private funding	69.1% (47)	30.9% (21)*
Public funding	51.4% (36)	48.6% (34)
Initial complaint		
Internal (noncosmetic)	63% (57)	37% (33)
External (cosmetic features)	100% (8)	0% (0)†
Well-care	45% (18)	55% (22)

*P = 0.051; †P < 0.01.

TABLE 2.—COMPARISON OF TRIAGE METHODS I AND II.

Variables	Method I (n = 138)	Method II (n = 83)
No show rate	39.8%	18.4%*
Sex		
Male	49.3%	45.1%
Female	50.7%	54.9%
Age (mean ± S.D.)	14.4 ± 1.7	14.7 ± 2.0
Grade	9.1 ± 1.7	9.5 ± 1.6
Miles to center	7.4 ± 4.0	6.5 ± 5.1
Funding		
Private	49.3%	46.5%
Public	50.7%	53.5%
Type of complaint		
Internal	65.2%	70.1%
External	5.8%	19.4%
Well care	28%	10.4%
Time to appointment (days)	39.9 ± 2.1	7.8 ± 0.4†

*$P < 0.0001$; †$P < 0.001$.

ments among teenagers with implementation of an initial screening form. The new system required involvement of both parents and adolescents in addition to family motivation. Use of a screening form may be beneficial in reducing broken appointments of new patients at other adolescent units. Broken appointments were not related to travel distance or waiting time in this study. Family characteristics and transportation issues may prove to be significant factors, however. Adolescent health care facilities should analyze factors in their own environments that may influence appointment-keeping behavior. Attention also should be given to follow-up appointments, block versus individual appointment methods, and the use of telephone or postcard reminders.

Why Teenagers Come for Treatment: 10-Year Prospective Epidemiologic Study in Woodlawn. Sheppard G. Kellam, Jeannette D. Branch, C. Hendricks Brown, and Gary Russell (Univ. of Chicago) followed up a cohort of first-grade children living in a black ghetto (Woodlawn) in Chicago in 1966 and 1967 with respect to help-seeking behavior. The cohort was assessed in third grade and recently at age 16 or 17 years, when they were offered an opportunity to seek help in a broad treatment program addressing the psychosocial needs of adolescents. The free program, which included transportation to and from home, was based on peer intervention and backup professional services. The follow-up rate at 10 years was 75%. A total of 685 teenagers were reassessed.

J. Am. Acad. Child Psychiatry 20:447–495, Summer 1981.

About 20% of the males and 25% of the females came for treatment. Neither the mothers' ratings of symptoms in first grade nor the teenagers' self-ratings of psychologic well-being predicted coming for treatment. The mother's evaluation of a teenager's psychologic well-being was also unrelated to coming for help. Children rated by their mothers as more aggressive in follow-up interviews were likelier to come for treatment. Family atmosphere variables could not be related to treatment intake. Some sessions had much higher or much lower proportions of teenagers coming for treatment than expected, and it was found that the primary assessors elicited different teenager responses.

The black college students who conducted reassessment sessions were a significant factor in determining which teenagers came for treatment. If similar findings are obtained in research on other populations, they will have an important impact on the design of mental health services and possibly human services in general. A basic part of the design of such services would be a central concern with how to structure the function of peer leaders within communities. In the present project, peer leaders operating at a highly community-integrated level were critical to the identification and involvement of those in need of treatment.

Mothers of Adolescent Mothers. Some workers have found that adolescent parenthood affects the mother-daughter relationship adversely, while others have found the relationship to be strengthened. Carol J. Poole, Mark Scott Smith and Martha A. Hoffman (Univ. of Washington, Seattle) examined the attitudes of 44 mothers of adolescent mothers (MAM) and the relationship between them and their adolescent daughters. The women had daughters who had delivered an infant when of junior high or high school age, and the granddaughter was aged 3 months to 3 years at the time of interviewing. A standardized open-ended interview technique was used.

More than half the study population was black; 37% were white. One-third were from the middle socioeconomic group, one-third from the low-middle, and one-third from the lowest. The mean ages of the MAM and their daughters were 42.6 and 15.9 years, respectively, and the infants had a mean age of 11.5 months. More than 80% of the adolescent mothers were primigravidas, and 91% were single. More than two-thirds lived with their mothers, and one-third were employed at the time of the study. One third of the MAM had themselves been pregnant when aged 17 or younger. Attitude scores of the MAM are given in the table.

Twenty-nine of the MAM did not feel that addition of the infant had significantly affected plans for their own lives, and 34 felt that the amount of time they had for themselves or others was not significantly affected. Only 3 MAM believed that they were somehow responsible for their daughters' pregnancies, but 6 believed others felt

J. Adolesc. Health Care 3:41–43, 1982.

MEAN ATTITUDES OF MOTHERS OF ADOLESCENT MOTHERS (n = 43)*

Attitudes	Mean[†]
Own life	3.5
Daughter	3.1
Infant	3.5
Grandmother role	3.3
Baby's father	2.3

*One questionnaire discarded because of major differences between questionnaire responses and interview.

[†]4 = very positive; 1 = very negative.

it to be their fault. The adolescent was the primary infant caretaker in 80% of the homes.

Half the MAM felt closer to their daughters than before the infant was born, while 19% felt less close. Some felt that a special bond now existed between them and their daughters that they wished could have developed before. The MAM had more negative feelings about the babies' fathers than in any other area.

In general, MAM are satisfied with their own life situation and believe that their daughters are trying to be mothers. Most believe their relationship with their daughters to be closer than before the infant was born. Addition of the infant to the family clearly is not necessarily detrimental, and it may frequently enhance the relationship between the MAM and her adolescent daughter.

Evaluation of Head Trauma: Efficacy of Skull Films. Skull films have reached a level of use that is nearly automatic in the evaluation of head trauma in most emergency rooms in the United States. Stuart J. Masters (Univ. of Massachusetts, Pittsfield) reviewed data on 1,845 patients to evaluate the efficacy of skull films in acute head trauma. Seventy-nine of the patients had skull fractures, but only 7 of 33 patients with significant intracranial sequelae of injury had fractures. In none of the 33 was the treatment or the outcome influenced by findings on skull films. Seven of the 1,845 patients (0.38%) had basilar skull fractures necessitating antibiotic therapy. These were the only patients whose management and outcome were altered by the radiographic findings. The predictive value of skull films for intracranial sequelae in this series is shown in the table.

Skull fracture alone seldom indicates more serious internal head injury, and routine skull films after head trauma do not contribute effectively to the management or outcome of acute intracranial injury. The author reports there is no reason to continue to order skull examinations after trauma in either pediatric or adult patients. After thorough clinical evaluation and probing of lacerations or puncture wounds for depression, patients should be observed, in the hospital if warranted. Further neurodiagnostic evaluation is generally indicated

AJR 135:539–547, September 1980.

PREDICTIVE VALUE OF SKULL FILMS FOR INTRACRANIAL SEQUELAE*

Skull Films	No. Patients		
	Alive	Dead	Total
Negative	17	9	26
Fracture	3	4	7
Total	20	13	33

*Yates correction of chi-square: $\chi^2 = 0.42; P < .55$.

when high-yield features for predicting significant intracranial sequelae are present. It is believed that computed tomography should be the primary noninvasive diagnostic procedure. When it is unavailable, a radionuclide scan or cerebral arteriogram can be obtained or surgical intervention carried out. Skull radiography may be of value as an adjunct to clarify equivocal computed tomography findings in some cases and to evaluate palpable depression or a clinically apparent basilar fracture.

▶ [Perhaps the ordering of skull films by the emergency unit should be restricted to the neurosurgeon who plans surgical intervention and feels the need for more definitive structural information.—D.K.W.] ◀

How Useful Is Skull X-ray Examination in Trauma? John de Campo and Peter G. Petty (Melbourne), in the belief that there is a low yield from skull x-ray examination in patients with suspected, and even known, head trauma, reviewed the findings in 1,053 injured patients with possible head trauma who underwent skull x-ray examination between 1978 and 1979. Only 24 patients (2.3%) had positive radiologic findings; 16 had linear vault fracture. Two patients each had suture separation, a depressed fracture, and a compound vault fracture, and 1 each had a basal fracture and pneumocephalus. Nine patients had clinical findings necessitating admission; in 6 of them, additional care was influenced by the radiologic findings. Six other patients were admitted, but only 1 had neurologic signs requiring evacuation of an intracerebral hematoma.

Thus, in only 0.6% of patients in this series was treatment influenced by the skull x-ray findings. These included patients with depressed and compound fractures. Management also may be influenced by the finding of a radiopaque foreign body. Patients without clinical criteria do not require skull x-ray examination. No legal indications exist for such studies unless there is a logical medical indication for an investigation. Over half of the present patients could have had computed tomographic studies for the same cost as all of the skull x-ray examinations, and much more useful information would have been obtained regarding the extent of intracranial injury.

▶ [The authors, a radiologist and neurosurgeon, verify the well-established fact that

Med. J. Aust. 2:553–555, Nov. 15, 1980.

skull x-ray films in the presence of trauma are an unnecessary procedure. Even the 0.6% patients who allegedly had treatment influenced by skull x-ray findings would undoubtedly have had more appropriate analysis of intracranial structural deficits by the use of CT scanning. The one exception may remain the intracranial metallic foreign body, where CT scatter in select instances may prevent accurate localization.— D.K.W.] ◄

Early Prediction of Outcome in Head-Injured Patients. Byron Young, Robert P. Rapp, J. A. Norton, Dennis Haack, Phillip A. Tibbs, and James R. Bean (Univ. of Kentucky) examined the relation between Glasgow Coma Scale (GCS) scores in the first week after head injury and the outcome at 1 year, and also the value of computerized tomographic (CT) scan data in predicting the outcome. Study was made of 170 prospectively selected patients with penetrating missile wounds, intracranial hematomas, depressed skull fractures, and blunt injuries causing major focal neurologic deficit or unconsciousness for 6 hours or longer. The 144 male and 26 female patients had an average age of 26.2 years. All patients required either surgery or treatment in an intensive care unit. All patients were seen within 12 hours after injury, and 90% of them within 6 hours.

The outcome at 1 year is related to initial GCS scores (table). Patients in the intermediate group with a midline shift of less than 4.1 mm on initial CT scanning had a significantly higher rate of favorable outcome than those with larger shifts, but predictions made by combining shift data with initial GCS scores were not significantly more accurate than those based solely on initial GCS scores. Age alone was a marginally significant predictive factor in the intermediate group. More accurate predictions were made by means of GCS scores alone if the scores changed later to more than 7 or less than 5. No patient who later worsened had a favorable outcome, whereas over 80% of those improving to a score higher than 7 had a favorable outcome. Only 21% of patients with scores of 5–7 persisting for 1 week had a favorable outcome. At later intervals, midline shift became an important factor in improving outcome predictions. Combining the 48-hour GCS scores with shift data significantly improved the accuracy of predictions. Data obtained by combining GCS scores at 72 hours and 1 week with shift data were marginally significant for predicting outcomes.

It is concluded that GCS scores and CT midline shift data are highly accurate indicators of outcome in head-injured patients. A short delay permits highly accurate predictions to be made for patients with intermediate initial GCS scores.

► [A favorite yardstick for measuring the head-injured patient is the Glasgow Coma Scale (GCS). The GCS is easily understood and relatively simple to remember. The authors point out that the main predictive value of the GCS lies in the comparative assessment between the initial emergency evaluation and that done 24 hours later. If CT evaluation of midline shift is added, long-range predictive outcome becomes even

J. Neurosurg. 54:300–303, March 1981.

OUTCOME AT 1 YEAR RELATED TO GCS SCORES[†]

Initial[*] GCS Score	No. of Cases	Favorable Outcome		Unfavorable Outcome		
		Good Recovery	Moderate Disability	Severe Disability	Vegetative State	Dead
8–15	76	63	9	3	0	1
5–7	73	28	8	9	4	24
3–4	21	1	0	0	1	19
total	170	92	17	12	5	44

[*]GCS = Glasgow Coma Scale.
[†]Courtesy of Young, B., et al.: J. Neurosurg. 54:300–303, March 1981.

more accurate. The role in the emergency unit is to provide the initial precise data base and not attempt long-term prognostications.—D.K.W.] ◄

Vomiting and Parotid Enlargement. An increasing number of girls and young women with multiple daily episodes of self-induced postprandial vomiting have been reported. When not associated with anorexia nervosa and cachexia the condition is termed "bulimia." Fred S. Herzon and Arthur Kaufman (Univ. of New Mexico, Albuquerque) describe 3 adolescent girls with long histories of self-induced postprandial vomiting and parotid enlargement as the chief physical abnormality. The patients, aged 15–19 years, had induced vomiting after meals for up to 2 years because of a fear of gaining excess weight. The parotid glands were diffusely enlarged, and in 1 case were mildly tender to palpation. Sialography in 2 cases was normal. One patient had mild ductal dilation and acute inflammation on parotid biopsy and underwent tympanic neurectomies to relieve discomfort.

Neither nutritional nor endocrinologic disorder appears to be a likely cause of parotid enlargement in these cases. Chronic autonomic stimulation of the salivary glands, by either the frequent vomiting itself or chronic stress, is a likelier cause. The vomiting reflex triggers parasympathetic stimulation of the salivary glands through direct stimulation of secretory cells. The stress reaction involves sympathetic stimulation of the glands via their vessels. Parotid enlargement may be the only presenting physical feature of bulimia, a condition that suggests substantial psychopathology.

► [Parotid enlargement accompanies dehydration and malnutrition, findings commonly associated with bulimia.—D.K.W.] ◄

Tetracycline-Induced Esophageal Ulcers: Report of Two Cases. Drugs rarely have been implicated as a cause of esophageal ulceration, but tetracycline and doxycycline recently have been reported to produce this lesion. Dinesh C. Khera, Barry R. Herschman, and Freddy Sosa (Providence Hosp., Southfield, Mich.) describe findings in 2 patients in whom odynophagia developed shortly after in-

South. Med. J. 74:251, February 1981.
Postgrad. Med. 68:112–115, October 1980.

gesting tetracycline. A boy aged 15 who was taking 250 mg of tetracycline twice daily for acne experienced retrosternal pain and odynophagia 4 hours after having taken a capsule of the drug with only a sip of water just before falling asleep. Endoscopy disclosed an ulcer 1 cm in size located 2 cm from the incisors; biopsy showed acute inflammation and necrotic debris. Antacids were given, and complete healing occurred within a week. Results of an esophageal motility study were normal. The second patient, a woman aged 35, was using tetracycline for a dermatologic condition; she experienced severe retrosternal pain and odynophagia about 3 hours after taking a tetracycline capsule with a small amount of water at bedtime. Symptoms lasted for about 5 days before subsiding spontaneously. Endoscopy was not performed.

Patients who experience the described symptoms usually take tetracycline with only a small amount of water, often at bedtime, with the result that retrosternal pain and odynophagia develop within hours. Esophageal mucosal injury from doxycycline is thought to be secondary to the drug's acidity. Also, the position of the patient after ingesting medication may affect the length of time the drug remains in the esophagus. Patients prescribed irritant drugs should be advised to take adequate water with these medications and to avoid taking them at bedtime. These drugs should not be given to patients having esophageal obstruction or motility disorders.

▶ [Perhaps the warning here should be expanded to any of the vast number of drugs with the suffix "hydrochloride."—R.W.A.] ◀

Functional Upper Airway Obstruction: New Syndrome. Functional upper airway obstruction is an uncommon condition that must be considered in adults with apparent airway distress and stridor without abnormal findings on laryngeal examination. Nancy Haley Appelblatt and Shan Ray Baker (Univ. of Michigan) report 3 cases of what is believed to be functional upper airway obstruction in women.

Woman, 23, previously well apart from a recent upper respiratory tract infection, awoke with considerable respiratory stridor. In the emergency room she exhibited continuous inspiratory and expiratory stridor with periods of apparently complete obstruction. Hypoxia was found, with an arterial P_{O_2} of 45 mm Hg and a pH of 7.55. Indirect laryngoscopy showed marked false and true vocal cord adduction. Tracheostomy was carried out; stridor ceased when anesthesia was induced. Direct laryngoscopy was negative. Further investigation was noncontributory. The patient had an eroding marital relationship, and psychoneuroticism with hysterical convergence reaction was diagnosed. Initial attempts at decannulation failed because of recurring stridorous episodes, but decannulation was achieved 2 weeks after tracheostomy.

Functional upper airway obstruction resembles psychogenic stridor with the addition of substantial respiratory tract obstruction. The sudden onset and absence of organic disease on extensive investigation suggest hysterical laryngeal spasm, possibly induced by emo-

---

Arch. Otolaryngol. 107:305–306, May 1981.

tional stress. Tracheostomy appears warranted if indicated on clinical grounds. One patient had positive pertussis titers and was known to have injected heparin and urine; psychiatric examination revealed severe emotional distress within the family. Colleagues have told of 5 similar cases, all requiring tracheostomy; all but 1 of the patients were young women. In another case the diagnosis of functional upper airway obstruction was made early and tracheostomy was averted. Functional airway obstruction should be considered in the differential diagnosis of airway obstruction in the adult.

Testicular Ultrasound for Trauma. Ultrasonography of the genitourinary tract has been an increasingly effective diagnostic measure. Gray-scale ultrasonography has been used to evaluate scrotal lesion. N. Erick Albert (Fort Hood, Texas) reports 3 cases in which testicular ultrasound study strongly suggested rupture, which was confirmed at operation. Salvage of the remaining testicular tissue was possible in 2 cases. A boy aged 15 years exhibited increased echoes within the tunica albuginea 6 hours after direct scrotal trauma, and at operation an expanding intratesticular hematoma was found, which was evacuated. A normal testis was present 6 weeks later. A man aged 23 showed loss of the normal ultrasonic pattern and disruption of the tunica albuginea 4 days after injury and was found to have an infarcted testicle with rupture at the epididymotesticular junction. The testis was removed. A man aged 23 who had findings of hematoma formation, underwent repair of a rupture of the lower half of the testis.

Surgery in 2 of these cases, in which symptoms resolved with only symptomatic care, might have been delayed had ultrasonographic examination not confirmed testicular rupture. In both cases, testicular tissue was preserved. Abnormal testicular architecture can be identified readily by ultrasonic comparison with the usually normal contralateral testis in cases of trauma. Areas of disruption and hemorrhage are seen as dense clusters of echoes.

Ultrasonography is useful in identifying rupture and intratesticular hematoma formation in patients with testicular trauma.

Additional Reading

Callaham, M.: Prophylactic antibiotics in common dog bite wounds: A controlled study. *Ann. Emerg. Med.* 9:410, 1980.

Daras, M., and Spiro, A. J.: "Stiff-man syndrome" in an adolescent. *Pediatrics* 67:725, 1981.

Ein, S. H., et al.: Ruptured spleen: When to operate? *J. Pediatr. Surg.* 16:324, 1981.

Fritz, G. K., et al.: Functional versus organic knee pain in adolescents. *Am. J. Sports Med.* 9:247, 1981.

Goldstein, E. J. C., et al.: Dog bite wounds and infection: Prospective clinical study. *Ann. Emerg. Med.* 9:508, 1980.

J. Urol. 124:558–559, October 1980.

Grossman, J. A. I., et al.: Prophylactic antibiotics in simple hand lacerations. *J.A.M.A.* 245:1055, 1981.

Irwin, C. E., Jr., et al.: Appointment-keeping behavior in adolescents. *J. Pediatr.* 99:799, 1981.

Kalter, N., and Rembar, J.: Significance of a child's age at the time of parental divorce. *Am. J. Orthopsychiatry* 51:85, 1981.

Mann, R. J.: Human bites of the hand. *Am. Fam. Physician* 23:110, 1980.

Peeples, E., et al.: Wounds of the hand contaminated by human or animal saliva. *J. Trauma* 20:383, 1980.

Rosa, R. M., et al.: Study of induced hyponatremia in prevention and treatment of sickle cell crisis. *N. Engl. J. Med.* 303:1138, 1980.

Infectious Diseases

"I remember my youth and the feeling that will never come back anymore, the feeling I could last forever, outlast the sea, the earth, and all men."—JOSEPH CONRAD

However, the "ole" germs spare no age group, and they inflict pain and suffering on the adolescent with great frequency. Sexually-transmitted diseases obviously constitute a large portion of diseases that plague the adolescent; but as we shall see in this section, infectious diseases of all kinds may affect young people.

Genital herpes has become a major issue in all ages in the 1980s. A number of articles in this section discuss the course of untreated herpes genital infections in young women, and it should be noted that recurrent genital herpes is sufficiently similar to recurrent oral herpes that the guidelines for topical antiviral therapy or oral herpes may be applied to genital herpes. Other articles included here discuss the role of various new agents such as acyclovir in the treatment of herpetic infections.

The article by Fiumara on the treatment of gonorrhea introduces the concept that there is ample evidence that the *Gonococcus* has recently become more sensitive to penicillin as well as to other antibiotics. This is encouraging to the health care professional who is working in this area. The article on nongonococcal urethritis by Kogan is worthy of attention in that this entity is also seen on a daily basis. The *Chlamydia* organism affects the genitourinary tract of adolescent and young adult males and females. Therefore it is important, as with the Fitz-Hugh–Curtis syndrome discussed below, that this organism be considered in the diagnosis of nongonococcal urethritis and that appropriate treatment be instituted.

The article on *Chlamydia trachomatis* infections in Fitz-Hugh–Curtis syndrome emphasizes the impact of sexually-transmitted diseases and various organisms. In the past, this syndrome was associated mainly with gonococcal infections; but according to the authors of this article, in a large percentage of cases the etiology of Fitz-Hugh–Curtis syndrome was associated with acute *Chlamydia* infections. A serodiagnosis of acute *C. trachomatis* infection was made in about 87% of the cases studied. It was noted that the clinician in viewing the Fitz-Hugh–Curtis syndrome should not solely attribute the infection to *Neisseria gonorrhoeae* but should also consider *Chlamydia* as a causative agent.

Toxic shock syndrome received a great deal of attention in the early

1980s. In this section are included many excellent articles on this particular topic. A number of them deal with identifying the exotoxin from *Staphylococcus aureus* which may be associated with the toxic shock syndrome, and treatment with various antibiotics is also discussed.

Finally, an article entitled "Should young adults with a positive tuberculin test take isoniazid?" challenges the concept of treating with isoniazid all those individuals whose tuberculin test is positive and who are indeed adolescents. It was noted that "among 100,000 subjects, treatment with isoniazid could prevent 168–910 cases of tuberculosis over a 20-year period, but 300–1,100 cases of isoniazid-related hepatitis would occur in the year of treatment." In this particular study, "the benefits of preventive therapy did not appear clearly to outweigh the risk of hepatic damage."

Histopathologic Evolution of Recurrent Herpes Simplex Labialis. J. Clark Huff, Gerald G. Krueger, James C. Overall, Jr., James Copeland, and Spotswood L. Spruance studied the natural history of recurrent herpes simplex labialis by examining hematoxylin-eosin-stained sections of biopsy specimens from lesions at various stages.

The earliest changes were noted within nuclei of keratinocytes. Two specific features of early herpes simplex infection, which increased in prominence in older lesions, were peripheral margination of chromatin and development of areas within the nucleoplasm that had a homogeneous, basophilic, "ground glass" appearance. These changes were frequently noted within nuclei with prominent nucleoli. Ballooning of nuclei, evidenced by rounding up of nuclei and foldings in the nuclear membranes, was not found in control biopsy specimens and progressed with age of the lesions. Enlargement of nucleoli and diffuse clumping of chromatin also were found to some extent in control specimens and did not prove to be consistently recognizable early changes. Absence of nucleoli could not be recognized in early lesions but was notable in the ballooned keratinocyte nuclei of vesicles and papules, as well as in crusted lesions. Eosinophilic intranuclear inclusion bodies (Cowdry A bodies) were unusual and occurred in late lesions.

Cytoplasmic changes tended to lag behind nuclear changes. Foamy vacuolization was the earliest cytoplasmic alteration within keratinocytes. Dyskeratosis and acantholysis followed in older lesions. Multinucleated giant cells, not noted in earlier lesions, were present in variable numbers in papules and vesicles, prominent in crusted lesions, and more numerous within the differentiating epidermal cell layers than within the basal cell layer. Nuclei in the giant cells demonstrated marked changes of herpes infection. As regards the formation of the multinucleated giant cells, the data are consistent with

J. Am. Acad. Dermatol. 5:550–557, November 1981.

syncytia formation. Mitotic figures were not found within giant cells or in adjacent epidermal cells.

The herpes-induced changes began focally along the basal cell layer. Early cytologic changes were present in specimens from patients who had prodromal symptoms without physical signs of a lesion. Within 24 hours of onset of the prodrome, herpes simplex virus-induced changes spread to involve larger areas, both in the basal cell layer and in overlying epidermal cells. The peripheral nucleated cells of sebaceous glands and the cells of the external root sheath of follicles were markedly affected. Within the dermis, no cells with typical herpes-induced changes were seen.

In early lesions, mononuclear and polymorphonuclear inflammatory cells were equally prominent; in later lesions neutrophils were more numerous. Necrosis of blood vessels was present to a minimal extent and only in older lesions.

Infection of epidermal cells probably occurs several hours prior to the onset of prodromal symptoms; the patchy distribution of early histologic changes and the speed with which lesions evolved are believed consistent with multicentric origin of the virus. Because biopsy was done on an individual only once, the "histopathologic evolution" observed in biopsy specimens from multiple subjects with lesions at different stages may not be representative of the evolution of a single lesion.

▶ [The histologic changes described correspond closely with those observed in cultured cells infected with herpesvirus. Of particular interest is the finding that the development of eosinophilic inclusions (Lipschütz or Cowdry A bodies) was a late phenomenon and was rarely seen. These inclusions have been shown to be Feulgen-negative, contain little or no DNA, and are now regarded as an artifact. This study also casts light on the mechanism of giant cell formation. Because cells infected with herpes are unable to synthesize DNA, nuclear division within an intact cytoplasm probably does not occur. Therefore, breakdown of cell membranes with subsequent cell fusion (syncytium formation) probably accounts for the appearance of multinucleated giant cells.—R.L.D.] ◀

Studies on Human Epidermal Langerhans' Cells: II. Activation of Human T Lymphocytes to Herpes Simplex Virus. Epidermal Langerhans' cells appear to play an important role in the human immune system. It has been shown that HLA DR-positive Langerhans' cells can stimulate allogeneic T lymphocytes. L. R. Braathen, E. Berle, U. Mobech-Hanssen, and E. Thorsby (Oslo) found that human Langerhans' cells can substitute for macrophages in inducing a herpes simplex virus-specific response of T cells from sensitized donors. Epidermis from patients with recurrent herpes labialis was separated from dermis by means of a suction blister device and trypsinized; the cell suspensions contained 3%–5% Langerhans' cells, as judged by immunofluorescence staining with a rabbit anti-DR antiserum. T lymphocytes from the same patients were cocultured with

Acta Derm. Venereol. (Stockh.) 60:381–387, 1980.

herpes simplex virus antigen (HSV-Ag) or live virus (HSV), with or without epidermal cells or macrophages.

A strong proliferative T cell response to both HSV-Ag and HSV was observed when the cultures also contained epidermal cells or macrophages. Pretreatment of the epidermal cells with rabbit anti-DR antiserum plus complement abolished these responses, while pretreatment with normal rabbit serum plus complement did not. Both HSV-Ag and HSV T cell responses were maximal with 10% macrophages added. Responses in cultures containing epidermal cells increased with the number of epidermal cells added up to the highest number tested (10^5). With epidermal cells present, a peak response was observed on day 7 for both HSV-Ag and HSV.

Human epidermal cells can replace macrophages in presenting HSV type I antigen and live HSV type I in an immunogenic manner to T lymphocytes. The findings may indicate a role for the Langerhans' cells in herpes simplex skin infections. It is possible that herpesvirus particles are bound to Langerhans' cells and then presented in association with HLA-D/DR molecules to T lymphocytes, constituting the afferent phase of the cutaneous immune response to HSV. The absence of Langerhans' cells from the cornea may be important in the pathogenesis of the often persistent and chronic herpes simplex infections of corneal epithelium.

▶ [The ability of epidermal Langerhans' cells to recognize and present antigens to T lymphocytes is certainly not restricted to herpes simplex virus. Langerhans' cells likely play a critical role in the body's natural defenses against various infectious and noninfectious agents and may be important in the recognition and destruction of neoantigen-bearing malignant keratinocytes.—R.L.D.] ◄

Transfer Factor in the Treatment of Herpes Simplex Types 1 and 2. Amanullah Khan, Beth Hansen, N. O. Hill, E. Loeb, A. S. Pardue, and J. M. Hill (Wadley Inst. of Molecular Medicine, Dallas) tried transfer factor (TF), a dialyzable extract obtained from human leukocytes that improves cellular immunity and induces interferon, in 17 patients with recurrent herpes simplex types 1 and 2. Eight patients had genital involvement. Transfer factor was administered in doses ranging from 5 to 10 units/sq m intramuscularly; in most patients, 10 units/sq m was given once a week for 4 weeks followed by the same dose given every 2 weeks for a total treatment period of 6–13 months. A unit of TF represented the amount obtained from 10^8 lymphocytes.

In 16 patients evaluated clinically, the recurrence rate decreased significantly from 10.7 ± 6.1 to 2.1 ± 2.5 (mean ± SD); 8 patients were completely free of disease and 8 had a reduced number of episodes during observation. Not only was the frequency reduced in the latter cases, but also the number of vesicles, area of involvement, and duration of the episodes.

In 7 patients who had abnormal T cell function as reflected by a low number of T cells or low lymphocyte transformation, statistically

Dermatologica 163:177–185, 1981.

significant improvement in T cell function was observed. The clinical response to TF was also statistically significant in 9 patients with normal immune responses. Delayed hypersensitivity skin test reactions improved significantly as well. Transfer factor treatment failed to cause significant changes in the immunoglobulin levels of patients treated for up to 6 months.

Transfer factor may be helpful in controlling recurrent herpes simplex. A controlled study should be conducted to prove or disprove the ultimate usefulness of this treatment.

▶ [Several other less complicated treatments (topical zinc sulfate or boric acid) have not yet been demonstrated to be ineffective in the treatment of herpes simplex. These are certainly worth trying before considering administration of transfer factor. We are willing to go out on a limb and predict that a controlled study with transfer factor will be unable to establish efficacy. Although profound immunologic changes can be induced with transfer factor, it is difficult to understand how defective cell-mediated immunity can lead to an exquisitely localized, self-limited infection. In the natural history of recurrent herpes simplex there is often an acceleration in the frequency and severity of attacks before the disease spontaneously abates. It is usually during this "crescendo" stage that patients are willing to try anything. This probably explains why treatment with agents now known to be ineffective (lysine, ether, levamisole etc., etc., etc.) produced such impressive initial results in uncontrolled studies.— R.L.D] ◀

Clinical Efficacy of Ribavirin in the Treatment of Genital Herpes Simplex Virus Infection. Stanley M. Bierman, William Kirkpatrick, and Humberto Fernandez conducted a double-blind placebo-controlled study in 48 patients to evaluate the efficacy of ribavirin, a synthetic nucleoside analogue, in the treatment of herpes simplex virus genital infection.

Ribavirin treatment (800 mg/day orally for 10 days) reduced disease severity and promoted recovery as compared with placebo treatment. New vesicles were fewer and ceased to appear earlier in ribavirin-treated patients, and their lesions healed faster. At the end of the 10-day period, the ribavirin group experienced disappearance of pain and had lesions that were healed or in crust phase; the placebo group continued to have new lesions appear and had persistent pain.

The only notable side effect observed was in a patient experiencing a fall in hemoglobin value from pretreatment levels of 12.6 to 9.9 gm/100 ml. The patient's hemoglobin level returned to prestudy values when the drug was withdrawn. The nature of the anemia is unknown. Two patients in the ribavirin group experienced slight, transient elevation of the total bilirubin level. Slight elevations of γ-glutamyl transpeptidase levels were seen in 2 patients in the ribavirin group and in 5 in the placebo group. Study design did not allow a conclusion regarding usefulness of the drug in preventing recurrences.

▶ [The "track record" of topical herpes simplex therapies is uninspiring. The results with ribavirin, although somewhat better than its placebo base, cannot be classified as a breakthrough. The problem, of course, is with the pathogenesis of the disease, not with the potency of the antiviral agent. Because involvement of the skin is sec-

Chemotherapy 27:139–145, 1981.

ondary, it is unlikely that topical therapy will be much more than palliative, and it cannot be expected to influence recurrence rates significantly.—R.L.D.] ◄

Topical Treatment of Recurrent Herpes Simplex and Postherpetic Erythema Multiforme With Low Concentrations of Zinc Sulfate Solution. Erythema multiforme is most commonly associated with a preceding herpes simplex (HS) infection. Isser Brody (Gen. Hosp., Eskilstuna, Sweden) investigated the preventive effect of low concentrations of zinc sulfate solution in recurrent HS of the skin and oral mucous membrane. The HS episodes with postherpetic erythema multiforme (PHEM) rashes were associated with upper respiratory tract infections of long duration (4–6 weeks), whereas HS episodes not preceding a PHEM rash were associated with upper respiratory tract infections of short duration (1–3 weeks).

METHOD.—For treatment of HS on the skin, a gauze compress soaked in a lukewarm zinc sulfate solution $(ZnSO_4 \cdot 7H_2O)$ was placed on the skin for about 10 minutes; for acute HS infection 0.025%–0.05% zinc sulfate solution was used and for the clinically normal skin at the site of the earlier HS lesion, 0.05% solution. Herpes simplex on the oral mucous membrane was treated with mouth rinses of zinc sulfate solution for 1–3 minutes in concentrations of 0.01%–0.025% for acute HS infection and 0.025% for a clinically normal mucous membrane. In 25 patients with recurrent HS on the skin and oral mucous membrane, treatment was started during an acute infection once a day until the lesions disappeared. Maintenance treatment was given first once a week for a month, and thereafter twice a month. In 5 patients with recurrent HS and PHEM, the initial treatment was given during a PHEM rash (at least 7–14 days after the preceding HS infection). The clinically normal skin at the site of the earlier HS lesion was treated once a week as long as the PHEM rash lasted. Maintenance treatment was given twice a month.

Treatment with low concentrations of zinc sulfate solution prevented relapses in all patients with recurrent HS on the skin and oral mucous membrane during an observation period of 16–23 months. Upper respiratory tract infections occurred as before. When the clinically normal skin at the site of the earlier HS lesions was treated in patients with recurrent HS and PHEM, there were no relapses of HS episodes associated with upper respiratory tract infections of short duration or of the PHEM rashes. However, the treatment did not prevent HS episodes occurring in association with upper respiratory tract infections of long duration. To prevent these, they had to be treated in an acute stage. With this treatment schedule, it was possible to keep the 5 patients with recurrent HS and PHEM lesion-free during a period of 17–22 months. However, they suffered from upper respiratory tract infections to the same extent as before treatment.

The recommended concentrations of zinc sulfate solution (0.2%–1%, *Merck Index,* 1968) for topical use cause severe irritation and dryness of the skin and oral mucous membrane and a strong emetic reflex. These side effects were not provoked by the low concentrations used in this study.

Br. J. Dermatol. 104:191–194, February 1981.

▶ [The efficacy of zinc sulfate solution has not been evaluated yet in a controlled, double-blind study. We can safely predict that it will not outperform a placebo. However, we recommend its use before it is proved to be ineffective.—R.L.D.] ◀

Recurrent Herpes Simplex: Outlook for Systemic Antiviral Agents. H. J. Field and P. Wildy (Univ. of Cambridge) discuss the future for systemic antiviral agents in the treatment of herpes simplex. The herpesviruses typically occur as an acute primary infection, subsiding after several days and conferring immunity on their host. However, once the clinical signs subside, there is no means of predicting whether the infection has been eradicated completely.

Idoxuridine and trifluorothymidine are useful in treating herpes in man. Both these compounds are "activated" by healthy cells, so their selectivity is poor and they are too toxic for systemic use. They are helpful in topical treatment, especially of ocular infections. Adenine arabinoside is suitable as a systemic drug, but it is not highly effective. Recently several new highly selective nucleoside analogues have been discovered that are extremely active against some herpesviruses in vitro yet appear to have very low toxicity in man. Foremost among these are acyclovir (acycloguanosine) and bromovinyldeoxyuridine.

The frequent observation that latent infections are refractory to systemic treatment is consistent with the concept of latently infected cells that contain virus in a resting state and that do not express the virus genome for long periods. One report described the detection of herpes thymidine kinase in dorsal root ganglia of latently infected mice for up to 60 days after inoculation. Whether herpes simplex virus or the cells that contain the latent infection become susceptible to nucleoside analogues during virus reactivation in vivo is not known; whether the natural reactivation event itself inevitably leads to lysis of the neurone containing the infection is also unknown.

Acyclovir and bromovinyldeoxyuridine appear to have low toxicity in mammalian systems and are expected to ameliorate the acute effects of herpes simplex virus infections by suppressing virus multiplication, both in the skin and in the nervous system.

▶ [Herpes simplex infections can range from the nuisance of recurrent cold sores to the considerable morbidity of recurrent genital herpes, to highly fatal herpes encephalitis. Relatively few treatments have been effective in the past, but some promising new developments suggest that antiviral compounds may change the outlook for severe herpetic infections.—L.E.H.] ◀

Protective Effects of Interferon, Various Antiviral Drugs, and Combinations of These on Herpes Simplex Virus Infection in Mice. The tendency of herpes simplex virus (HSV) infections to recur because of latency of the virus makes treatment difficult. There is evidence that interferon (IF) or interferon inducers are therapeutically effective in both human subjects and experimental animals. Motoo Matsubara (Kyoto Univ.) evaluated the possibility of a synergistic effect of IF with other agents on HSV infection in mice. Young adult

Br. Med. J. 282:1821–1822, June 6, 1981.
J. Dermatol. (Tokyo) 8:31–42, February 1981.

mice were inoculated intraperitoneally with 30 LD_{50} of HSV type 1 (Miyama strain). They died within 2 weeks after inoculation.

The mice were equally protected by intraperitoneal injection of L cell interferon (L-IF) and mouse brain IF, given 1 day before, simultaneously with, and 1 day after HSV inoculation. Mice were also protected when 100 μg of polyinosinic acid-polycytidylic acid (Poly I:C) was given intraperitoneally 1 day before or on the same day as virus inoculation, but not when it was given the next day. Protection was afforded when adenine arabinoside was given from day 1 to day 4 after virus inoculation. Mortality was not reduced by lipopolysaccharide, amphotericin B methyl ester, or γ-globulin. A protective effect was observed when poly I:C and L-IF were combined in doses that were individually ineffective. No synergism between L-IF and adenine arabinoside was seen. The clinical applications of combined therapy in the treatment of virus diseases has not been established.

▶ [Studies of this type may well lead to more effective prophylaxis of herpes simplex infections in high-risk patients.—R.L.D.] ◀

The Course of Untreated Recurrent Genital Herpes Simplex Infection in 27 Women. Genital herpes simplex infection affects an ever-increasing number of persons in the United States. Women, who are particularly burdened with this infection, may incur an increased risk of cervical cancer and may transmit herpes infection to their offspring. Mary E. Guinan, Janet MacCalman, Earl R. Kern, James C. Overall, Jr., and Spotswood L. Spruance (Univ. of Utah) studied 27 women with a recurrence of genital herpes.

Seven women also had recurring oral herpes simplex, but none had concomitant oral and genital recurrences. Twenty-three patients usually had prodromal symptoms, which in 19 were itching, tingling, burning, or tenderness at the site of subsequent eruption; 5 described radiating pain consistent with neuralgia. Sixteen had recurrences every 2 months or more frequently, 7 had lesions every 3–6 months, and 3 had them once a year; 8 reported emotional stress, 5 reported menses, and 1 reported physical trauma as precipitating factors for recurrence. In 13 of 19 patients studied, the recurrence began 5–12 days before menses; assuming a random distribution of recurrences throughout 28 days, this was statistically significant. Seven women noted vaginal discharge coincident with the onset of herpes lesions. Twenty-one patients had only one lesion throughout the episode observed. Lesion location included the labia minora (9 patients), labia majora or perineum (5), mons pubis (4), perianal area (3), buttocks (1), and coccyx (1).

Maximum pain (usually mild), lesion size, and maximum viral titers in lesions (mean, $10^{3.2}$ plaque-forming units) occurred within 2 days of onset. Mean duration of virus shedding from lesions was 4.8 ± 2.7 SD days, and mean healing time was 8.0 ± 2.8 days (Fig. 1); 16% of women shed virus from lesions after 6 days. A vesicle stage

N. Engl. J. Med. 304: 759–763, Mar. 26, 1981.

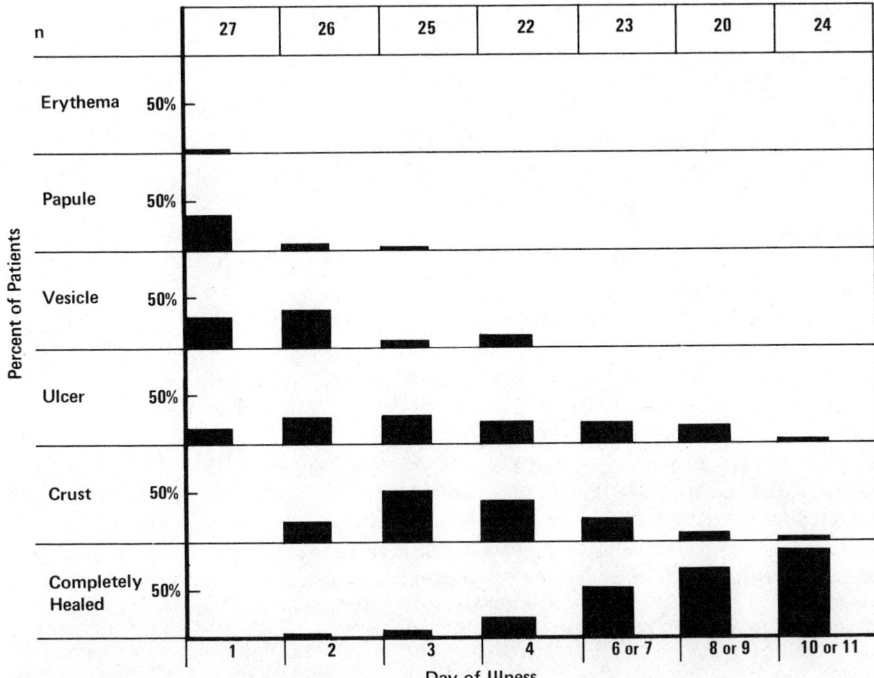

Fig 1.—Frequency of appearance of lesion stages during illness in women with recurring genital herpes simplex virus infection. Letter *n* denotes number of patients examined on day or days indicated. (Courtesy of Guinan, M. E., et al.: N. Engl. J. Med. 304:759–763, Mar. 26, 1981.)

was not observed in 6 patients, and an ulcer stage was not seen in 12. Healing times were shorter in those with single lesions than in those with multiple lesions and shorter for lesions in moist skin areas, such as the labia minora, than for lesions on dry areas, such as the mons pubis. Persistence of virus was not associated with the number or size of lesions. Eighteen herpes simplex virus (HSV) isolates typed were all type 2. Cervical or vaginal lesions were not observed, but cervical shedding of HSV was noted in 33% of patients during recurrence. Between recurrences, only 1 of 64 cervical cultures was positive for HSV.

The rarity of internal lesions and the low viral titers in the absence of lesions suggest the risk of HSV transmission through sexual intercourse during asymptomatic periods is small. Recurrent genital herpes is sufficiently similar to recurrent oral herpes so that the guidelines developed for topical antiviral therapy of oral herpes may be applied to genital herpes.

▶ [This relatively small, but carefully done, study adds to our knowledge of the natural history of recurrent genital herpes infection. No vaginal or cervical lesions were noted during the acute episodes, but 30% of patients had positive viral cultures from the cervix on day 1. In contrast, only 1 of 64 cervical cultures was positive in the asymptomatic period between recurrences.—R.M.P.] ◀

Acyclovir in Herpes Zoster. N. A. Peterslund, J. Ipsen, H. Schonheyder, K. Seyer-Hansen, V. Esmann, and H. Juhl (Marselisborg Hosp., Denmark) describe a double-blind, randomized trial in which nonimmunocompromised patients older than age 30 who had acute herpes zoster and were free of malignant disease received acyclovir, 5 mg/kg (27 patients), or placebo (29 patients), 3 times daily for 5 days as an intravenous bolus injection. Acyclovir, a guanine derivative, is selectively monophosphorylated in herpes simplex virus-infected cells by a virus-specific thymidine kinase, and the resultant triphosphate derivative specifically inhibits the DNA polymerase of herpes simplex virus.

Acyclovir significantly improved the rate of healing of the skin lesions and shortened the period of pain in the acute phase of zoster. Particularly responsive patients were those older than age 67 years, those with fever, and those with less than 4 days of pain before treatment. No adverse effects were observed.

The study shows that acyclovir is highly effective and nontoxic when used systemically in the treatment of acute herpes zoster. The need for intravenous administration limits the use of the drug for treatment of local herpes zoster in the nonimmunocompromised host.

▶ [Acyclovir is truly a masterpiece of pharmacologic engineering. In effect, the drug is manufactured by the virus to cause its own destruction. This study, as well as several others, establishes the remarkable efficacy of acyclovir in the treatment of both herpes simplex and herpes zoster, particularly in high-risk, immunocompromised patients. Now for the bad news! Resistance to acyclovir has been reported (Crumpacker, C., et al.: *N. Engl. J. Med.* 306:343, 1982). A herpes simplex virus deficient in thymidine kinase has been isolated from an immunodeficient child who received three courses of acyclovir. It is, therefore, strongly recommended that acyclovir not be used for patients with the usual recurrent herpes simplex or with uncomplicated herpes zoster. To do so will undoubtedly induce the development of many resistant strains and seriously limit the utility of acyclovir in life-threatening infections.—R.L.D.] ◀

Treating Gonorrhea. Nicholas J. Fiumara (Boston) evaluated the effectiveness of current therapy used for treating gonorrhea in Massachusetts. Patients suspected of having gonoccocal proctitis (alone or in combination with urethritis, pharyngitis, or cervicitis) are usually given 4.8 million units of aqueous procaine penicillin G intramuscularly. This is followed by 4 days of ampicillin, 500 mg orally four times daily. If the patient is allergic to penicillin, spectinomycin, 4 gm intramuscularly, is administered. Complications of gonorrhea, such as pelvic inflammatory disease, are treated with procaine penicillin G, 4.8 million units intramuscularly, followed by ampicillin, 500 mg orally four times daily for the next 9 days. Patients allergic to penicillin are given oral tetracycline, 500 mg orally four times daily for 10 days, for a total of 20 gm. The study included 1,381 patients treated for laboratory-confirmed gonorrhea during 3 months in 1979.

Lancet 2:827–830, Oct. 27, 1981.
Am. Fam. Physician 23:123–126, May 1981.

A total of 780 patients with urethritis were treated with 4.8 million units of aqueous procaine penicillin G. Of these, 761 (98%) had post-treatment negative smears and cultures. Of the 266 patients who returned for posttreatment checkup among 271 treated with penicillin for cervicitis, all had negative smears and cultures. Five patients were considered to be reinfected. Of 34 returning patients among 38 treated for pharyngitis, 33 had negative cultures (97% cure rate). Of 78 returning patients treated with penicillin for gonococcal proctitis, all had negative posttreatment cultures. All 18 patients treated for pelvic inflammatory disease as a complication of gonorrhea had negative posttreatment cultures and were symptomatically improved.

There is ample evidence that gonococcus has recently become more sensitive to penicillin as well as other antibiotics. During one month's time in 1980, 54% of gonococcal cultures collected from the clinics had minimal inhibitory concentrations of 0.03 µg or less of penicillin G per ml. Another 24% required 0.06 µg/ml.

▶ [For a while, resistant strains of gonococci seemed to be an imminent threat. It is now good news that the reverse is the case; the *Gonococcus* is more sensitive than before to commonly used antibiotics. The success rate in the present series is impressive. The Center for Disease Control recommends 1 gm of probenecid by mouth along with penicillin, but otherwise treatment regimens were similar (*Arch. Dermatol.* 115:993, 1979). It is important to rule out other sexually acquired diseases in any patient who presents with gonorrhea.—L.E.H.] ◄

Etiology of Anorectal Infections in Homosexual Men. Several enteric infectious agents have become increasingly evident in homosexual men. Enteric pathogens may be transmitted by ingestion during oral-anal exposure or when fellatio or anal insertive intercourse occurs with a partner contaminated by previous anal intercourse. Thomas C. Quinn, Lawrence Corey, Robert G. Chaffee, Michael D. Schuffler, Frank P. Brancato, and King K. Holmes (Univ. of Washington) examined the infectious causes of symptomatic anorectal disease in 52 homosexual men, seen between 1976 and 1979, who did not have gonococci on initial Gram staining of anorectal exudate. All patients had had anorectal symptoms for less than 3 weeks. None had received antibiotics in the prior 6 weeks. Mean age was 26.4 years. The average number of sexual contacts over a 6-month period was about 6 per month.

Herpes simplex virus (HSV) was recovered from the rectal mucosa of 29% of patients. *Neisseria gonorrhoeae* was recovered from rectal cultures of 14% of patients. Two patients with gonorrhea also had anorectal HSV infection, and 2 had syphilis. Three patients had *Giardia lamblia* or *Entamoeba histolytica* infection, or both. More than one pathogen was found in 6 patients. In 22 patients no pathogen was identified. About 40% of patients had a history of similar acute, self-limited illness. The most common symptoms were anorectal discharge and pain, diarrhea, and constipation. Perianal chancres were seen in 2 patients with positive serologic tests for syphilis. A pathogen was

Am. J. Med. 71:395–406, September 1981.

isolated from 5 of 8 patients with sigmoidoscopic evidence of acute proctitis and from 13 of 18 with evidence of proctitis, anorectal leukocytes, or both.

Gram staining of rectal exudate is insensitive for diagnosis of rectal gonorrhea. Herpes simplex virus is still an infrequent cause of anorectal disease in homosexual men. Nearly half of reported cases of early syphilis in the United States occur in homosexual or bisexual men. Noninfectious causes of anorectal disease include trauma from anal intercourse and anal passage of foreign objects. Sigmoidoscopy and repeated cultures are indicated in patients who still have symptoms after treatment for gonorrhea or syphilis. If a specific pathogen is identified, all sexual contacts in the past month should be evaluated. If no pathogen is found and polymorphonuclear leukocytes are found on a rectal swab, rectal biopsy and full gastroenterologic evaluation are indicated.

▶ [It is clear that a variety of anorectal infections are prevalent in homosexual men. The approach of Quinn et al. to homosexual men who present with anorectal symptoms (anorectal pain or discomfort, rectal discharge, tenesmus, change in bowel habits, or perianal lesions) is as follows: (1) A careful history should be obtained from each patient concerning present symptoms and their duration, sexual activity, and knowledge of any recent illness in sexual contacts. (2) A thorough and detailed physical examination, including anoscopy, should be performed. (3) Initial laboratory tests should include Gram staining of rectal exudate, a serologic test for syphilis, dark-field examination of any ulcers, and a rectal culture for *N. gonorrhoeae*. (4) If a diagnosis of gonorrhea is made by a positive Gram stain or culture, or if syphilis is confirmed by dark-field examination or serology, treatment with penicillin should be instituted. (5) If cultures are negative or if the patient remains symptomatic after treatment for gonorrhea or syphilis, he should undergo sigmoidoscopy. Repeat cultures for *N. gonorrhoeae* and cultures for herpes simplex virus, *Chlamydia trachomatis, Shigella, Salmonella,* and *Campylobacter* should be obtained along with stool specimens for ova and parasites. (6) Specific treatment should be based on identification of the infectious pathogens. (7) When a specific pathogen is identified, epidemiologic investigation of all sexual contacts within the past month should be performed and diagnostic tests obtained. This is especially important for those diseases that can be eliminated by treatment, such as gonorrhea, *C. trachomatis* infections, syphilis, and infections caused by enteric pathogens. (8) If no pathogen is identified and a Gram stain of a rectal swab reveals polymorphonuclear leukocytes, the patient should undergo rectal biopsy and full gastroenterologic evaluation to exclude other inflammatory bowel diseases.—N.J.G.] ◀

Nongonococcal Urethritis is reviewed by Barry A. Kogan (Univ. of Michigan). The term "nongonococcal urethritis" refers to cases of urethritis not attributable to recognized causes such as infection by *Neisseria gonorrhoeae* or the presence of a urethral catheter. In England, where nongonococcal urethritis has been reportable since 1951, the incidence has increased tenfold from 1951 to 1978. Gonorrhea has increased just more than fourfold in the same period. Nongonococcal urethritis is characterized by gradual onset of mild dysuria. Urinary frequency and pruritus also can occur, and there may be a clear mucoid urethral discharge. The diagnosis is made by excluding *N. gonorrhoeae* on Gram staining and culture of the urethral

Urology 17:219–222, March 1981.

discharge. *Chlamydia trachomatis, Ureaplasma urealyticum,* and *Trichomonas vaginalis* recently have been implicated as causal agents. *Chlamydia trachomatis* or *T. vaginalis* may be responsible for 40% to 50% of cases. Evidence for trauma, allergy or viral or fungous infection as causes is lacking.

Most studies suggest a beneficial effect of tetracycline in nongonococcal urethritis, but many cases may resolve spontaneously. Alternative treatments include erythromycin and trimethoprim-sulfamethoxazole. Penicillin is of no benefit. Apparent nongonococcal urethritis is seen in some patients after seemingly adequate treatment of gonococcal urethritis, and treatment with tetracycline eradicates the condition in most instances. If symptoms recur and no discharge is ever documented and no organic cause can be found, psychogenic urethritis should be considered. Recent evidence indicates that nongonococcal urethritis can be involved in epididymitis, pelvic inflammatory disease, and infantile pneumonia.

▶ [*Chlamydia trachomatis* is a ubiquitous organism in genitourinary diseases. Its involvement in the female urethral syndrome is discussed elsewhere in this chapter. *Chlamydia trachomatis* has a predilection for cervical colonization of female consorts of patients with nongonococcal urethritis, and this cervical colonization may produce chronic cervicitis, endometritis, or salpingitis in the female. *Chlamydia* also may be passed to the newborn as it traverses the birth canal and may become the causative agent for conjunctivitis or a pneumonia syndrome, called by some the "afebrile pneumonia syndrome," in the infant at 3–4 weeks of age. This pneumonia and conjunctivitis are best treated with sulfamethoxazole or erythromycin to shorten the duration of symptoms.

An entire issue of the journal *Cutis* was devoted to sexually transmitted diseases. In that issue, Hansfield (*Cutis* 27:268, 1981) further characterizes nongonococcal urethritis as the most common sexually transmitted disease syndrome in the United States and Western Europe. The author further points out the occurrence of acute perihepatitis (Fitz-Hugh–Curtis syndrome) as a resultant complication of *Chlamydia* infection. Other studies have linked *Chlamydia* infection with precancerous cervical dysplasia, midtrimester abortion and stillbirth, endocarditis, and acute proctocolitis in homosexual men. To believe that nongonococcal urethritis is a clinically unimportant syndrome without serious threats to health is inappropriate. Tetracyclines are the agent of choice for the treatment of nongonococcal urethritis; a dose of 500 mg 4 times per day for 7 days is recommended. Doxycycline and minocycline, 100 mg daily for 7 days, have the important advantage of having a once-daily dosage but are no more effective than generic tetracycline and are much more expensive. In addition, these more potent tetracyclines are associated with an increased frequency of side effects. When tetracycline cannot be given, 500 mg of erythromycin, 4 times a day for 7 days, is the treatment of choice. All sexual partners should be treated.—C.E.D.] ◀

"Borderline" Smear in Men With Urethritis. In men with signs and symptoms of urethritis, the diagnosis is made by examination of a stained slide of urethral exudate. A "positive" slide shows typical gram-negative diplococci with rounded external and flattened internal contours within polymorphonuclear leukocytes, which are considered to be diagnostic of gonorrhea. A "negative" slide shows no typical gram-negative diplococci, indicating nonspecific urethritis. A "borderline" slide shows typical gram-negative extracellular diplococci, either alone or among pleomorphic diplococci. To determine whether these borderline slides represent gonorrhea or nonspecific urethritis, Alan J. Arnold and George S. Kleris (Emory Univ.) examined stained slides and cultures of urethral exudate from 403 consecutive male patients with dysuria, urethral discharge, or both.

Of the 403 smears, 57 (14.1%) were interpreted as borderline. Of these 57, only 10.5% correlated with positive cultures, whereas 86.3% of the positive smears and 5.7% of the negative smears correlated with positive cultures. In a second study with full Gram stain and cultures performed by a single examiner, 12 more borderline slides were obtained, of which only 1 was culture positive. Thus, the overall correlation of borderline smears with positive cultures was 10.1%.

Patients with urethritis and borderline slides should be treated for nongonococcal urethritis with tetracycline hydrochloride rather than with aqueous penicillin G procaine.

▶ [Tetracycline, 500 mg four times daily for 5 days, is as effective in treating gonorrhea as is procaine penicillin G, 4.8 million units intramuscularly plus 1 gm of probenecid (Benemid) orally. This same dose of tetracycline for 2 additional days (i.e., a total of 7 days) is recommended for treating nonspecific urethritis. When in doubt, use tetracycline, *not* penicillin, which is useless against nonspecific urethritis.— L.C.L.] ◀

Metronidazole for Vaginal Trichomoniasis: Seven-Day Versus Single-Dose Regimens. W. David Hager, Stuart T. Brown, Stephen J. Kraus, George S. Kleris, Goldie J. Perkins, and Musetta Henderson (Center for Disease Control, Atlanta) undertook a randomized double-blind evaluation of metronidazole therapy for trichomonal vaginitis to compare the efficacy and side effects of the single 2-gm dose and the standard 7-day (250 mg 3 times daily) regimens. The study group included women attending venereal disease clinics who had signs and symptoms of vaginitis and who had motile trichomonads in material obtained from the posterior vaginal fornix. Patients were requested to abstain from coitus and use of alcohol and to return 7–21 days after completing therapy. Patients with negative wet mounts and cultures were classified as cured.

Of 468 infected women who entered the study, 176 (37.6%) returned for reevaluation. Of these, 93 were assigned randomly to the 2-gm dose regimen and 83 to the standard 7-day regimen. There were 73 (79%) women in group A (single dose group) and 72 (87%) in group B (standard dose) who had symptoms of vaginal infection, e.g., discharge, pruritis, and dysuria. The remaining 31 women, examined because of histories of contact with men with gonorrhea or nonspecific urethritis, had abnormal vaginal discharges detected at that time. Eighty (86%) of the 93 women examined 7–21 days after therapy with the 2-gm regimen and 76 (91.6%) of 83 examined after the 7-day regimen were cured. These cure rates were not significantly different. In addition, symptom duration and the occurrence of side effects and yeast infection were not significantly different for the two groups. No

JAMA 244:1219–1220, Sept. 12, 1980.

significant difference was found in reports of sexual partner treatment with metronidazole between patients who failed treatment, compared with those who were cured. Nausea, vomiting, or both were reported by 22 patients (12%), but only 1 patient receiving the standard regimen had sufficiently severe problems to interrupt therapy. Whereas side effects between the treatment groups did not differ significantly, vertigo and headache were noted only in those taking the single 2-gm dose.

These findings support the single-dose regimen as a safe, effective treatment, but poor follow-up (38%) limits the confidence of this conclusion. More research on the safety and efficacy of this dose is required.

The vaginal pool wet mount is helpful in evaluating vaginitis; the test is rapid, simple, and highly specific, although its sensitivity is related to the number of organisms present. In the present study, the culture was positive in 466 (99.5%) of 468 women having a positive pretreatment wet mount; however, the wet mount was less useful as a test of cure, perhaps because of fewer organisms. Because patients will be more likely to comply with a single dose of medication than with 7 days of treatment, and because this regimen is less expensive, the 2-gm dose schedule is recommended.

▶ [Single-dose therapy was as effective as a standard 7-day metronidazole regimen in this placebo controlled, double-blind study of the treatment of vaginal trichomoniasis. Although there were no statistically significant differences in side effects, nausea and vomiting were more frequently reported by patients assigned to the single-dose regimen. The authors of this report acknowledge the high " lost to follow-up" rate (62%) in the study, which limits interpretation. Nonetheless, the results do suggest this matter should be looked at further; more convenient regimens using less total drug probably will replace the therapeutic plans most of us currently prescribe.

The efficacy of the single 2-gm dose was confirmed by Lossick (*Obstet. Gynecol.* 56:508, 1980). Side effects were reportedly not a problem.—R.M.P.] ◀

Pelvic Inflammatory Disease and the Intrauterine Device: Findings in a Large Cohort Study. M. P. Vessey, D. Yeates, Rosemary Flavel, and Klim McPherson (Oxford) investigated the incidence of pelvic inflammatory disease among parous women in the Oxford-Family Planning Association contraceptive study.

Hospital admission rates for "acute definite" disease were 1.51/1,000 woman-years among those currently using an intrauterine device (IUD) and 0.14/1,000 woman-years among those using other birth control methods (age-standardized relative risk, 10.5 to 1 with 95% confidence limits of 5.4 to 1 and 32 to 1). There was also a suggestion that the risk might be slightly raised in ex-users. However, hospital admission for "chronic definite" disease was more common in ex-users of an IUD than in current users (table); women with "other" disease had no confirmatory evidence and may have had noninflammatory pelvic or abdominal disorders. No disease category showed a strong relation to age, though rates declined in women older than age 40. Acute definite disease occurred somewhat more frequently in

Br. Med. J. 282:855–857, Mar. 14, 1981.

INCIDENCE RATES PER 1,000 WOMAN-YEARS OF OBSERVATION FOR THE
THREE CATEGORIES OF PELVIC INFLAMMATORY DISEASE (PID) IN RELATION
TO IUD USE*

	Woman-years of observation	PID category		
		Acute definite	Chronic definite	Other
Current users of an IUD	20 482	1·51 (31)	0·54 (11)	0·54 (11)
Ex-users of an IUD	4 210	0·48 (2)	0·95 (4)	0·48 (2)
Non-users of an IUD	65 259	0·14 (9)	0·23 (15)	0·25 (16)

*Numbers in parentheses indicate number of patients with PID.

Note: current users vs. nonusers: acute definite $x^2_{(1)} = 60.27$, $P < .001$; chronic definite $x^2_{(1)} = 3.89$, $P = .05$; other, not significant. Ex-users vs. nonusers: acute definite, not significant; chronic definite $x^2_{(1)} = 511$, $P < .05$; other, not significant.

early months of IUD use than in later months, though a steady downward trend in incidence was interrupted by a high rate in those using an IUD for more than 6 years. While the rate of such disease was increased in users of each type of device, the highest rate (8.1/1,000 woman-years) was observed in Dalkon shield users, but this rate was based on only 3 affected women. Chronic definite disease showed little relation to duration of use, but numbers were very small.

Since the "control" group consisted largely of women using the pill and diaphragm for contraception, and there is evidence that these methods may reduce the risk of pelvic inflammatory disease (compared with no method), this may in part explain the high relative risk of acute definite disease observed in current IUD users as compared with nonusers. Another possible reason for the high relative risk in this study were the stringent criteria applied in allocating cases to the acute definite disease category. Women in this study represented a selected group with a more positive attitude to health than average: at the time of the study, the participants were at least 25 years old, married, and had no known history of pelvic inflammatory disease; all these factors probably contributed to the generally low rate of disease and to the fact that little relation was observed between risk of disease and age or social class. The relative risk of acute pelvic inflammatory disease associated with IUD use has been found to be much higher in nulliparous than in parous women (Westrom et al., *Lancet,* 1976); the present study leaves little doubt of a substantially increased risk in parous women. The progressive decline in acute definite pelvic disease rates may reflect selective IUD discontinuation by women at risk. The possibility of an association between the apparent increase in acute definite disease risk in women using an IUD for more than 6 years and IUD replacement cannot be excluded.

▶ [This paper is representative of a number in the recent literature that strongly suggest a relationship between IUD usage and pelvic inflammatory disease. Acute infections were found significantly more frequently in users than in either ex-users or nonusers, whereas chronic disease occurred more often in ex-users than in the other two groups. The overall risk of acute pelvic inflammatory disease seemed to be increased about tenfold with the IUD, assuming that users and nonusers are otherwise similar.—R.M.P.] ◀

***Chlamydia trachomatis* Infection in Fitz-Hugh–Curtis Syndrome.** *Chlamydia trachomatis* now is recognized as a common cause of pelvic inflammatory disease (PID). Perihepatitis, or the Fitz-Hugh–Curtis (FHC) syndrome, has been considered a complication of gonococcal PID. San-Pin Wang, David A. Eschenbach, King K. Holmes, Gael Wager, and J. Thomas Grayston (Univ. of Washington, Seattle) studied 23 patients with PID associated with pleuritic upper abdominal pain, a combination characteristic of FHC syndrome. Seventeen patients were among 442 seen in a 6-year period with 523 episodes of PID. Six other women with recent or current PID were referred specifically because of suspected FHC syndrome. Control subjects included 19 PID patients without FHC syndrome and 18 women without evidence of PID who were seen at a venereal disease clinic.

Only 4 study patients were older than age 25. Pleuritic pain was noted either at the same time as or subsequent to the onset of PID. Laparoscopies performed in 5 cases showed evidence of salpingitis and signs of edema of the liver capsule in all; only 1 patient had typical adhesions between the liver capsule and peritoneum. *Neisseria gonorrhoeae* was isolated from the cervix in 7 cases (30%), and *C. trachomatis* in 3 of the 10 patients studied (30%). A serodiagnosis of acute *C. trachomatis* infection was made in 20 cases (87%). A significant titer change was found in 14 of 18 evaluable patients. Seven of 11 patients with IgM antibody had an immunotype specificity different from the corresponding predominant IgG antibody type. A serodiagnosis of acute *C. trachomatis* infection was made in 47% of control PID patients, but the titers were lower than in study patients.

Fitz-Hugh–Curtis syndrome is not solely attributable to infection with *N. gonorrhoeae*. Most cases appear to be associated with acute *C. trachomatis* infection. The microimmunofluorescence test is of value in the serodiagnosis of *C. trachomatis* infection in cases of FHC syndrome.

▶ [Nongonococcal urethritis is now recognized to lead to nongonococcal salpingitis or *Chlamydia trachomatis* PID in women. In this series, chlamydial infections were far more common than those caused by the gonococcus.—S.J.D.] ◀

***Chlamydia Trachomatis* in Acute Salpingitis.** Classically, acute salpingitis has been divided into gonococcal and nongonococcal forms, based on recovery or nonrecovery of *Neisseria gonorrhoeae* from the lower genital tract. Recently, however, the most common cause of sexually transmitted diseases in many western societies has been *Chlamydia trachomatis*. Jorma Paavonen (Univ. Central Hosp., Helsinki) assessed the extent of chlamydial involvement in acute salpingitis in a prospective study of 228 women hospitalized with the disorder. Abscess formation was present in 86 cases.

Lower genital tract cultures for *C. trachomatis* and *N. gonorrhoeae* were positive in 69 and 60 patients, respectively (table). Seventeen patients had cultures positive for both microorganisms. Antichlamy-

Am. J. Obstet. Gynecol. 138:1034–1038, Dec. 1, 1980.
Ibid., 957–959.

RESULTS OF CULTURES FOR *C. TRACHOMATIS* AND *N. GONORRHOEAE* FROM LOWER GENITAL TRACT OF 228 PATIENTS WITH ACUTE SALPINGITIS

Culture for N. gonorrhoeae	*Culture for C. trachomatis*		
	Positive	*Negative*	*Total*
Positive	17	43	60
Negative	52	116	168
Total	69	159	228

dial IgG antibody titers equal to or greater than 512 were found in 56 patients. The mean antibody titer was 264 in serums from patients with cultures positive for *C. trachomatis,* but only 49 in patients with negative cultures. In 167 patients with paired serums, marked titer changes were observed in 17 of 54 (32%) with cultures positive for *C. trachomatis* and in 15 of 113 (13%) with negative cultures. Patients with abscess formation had a higher mean antichlamydial antibody titer (192) than those without pelvic mass (53), as well as a longer mean duration of symptoms. However, there was no correlation between a positive culture for *C. trachomatis* and abscess formation.

The results indicate that *C. trachomatis* is a common etiologic agent in acute salpingitis, which underscores the need to treat chlamydial cervicitis before it develops.

▶ [Cultures of the purulent peritoneal exudate in cases of acute salpingitis often indicate infection with several different species of aerobic and anaerobic organisms. *Neisseria gonorrhoeae* usually is recovered from only a minority of these patients. The polymicrobial nature of established pelvic inflammatory disease (PID) is generally accepted (1980 YEAR BOOK OF OBSTETRICS AND GYNECOLOGY pp. 346–348). What remains somewhat controversial is the role of *N. gonorrhoeae* as the initiating agent. Some suggest that the gonococcus is nearly always the primary pathogen that paves the way for secondary infection by a variety of other organisms. Others think that nongonococcal salpingitis as a primary process is common. This latter view is prevalent in Scandinavia, where the number of cases of PID is increasing in the face of a decline in lower genital tract gonorrhea. *Chlamydia trachomatis* is considered by the author of this report to be a common etiologic agent in acute salpingitis. The significant titer changes in one third of tested patients with positive cervical cultures is suggestive. The relative importance of chlamydia versus gonococci in acute salpingitis may vary with the patient population being investigated.—R.M.P.] ◀

Treatment of Acute Urethral Syndrome. Walter E. Stamm, Kate Running, Mary McKevitt, George W. Counts, Marvin Turck, and King K. Holmes (Seattle) conducted a randomized, double-blind comparison of the effectiveness of doxycycline and placebo in the treatment of 62 women, aged 19 to 73 years, who had acute urethral syndrome without bacterial cystitis or vaginitis.

Patients received treatment for 10 days with either doxycycline (100 mg twice daily by mouth) or placebo (1 tablet twice daily). They were examined periodically for 3 months after completion of treatment.

N. Engl. J. Med. 304:956–958, Apr. 16, 1981.

CLINICAL AND MICROBIOLOGIC RESPONSE TO THERAPY

RESPONSE	DOXYCYCLINE GROUP (N = 32)	PLACEBO GROUP (N = 30)	P VALUE *
	no. cured/no. treated		
Clinical cure			
Bladder bacteriuria †	11/12	4/10	0.016
Sterile pyuria ‡	10/10	3/9	0.003
No pyuria	7/10	8/11	0.63
All cases	28/32	15/30	0.002
Microbiologic cure			
Esch. coli/Staph. saprophyticus	11/12	3/10	0.005
C. trachomatis	4/4	0/3	0.03
Resolution of pyuria			
Bladder bacteriuria	8/12	3/10	0.09
Sterile pyuria	9/10	2/9	0.005

*Fisher's exact test, one tailed.

†Urine obtained by suprapubic aspiration or catheterization contained *Escherichia coli* or *Staphylococcus saprophyticus,* although two consecutive cleancatch, midstream urine specimens contained less than 10^5 uropathogens per ml.

‡Urine obtained by suprapubic aspiration or catheterization was sterile but contained at least 8 WBCs per cu mm; 11 of the 19 women were infected with *C. trachomatis,* as measured by microimmunofluorescence assay.

Clinical cure occurred in 28 of 32 women given doxycycline but in only 15 of 30 given placebo (table). Doxycycline was significantly more effective than placebo in eradicating urinary tract symptoms, pyuria, and the infecting microorganism among women with the urethral syndrome due to coliforms, staphylococci, or *Chlamydia trachomatis.* In women with acute urethral syndrome and no pyuria, however, no benefit could be ascribed to antibiotic therapy. Side effects were infrequent and mild in both treatment groups.

▶ [Women with dysuria and increased urinary frequency who do not have vaginitis may have "infected" urine in the absence of the traditional 10^5 organisms per ml. Those patients with pyuria (defined as 8 or more white blood cells per cu mm of unspun urine) and colony counts $<10^5$ tended to have either lower numbers of bladder bacteria or evidence of chlamydial infection. Our standard criteria for evaluating patients with these symptoms may well require revision.

If the symptoms are due to infection, antimicrobial therapy should help. Doxycycline was more effective than a placebo, according to this article by Stamm et al., except in patients who did not have pyuria. Another view emphasizing psychodynamic rather than microbiologic factors follows.—R.M.P.] ◀

Toxic Shock Syndrome, A Newly Recognized Disease Entity: Report of 11 Cases. Only recently has toxic shock syndrome been recognized as a disease entity. Ursula G. McKenna, J. Allen Meadows III, Nelson S. Brewer, Walter R. Wilson, and Jean Perrault (Mayo Clinic) report the clinical features and laboratory findings in 11 female patients with toxic shock syndrome seen at the Mayo Clinic since August 1975. The patients ranged in age from 13 to 43 years, with a median of 17 years; only 3 patients were 21 years of age or

Mayo Clin. Proc. 55:663–672, November 1980.

CRITERIA FOR TOXIC SHOCK SYNDROME*

All five of the following:
1. Hypotension (blood pressure <90 mm Hg)
2. Fever (≥38.9°C)
3. Erythematous rash followed by desquamation
4. Involvement of at least four organ systems
5. Reasonable evidence for absence of other well-known causes

*Note that these criteria have been modified slightly from those currently formulated by the Center for Disease Control.

---

older. Four patients had 1 episode of toxic shock syndrome, 6 had 2 episodes, and 1 had 3 episodes. One patient died. All of the cases met the criteria for toxic shock syndrome (table.)

The syndrome was often life-threatening, developed shortly before or after the onset of menstruation, and was characterized by transient prodromal illness involving high fever, vomiting, diarrhea, conjunctivitis, headache, irritability, sore throat, myalgias, abdominal tenderness, and erythematous rash. The syndrome can progress to include hypotension or prolonged refractory shock, adult respiratory distress syndrome, diffuse intravascular coagulation with severe thrombocytopenia, and kidney failure. Pancreatitis developed in 2 patients, which may suggest an explanation for the persistent, generalized abdominal tenderness observed throughout the course of the illness and the intercurrent hypotension, hypocalcemia, and hyperglycemia. Pronounced desquamation and peeling of the skin occurred during convalescence. Numerous laboratory abnormalities were observed, including normocytic, normochromic anemia, hypokalemia, abnormal liver function tests, elevated creatine kinase levels, and metabolic acidoses. *Staphylococcus aureus* was isolated from the conjunctiva, throat, hard palate, nares, vagina, cervix, or stool in 5 of 11 patients. Vaginal or cervical cultures performed in 6 patients were positive for *S. aureus* in 4. A recently identified pyrogenic staphylococcal exotoxin was found in the isolates of 3 patients, though its etiologic significance remains unknown. Therapy consists mainly of supportive measures. Antistaphylococcal therapy did not appear to influence the course or outcome of the illness.

All of the patients in this series used tampons of various manufacture, although the role of vaginal tampons, if any, in the pathogenesis of toxic shock syndrome remains to be demonstrated.

▶ [No medical condition in recent times has received as much notoriety as has the toxic shock syndrome. This report of 11 cases from the Mayo Clinic is the largest series reported to date from a single institution, and it details the clinical and laboratory features.

These cases of toxic shock syndrome associated with tampon usage were reported by Watsky and Iannini (*Conn. Med.* 44:776, 1980). Vaginal cultures consistently grew *Staphylococcus aureus*. A similar association with *S. aureus* was made in a much larger series by Shareds and associates (*N. Engl. J. Med.* 303:1436–1442, 1980).— R.M.P.] ◀

Clinical Manifestations of Toxic Shock Syndrome. P. Joan Chesney, Jeffrey P. Davis, William K. Purdy, Phillip J. Wand, and Russell W. Chesney reviewed the findings in 22 patients seen during 1977–1980 in Madison hospitals with a diagnosis of toxic shock syndrome (TSS). All were female, and all but 1 had onset of disease during menses. The mean age was 22 years. All but 1 of 12 patients studied before antimicrobial therapy had cervical or vaginal cultures positive for coagulase-positive staphylococci. The time sequence of clinical manifestations is outlined in Figure 2, and the dermatologic features are listed in the table. All the patients were previously healthy. All had vomiting; diarrhea tended to occur later. Confusion, disorientation, or hallucinations were noted in all patients. Four had joint abnormalities. All had sinus tachycardia, 2 had aberrant cardiac beats of bundle origin, and 1 had premature ventricular beats on exertion.

Seventeen patients received a β-lactamase-resistant antimicrobial for 3 to 14 days, whereas 2 received no antibiotics. All patients required intravenous fluids, and 7 required dopamine to maintain a low-normal blood pressure. One patient required hemodialysis. Eight patients received one to three doses of intravenous steroid therapy in the first 24 hours. Ventilatory support was necessary in 2 patients.

Fig 2.—Composite drawing of major systemic, skin, and mucous membrane manifestations of toxic shock syndrome. (Courtesy of Chesney, P. J., et al.: JAMA 246:741–748, Aug. 14, 1981; copyright 1981, American Medical Association.)

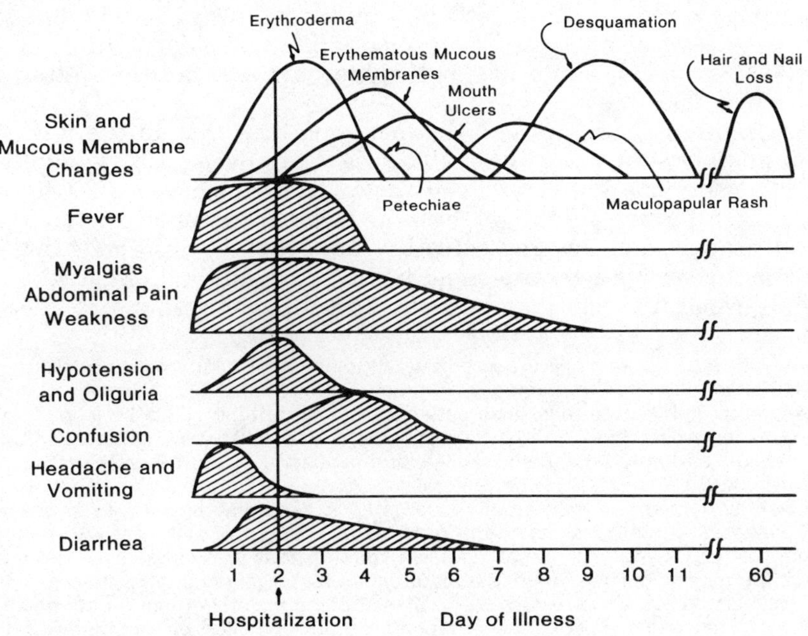

JAMA 246:741–748, Aug. 14, 1981.

DERMATOLOGIC MANIFESTATIONS OF TOXIC SHOCK SYNDROME IN 22 PATIENTS

No. of Patients

Mucous Membrane	Skin
Early, Days 1-4	
Eye	Erythroderma
Scleral injection with photophobia (20)	Diffuse involving chest, abdomen
Subconjunctival hemorrhages (7)	or back, and extremities (22)
Discharge (3)	Primarily lower abdomen and thighs (5)
Ear	Primarily extensor surfaces of
Inflamed tympanic membrane (5)	joints (1)
Oropharynx	Petechiae
Erythema, pain (2)	Primarily on extremities (6)
Strawberry tongue (18)	Localized abscesses (10)
Vulva	Severe acne (2)
Erythema, swelling (5)	Infected extremity lesions (5)
	Impetiginous lesions of mouth (1)
	Purulent conjunctivitis (3)
	Lesions on neck, chin (1)
	Perirectal
	Erythema (5)
	Excoriations (4)
	Vesicles (1)
	Nikolsky's sign (2)
Late, Days 4-14	
Oropharynx	Maculopapular
Ulcers (12)	Total body, pruritic (7)
Swollen, denuded tongue (15)	Desquamation
	Palms, soles, tips of fingers and toes (22)
Delayed, Days 60-90	
None	Telogen effluvium
	Loss of hair and nails ($>$10)

All patients recovered, but all had prolonged fatigue and weakness for up to several months. Two patients had transient neurologic sequelae. Several patients had reversible hair and nail loss after the episode of TSS.

Toxic shock syndrome is a distinct syndrome that in the past has been mistaken for many other illnesses. Coagulase-positive staphylococci and tampon use have been shown to be important in TSS, but the reason for the recent increase in incidence is unclear. Rapid removal of tampons, sponges, or other intravaginal absorbent materials, vaginal irrigation, and rapid intravenous fluid administration to restore renal function may be critical in the management of affected patients.

▶ [As with most illnesses, the cases that call toxic shock syndrome to attention are dramatic, serious, life-threatening syndromes. Such is true here. However, Chesney et al. are careful to note that these patients may flag but the tip of the iceberg. Two of the patients described here had experienced milder episodes characterized by fever, myalgia and arthralgia, rash, nausea, and headache of 3 to 7 days' duration during prior menses.

The most impressive physiologic aspect of this syndrome appears to be massive vasodilation and rapid loss of serum proteins and fluid into extravascular compartments. Oliguria, hypotension, edema, low central venous pressures, and hypoproteinemia are common. Thus, there is a requirement for large amounts of fluid, colloids, and vasopressor drugs to restore blood pressure and maintain renal function.

Keep in mind that most of these patients do not complain of vaginal symptoms. Vaginal discharge may be minimal or absent, so the genital tract is not suspected immediately as an initiating focus. However, red, swollen, and tender labial, vaginal, and perirectal tissues are frequent findings on examination.

For other nice articles appearing this year that gradually unravelled certain facets of the syndrome see the following.

1. Davis, J.P., et al.: Toxic shock syndrome: Epidemiologic features, recurrence, risk factors, and prevention. *N. Engl. J. Med.* 303:1429–1435, 1980.

2. Shands, K.N., et al.: Toxic shock syndrome in menstruating women: Association with tampon use and *Staphylococcus aureus* and clinical features in 52 cases. *N. Engl. J. Med.* 303:1436–1442, 1980.

3. Toffe, R.W., and Williams, D.N.: Toxic shock syndrome: Clinical and laboratory features in 15 patients. *Ann. Intern. Med.* 94:149–156, 1981.

4. Fisher, R.F., et al.: Toxic shock syndrome in menstruating women. *Ann. Intern. Med.* 94:156–163, 1981.

It now generally is agreed that this is not a new syndrome. While first reported in its current form by Todd and his associates in 1978, the occurrence of a scarlatiniform rash with staphylococcal infection has been reported occasionally since 1927. The patients with toxic shock syndrome are not bacteremic, and all evidence points to the fact that a previously unidentified toxin plays an important, though as yet incompletely formulated, role.—D.E.R.] ◄

Toxic Shock Syndrome: Epidemiologic Features, Recurrence, Risk Factors, and Prevention. Jeffrey P. Davis et al. (Madison, Wis.) report the findings of a toxic shock syndrome (TSS) surveillance program and associated case-control study in Wisconsin regarding the epidemiologic features, risk factors, and recurrence of TSS.

Thirty-eight cases with onsets from September 1975 through June 1980 were reported, 37 of which occurred after Jan. 1, 1979. All but 1 of the patients were women. In 35 of the 37 women, onset of TSS was during the menstrual period or within 2 days of the end of menses (Fig 3). The only male patient had a staphylococcal pustule in the left axilla at onset. There was 1 death. Of 23 cervical or vaginal cultures obtained before antibiotic treatment, 17 grew *Staphylococcus aureus*. Type I herpes simplex virus was isolated from oral lesions of 2 patients. Ten women had recurrent illness during subsequent men-

Fig 3.—Days from onset of menstrual bleeding to onset of toxic shock syndrome among women in Wisconsin. All women depicted were menstruating at onset. Two women with onsets within 48 hours of end of menses and 1 woman with onset during menses are not depicted. (Courtesy of Davis, J. P., et al.: N. Engl. J. Med. 303:1429–1435, Dec. 18, 1980.)

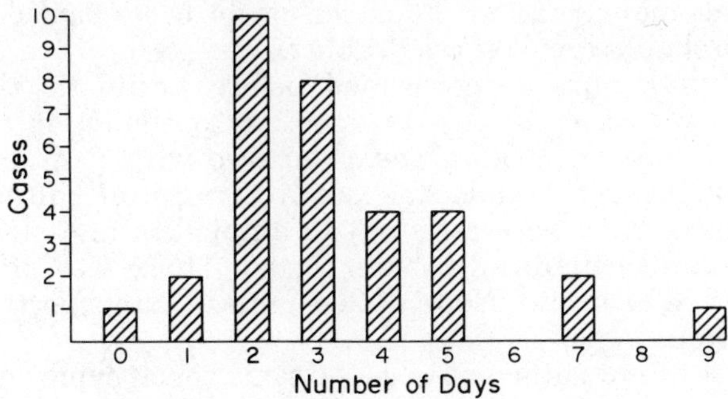

ses; 5 had two episodes and 5 had three or more. In 8 of these women the first occurrence was the most severe. The rate of recurrence was markedly lower in patients who had been treated with β-lactamase-resistant antibiotics.

In the case-control study, 35 patients were matched for age and menstruation with 105 controls. Thirty-four patients and 80 controls used tampons during every menstrual period (P <.01) and 9 patients and 64 controls used contraceptive methods (P <.001). In Wisconsin, the overall minimum crude rate of TSS as defined by clinical criteria was 6.2 cases per 100,000 menstruating women per year. Among regular tampon users, the rate was 8.8/100,000 per year. Among menstruating women, the rate of TSS in those under age 30 years was 2.4 to 3.3 times the rate among those aged 30 years or older.

Although it is not known why the incidence of TSS has increased in recent years, the possible influence of immune mechanisms, materials in recently marketed tampons, contraceptive methods, and other factors requires further study.

▶ [The finding of fever, diarrhea, vomiting, hypotension with mental confusion, decreased renal output and a scarlatiniform rash in a young lady should suggest the diagnosis of toxic shock syndrome. Unless it is recognized and properly treated, about one fourth of patients will have recurrences. The episodes usually are associated with menses and are probably due to a toxin elaborated by a *Staphylococcus aureus* organism.—P.G.C.] ◄

Toxic Shock Syndrome in Menstruating Women: Association With Tampon Use and *Staphylococcus aureus* and Clinical Features in 52 Cases. Kathryn N. Shands et al. (Center for Disease Control, Atlanta) conducted a retrospective telephone study of 52 cases and 52 age-matched controls to determine risk factors associated with toxic shock syndrome in menstruating women.

Mean age was 27 years. Features of the syndrome are listed in Table 1. Tampons were used in 52 cases and 44 controls. In case-control pairs in which both women used tampons, cases were more likely than controls to use tampons throughout menstruation (P <.05). There were no significant differences in brand of tampon used, degree of absorbency specified on label, frequency of tampon change, type of contraceptive used, frequency of sexual intercourse, or sexual intercourse during menstruation. Fourteen of 44 cases had one or more definite or probable recurrences (Table 2).

Of 16 vaginal cultures performed before antibiotic therapy, all yielded *Staphylococcus aureus*. In nonstudy patients, 46 (96%) of 48 vaginal cultures yielded *S. aureus*, compared with 7 of 71 in healthy controls; 4 of these 7 women had positive introital cultures. Of the isolates studied, 92% were resistant to ampicillin and penicillin and sensitive to 20 other antimicrobials tested. There was no characteristic phage type or group. None of 264 unused tampons was found to harbor *S. aureus*.

Tampon use is not sufficient to cause toxic shock syndrome, because

N. Engl. J. Med. 303:1436–1442, Dec. 18, 1980.

TABLE 1.—FREQUENCY OF SIGNS, SYMPTOMS, AND LABORATORY ABNORMALITIES IN 52 PATIENTS WITH TOXIC SHOCK SYNDROME*

CLINICAL SIGN OR SYMPTOM	PERCENTAGE	LABORATORY FINDING	PERCENTAGE
Diarrhea	98	Elevated serum creatinine §	69
Myalgia	96		
Vomiting	92	Thrombocytopenia †	59
Temperature ≥40°C	87	Hypocalcemia ‡	58
Headache	77	Azotemia §	57
Sore throat	75	Hyperbilirubinemia §	54
Conjunctival hyperemia	57	Elevated hepatic enzymes §	50
Decreased sensorium	40	Leukocytosis ¶	48
Vaginal hyperemia	33	Abnormal urinary sediment ‖	46
Vaginal discharge	28		
Rigors	25	Elevated CPK §	41
		Immature leukocytes ≥50%	36

*All patients had fever, rash, desquamation of palms and soles, and hypotension.

†Platelet count < 100,000/ml.

‡Serum calcium concentration no more than 7.5 mg/dl.

§Value greater than or equal to twice upper limit of normal for laboratory.

¶White blood cell count at least 15,000/cu mm.

‖At least 5 WBC per high-power field; at least 2 RBC per high-power field, or presence of RBC casts.

TABLE 2.—RECURRENCE CATEGORIES FOR TOXIC SHOCK SYNDROME

Major criteria
    Temperature ≥38.9°C
    Rash
    Vomiting or diarrhea
    Myalgia

Definite recurrence
    Desquamation and at least three of four major criteria

Probable recurrence
    Desquamation and two of four major criteria or
    Three of four major criteria

No recurrence
    Two major criteria or fewer; no desquamation

tampon use is extremely common, and the incidence of the disease is low. It is likely that the syndrome is produced by a toxin elaborated by *S. aureus*. A blood-soaked tampon at body temperature is a suitable culture medium for *S. aureus* and may enhance toxin production.

Women who have not had toxic shock syndrome are at low risk of its development and probably need not change their pattern of tampon use. However, if they want to reduce an already small risk, they might use tampons for only part of the day or night or for only part of the period. Women who have had the syndrome are at considerable risk of recurrences and should not use tampons, aͬ least until *S. aureus* has been eradicated from the vagina. The possibility that a toxigenic strain of *S. aureus* can be carried elsewhere and lead to vaginal reinfection needs further assessment.

▶ [*Morbidity and Mortality Weekly Report* (30:25, 1981) documented 941 confirmed cases of toxic shock syndrome (TSS) that have been reported to the Center for Disease Control (CDC). Ninety-nine percent of these cases were in women, and 98% (905) had their onset during a menstrual period. Eleven cases occurred in the postpartum time frame. The cases reported over the past decade are from 48 states, Vermont and Alaska reporting none. In late 1978, the incidence of reported cases began to increase and underwent a rapid upward trend that continued through August of 1980. Now, however, a sudden decrease in the number of cases has occurred. The first medical article on TSS was published in November of 1978. Increased publicity has occurred since that time. The increase in cases that was expected as a result of the publicity did not occur. The most likely explanation for the decline in numbers of cases is that women have changed their tampon wearing habits. Women with early symptoms of TSS realize what has happened, remove their tampons, and seek the attention of physicians more quickly. It is still true that women can eliminate their risk of TSS almost entirely by not wearing tampons and women who do choose to use them can reduce their risk by intermittently using them during each menstrual period. Cases not associated with menstruation will continue to occur, but at a very low rate.

Davis et al. (*N. Engl. J. Med.* 303:1429, 1980) reported 38 cases of TSS detected in Wisconsin from 1975 through 1980. Ten of the patients had at least one recurrent episode during subsequent menstrual periods. The recurrence rate seems to be lower in patients who had been treated with β-lactamase-resistant antibiotics. McKenna et al. (*Mayo Clin. Proc.* 55:663, 1980) describe several newly identified features of TSS, including a high recurrence rate associated with initial episodes that are mild. They also noted the frequent involvement of *Staphylococcus aureus* infection of the conjunctiva and implicated this as the possible source of TSS.—C.E.D.] ◀

A New Staphylococcal Enterotoxin, Enterotoxin F, Associated With Toxic-Shock-Syndrome *Staphylococcus aureus* Isolates. Over 400 cases of toxic shock syndrome (TSS) were reported to the Centers for Disease Control by October 1980. Symptoms characteristically associated with enterotoxins have been noted in TSS. Merlin S. Bergdoll et al. (Madison, Wis.) examined 65 *S. aureus* strains isolated from TSS patients for enterotoxigenicity. Diagnostic criteria for TSS included fever above 38.9 C, hypotension or orthostatic dizziness, diffuse or palmar erythroderma followed by desquamation, and multisystem dysfunction.

All but 4 of the 65 *S. aureus* strains (94%) produced an enterotoxinlike protein, tentatively identified as staphylococcal enterotoxin F (SEF). Another strain produced staphylococcal enterotoxin B, and another, enterotoxin C. All 34 TSS-associated *S. aureus* strains examined and 3 of 26 control strains (11.5%) produced SEF. Two of the control strains were from the vaginas of women with no history of TSS. Only 4.6% of 87 *S. aureus* strains from other sources produced SEF. Five of 29 TSS patients with acute serums available had anti-SEF antibody present in titers of 1:100 and above, compared with 79% of 56 control subjects.

Lancet 1:1017–1021, May 9, 1981.

Staphylococcal enterotoxin, particularly SEF, may be a cause of the clinical features of toxic shock syndrome, but SEF appears to be associated with very few *S. aureus* strains isolated from other sources. Although SEF itself has not been tested in a suitable animal model, the present evidence strongly implicates it as a causative agent in TSS.

▶ [The identification of staphylococcal enterotoxin F seems to be a major step forward in our understanding of the toxic shock syndrome.—P.G.C.] ◀

Toxic Shock Syndrome: Possible Confusion With Kawasaki Disease. Toxic shock syndrome (TSS) is a recently recognized disorder associated with strains of *Staphylococcus aureus* that produce a unique epidermal toxin. Affected patients have multisystemic complaints including fever, headache, subcutaneous edema, myalgia, scarlatiniform rash, conjunctival hyperemia, confusion, diarrhea, oliguria, hypotension, and shock. This is followed by palmoplantar desquamation. Most reported cases have been in young, menstruating women who used vaginal tampons regularly. Sharon S. Raimer, Eduardo H. Tschen, and Martha K. Walker (Univ. of Texas, Galveston) report a case of TSS that was originally misdiagnosed as mucocutaneous lymph node syndrome (MLNS or Kawasaki disease).

Woman, 26, noticed pruritus in the vaginal and groin area during the latter part of a slightly prolonged menstrual cycle. Two days later, she had severe pruritus of the palms and soles. A faint erythematous macular eruption was evident on both hands 2 hours later. Shortly thereafter, examination showed a macular, patchy, erythematous eruption that was particularly prominent over the lower part of the trunk. Bright red erythema of the palms, soles, and flexural creases also was seen. Later in the day, she began to have chills and her temperature rose to 40 C and remained high despite aspirin and acetaminophen therapy. The following day, she continued to have a high fever with shaking chills and developed severe myalgias, arthralgias, and vomiting. Examination on admission that evening revealed fever, tachypnea, tachycardia, and a generalized erythematous macular skin eruption. She also had an erythematous pharynx with dry mucous membranes, bilateral carpal-pedal spasm, and marked erythema and edema of the hands and feet. Blood pressure was 100/80 mm Hg. Abnormal laboratory findings included elevated levels of serum glutamic oxaloacetic transaminase, serum glutamic pyruvic transaminase, and alkaline phosphatase. Throat and multiple blood cultures were negative. The patient remained feverish, with a marked increase in arthralgias and peripheral swelling. Episodic vomiting persisted. On the fifth day of illness, she was noted to have bilateral conjunctival injection, watery diarrhea, serous otitis media, and severe laryngitis. A beefy red tongue with prominent papillae was also seen. On the sixth day of illness, her temperature returned to normal and she was discharged the following day in good condition. At discharge, the scarlatiniform eruption had faded, the sclera had cleared, and the myalgias were markedly improved. Early periungual desquamation of the palms and soles was evident. Based on the presence of injected sclera, "strawberry tongue," and desquamated, edem-

---

Cutis 28:33–36, July 1981.

atous palms and soles, a discharge diagnosis of MLNS was made. The diagnosis was later changed to TSS.

The symptoms shown by this patient are typical of those associated with TSS, except for the absence of profound shock, which may have been obviated by early institution of intravenous fluid therapy. Because there are similarities between TSS and MLNS, as well as other conditions, early recognition and treatment of TSS are essential.

▶ [Some of the previously reported cases of Kawasaki disease in young women were, in retrospect, probably TSS (Everett, E.: *JAMA* 242:542, 1979; Schlossberg, D., et al.: *Arch. Dermatol.* 115:1435, 1979; and Milgrem, H., et al.: *Ann. Intern. Med.* 92:467, 1980). Signs common to both conditions include desquamation of the palms and soles, an erythematous tongue with prominent papillae, and injected sclera. In Kawasaki disease, a maculopapular eruption is seen; however, in TSS there is diffuse erythroderma. Other features of TSS (Shands, K., et al.: *N. Engl. J. Med.* 303:1436, 1980), including myalgias, abdominal pain, hypertension, adult respiratory distress syndrome, renal insufficiency, and thrombocytopenia, are absent or rare in Kawasaki disease. Lymphadenopathy, which is present in more than 90% of patients with Kawasaki disease, is absent in TSS.

The differential diagnosis of TSS includes, in addition to Kawasaki disease, staphylococcal scalded skin syndrome, scarlet fever, Rocky Mountain spotted fever, leptospirosis, and early erythema multiforme.—R.L.D.] ◀

Should Young Adults With a Positive Tuberculin Test Take Isoniazid? The American Thoracic Society and the Centers for Disease Control have recommended isoniazid for prevention of tuberculosis in adults under age 35 years without other risk factors, because the benefit outweighs the risk of hepatitis. William C. Taylor et al. (Boston) used decision analysis to evaluate this contention with respect to young adults whose only risk factor for active tuberculosis was a positive tuberculin skin test. Subjects aged 20–34 years were considered in the analysis. The decision considered was whether to initiate a year of preventive therapy with isoniazid.

It was assumed that the risk of active tuberculosis developing over 20 years ranged from 0.56% to 1.30%, that isoniazid can reduce the risk by 30%–70%, and that the risk that isoniazid-related hepatitis would develop ranged from 0.3% to 1.1%. Among 100,000 subjects, treatment with isoniazid could prevent 168–910 cases of tuberculosis over a 20-year period, but 300–1,100 cases of isoniazid-related hepatitis would occur in the year of treatment.

In this analysis, the benefits of preventive therapy did not appear clearly to outweigh the risks, and the authors conclude that the recommendation that all young adults with a positive tuberculin skin test take isoniazid is unwise. Some such subjects may choose to take isoniazid for a year under supervision by a physician, whereas others may choose to refuse prophylaxis. At present, the latter choice appears to be entirely reasonable and for many is preferable to the risks of isoniazid. Economic costs, public health implications, or different considerations for tuberculin reactors in nonindustrialized societies were not addressed.

Ann. Intern. Med. 94:808–813, June 1981.

▶ [The authors estimate that isoniazid could reduce deaths from tuberculosis by 2–33 during a 20-year period, but estimate that 0–51 deaths would be caused by hepatotoxicity during 1 year of isoniazid treatment. They do not feel that the benefits of isoniazid therapy outweigh the risks.—R.E.R.] ◀

Additional Reading

Antonioli, D. A., et al.: Natural history of diethylstilbestrol-associated genital tract lesions: Cervical ectopy and cervicovaginal hood. *Am. J. Obstet. Gynecol.* 137:847, 1980.

Bierman, S. M., et al.: Clinical efficacy of ribavirin in treatment of genital herpes simplex infection. *Chemotherapy* 27(2):139, 1981.

Blaser, M. J., et al.: *Salmonella typhi:* The laboratory as a reservoir of infection. *J. Infect. Dis.* 142:934, 1980.

Buchanan, T. M., et al.: Gonococcal salpingitis is less likely to recur with *Neisseria gonorrhoeae* of same principal outer membrane protein antigenic type. *Am. J. Obstet. Gynecol.* 138:978, 1980.

Carson, C. C., et al.: Evaluation and treatment of female urethral syndrome. *J. Urol.* 124:609, 1980.

Collum, L. M. T., et al.: Randomized double-blind trial of acyclovir and idoxuridine in dendritic corneal ulceration. *Br. J. Ophthalmol.* 64:766, 1980.

Crosnier, J., et al.: Randomized placebo-controlled trial of hepatitis B surface antigen vaccine in French hemodialysis units: II. Hemodialysis patients. *Lancet* 1:797, 1980.

Doroghazi, R. M., et al.: Invasive external otitis: Report of 21 cases and review of the literature. *Am. J. Med.* 71:603, 1981.

Farrell, M. K., et al.: Prepubertal gonorrhea: A multidisciplinary approach. *Pediatrics* 67:151, 1981.

Ginsburg, C. M., et al.: Treatment of group A streptococcal pharyngitis in children: Results of a prospective, randomized study of four antimicrobial agents. *Clin. Pediatr. (Phila.)* 21:83, 1982.

Gislason, T., et al.: Acute epididymitis in boys: A five-year retrospective study. *J. Urol.* 124:533, 1980.

Gumpel, J. M., et al.: Reactive arthritis associated with *Campylobacter* enteritis. *Ann. Rheum. Dis.* 40:64, 1981.

Hadler, S. C., et al.: Outbreak of hepatitis B in a dental practice. *Ann. Intern. Med.* 95:133, 1981.

Harding, G. K. M., et al.: Prospective, randomized comparative study of clindamycin, chloramphenicol, and ticarcillin, each in combination with gentamicin, in therapy for intra-abdominal and female genital tract sepsis. *J. Infect. Dis.* 142:384, 1980.

Hoffnagle, J. H., et al.: Seroconversion from hepatitis B e antigen to antibody in chronic type B hepatitis. *Ann. Intern. Med.* 94:744, 1981.

Immunization Practices Advisory Committee: Rubella prevention. *Morbid. Mortal. Weekly Rep.* 30:37, 1981.

Johannisson, G., et al.: Genital *Chlamydia trachomatis* infection in women. *Obstet. Gynecol.* 56:671, 1980.

Kaufman, R. H., et al.: Herpesvirus-induced antigens in squamous cell carcinoma in situ of the vulva. *N. Engl. J. Med.* 305:483, 1981.

Kernbaum, S., and Hauchecorne, J.: Administration of levodopa for relief of herpes zoster pain. *J.A.M.A.* 246:132, 1981.

Lyng, J., and Christensen, J.: A double-blind study of the value of treatment with a single-dose tinidazole of partners to females with trichomoniasis. *Acta Obstet. Gynecol. Scand.* 60:199, 1981.

McCormick, R., and Maki, D. G.: Epidemiology of needle-stick injuries in hospital personnel. *Am. J. Med.* 70:928, 1981.

Mitchell, C. D., et al.: Acyclovir therapy for mucocutaneous herpes simplex infections in immunocompromised patients. *Lancet* 1:1389, 1981.

Morens, D. M., et al.: Surveillance of Reye's syndrome in the United States, 1977. *Am. J. Epidemiol.* 114:406, 1981.

Offit, P. A., et al.: Severe Epstein-Barr virus pulmonary involvement. *J. Adolesc. Health Care* 2:121, 1981.

Peacock, J. E., Jr., et al.: Methicillin-resistant *Staphylococcus aureus:* Introduction and spread within a hospital. *Ann. Intern. Med.* 93:526, 1980.

Preblud, S. R., et al.: Fetal risk associated with rubella vaccine. *J.A.M.A.* 246:1413, 1981.

Quinn, T. C., et al.: *Chlamydia trachomatis* proctitis. *N. Engl. J. Med.* 305:195, 1981.

Rubin, R. H., et al.: Single-dose amoxicillin therapy for urinary tract infection: Multicenter trial using antibody-coated bacteria localization technique. *J.A.M.A.* 244:561, 1980.

Schlievert, P. M., et al.: Identification and characterization of exotoxin from *Staphylococcus aureus* associated with toxic shock syndrome. *J. Infect. Dis.* 143:509, 1981.

Sotman, S. B., et al.: *Staphylococcus aureus* bacteremia in patients with acute leukemia. *Am. J. Med.* 69:814, 1980.

Spiegel, C. A., et al.: Anaerobic bacteria in nonspecific vaginitis. *N. Engl. J. Med.* 303:601, 1980.

Stamm, W. E., et al.: Causes of the acute urethral syndrome in women. *N. Engl. J. Med.* 303:409, 1980.

Sweet, R. L., et al.: Microbiology and pathogenesis of acute salpingitis as determined by laparoscopy: What is the appropriate site to sample? *Am. J. Obstet. Gynecol.* 138:985, 1980.

Szmuness, W., et al.: Hepatitis B vaccine: Demonstration of efficacy in a controlled clinical trial in a high-risk population in the United States. *N. Engl. J. Med.* 303:833, 1981.

van Buchem, F. L., et al.: Therapy of acute otitis media: Myringotomy, antibiotics, or neither? A double-blind study in children. *Lancet* 2:883, 1981.

Ware, A. J., et al.: Prospective trial of steroid therapy in severe viral hepatitis: Prognostic significance of bridging necrosis. *Gastroenterology* 80:219, 1981.

Dermatology

"Ode To Zits"
*"I think that I shall never see a sight as ugly as a zit, a reddish,
whitish, smelly thing that grows and grows from ear to ear. A zit
that sits for all to see why couldn't God just have made trees?"*—UN-
KNOWN (You don't think I would take credit for this do you?)

For the adolescent, dermatology involves primarily the treatment
of acne vulgaris. However, as noted in this section, the health care
professional needs to be concerned with a number of different skin
conditions that affect the adolescent.

With respect to acne vulgaris, I have included several articles on
the use of tetracycline and other topical antibiotics. The article by
Padilla and associates comparing topical treatment with tetracycline
or clindamycin offers a number of interesting observations. In this
group of 52 subjects, clindamycin phosphate was significantly more
effective than tetracycline hydrochloride in reducing lesion counts.
Also, the use of 13-*cis*-retinoic acid to reduce bacterial skin flora is
interesting. As noted in several articles, it is unclear whether the
change in skin bacteria is merely secondary to marked suppression of
sebum excretion or whether there is actual clinical improvement. In
some cases, 13-*cis*-retinoic acid tends to improve the acne condition,
especially in those individuals with severe acne vulgaris. The exact
mechanism of its action still remains debatable. The articles in this
section dealing with acne and its treatment should provide the clinician with a good basis for caring for his patients.

There is also a broad range of skin manifestations of systemic diseases which the health care professional may see in adolescents. Histiocytosis X, for example, can present in the adolescent as chronic
inflammation and ulceration *or* as an eosinophilic lesion. The article
by Fitzpatrick et al. discusses the cutaneous and oral findings in 59
patients who had histologically confirmed histiocytosis X. In working
with adolescents it is important to remember that this condition can
present as an oral lesion as well as a dark skin manifestation.

I have included two articles dealing with systemic lupus erythematosus. Especially helpful is the article by Caeiro and associates
which reviews the various clinical presentations of lupus in children
and adolescents. This disease must be considered in any adolescent
who presents with a chronic dermatologic lesion and other systemic
signs. An excellent article on muscle involvement in systemic lupus
erythematosus is included in the reading list.

Johansson et al. discuss the syndrome of mixed connective tissue disease (MCTD) in 12 patients aged 17–41 years at onset. The common manifestations for this were Raynaud's phenomenon and cold sensitivity. In adolescents and young adults presenting with these signs, we must suspect collagen vascular disease, especially MCTD.

Acne Vulgaris—Its Etiology and Treatment: Review. W. J. Cunliffe, A. D. Clayden, D. Gould, and N. B. Simpson (Leeds, England) report that up to 30% of teenagers have acne severe enough to require treatment. Acne is rarely life-threatening, but its cosmetic effects often produce social problems, which in extreme cases have led to suicide.

In a study of 157 patients given erythromycin, 250 mg twice daily, and a topical benzoyl peroxide preparation twice daily, mean improvements were 22% after 2 months, 27% after 4 months, and 49% at 6 months. After 6 months of therapy, improvement of 50% or more had occurred in 62% of the patients. Failure to exhibit 50% improvement at 6 months correlated with an earlier age of onset of acne. There was no statistical difference between responders and nonresponders with regard to duration or initial grade of acne, family acne history, oral contraceptive use, or age of onset of acne with relation to menarche. By the end of 10 months, in 73% of patients who discontinued erythromycin therapy the disease had relapsed to within 50% of its original grade. No significant correlation was found with possible "risk" factors. In a study of 278 individuals, females had a significantly better response rate than males. Females aged 14–15 years and males aged 16–17 and 22–29 years had a poor response. Perhaps such patients should be given a larger initial antibiotic dose than would normally be prescribed for their acne grade.

Gastrointestinal side effects of treatment always responded to antispasmodics, and vaginal candidiasis responds to nystatin. Side effects (a maculopapular eruption due to erythromycin) required treatment withdrawal in only 1 patient. The initial high incidence of side effects from topical benzoyl peroxide decrease with continued application.

▶ [These data provide the results of the long-term treatment of acne with conventional therapy. Of particular interest was the poor response of certain age groups. Although, to our knowledge, this has not been reported previously, its significance is questionable. The major problem with studies of this type is that a standardized regimen was used. With individualized therapy, such as usually is used in practice, lack of response is encountered less commonly.—R.L.D.] ◀

The Menstrual Cycle and Plasma Testosterone Levels in Women With Acne. E. Steinberger, L. J. Rodriguez-Rigau, K. D. Smith, and B. Held prospectively studied ovarian function and plasma testosterone levels in 139 women with a chief complaint of acne without other medical problems, with unsatisfactory response of the acne to routine dermatologic therapy. They received no hormone therapy before study. The women were of reproductive age, of

Clin. Exp. Dermatol. 6:461–469, September 1981.
J. Am. Acad. Dermatol. 4:54–58, January 1981.

average height and weight, and had experienced menarche at the expected age.

In 90% of the patients, plasma testosterone levels were above normal mean; 97.1% of patients had masculine-type hair growth in 1 or more areas. Amenorrhea was present in 17.2%, anovulation in 18.4%, and variable degree of ovulatory dysfunction in 57.2%. In patients with ovulatory changes, the mean follicular phase length was 20.2 ± 0.8 days (abnormally long), and the mean luteal phase length was 12.1 ± 0.3 days (abnormally short). The duration of both phases of the menstrual cycle was within normal range in only 7.2% of patients. The severity of ovarian dysfunction was directly proportional to plasma testosterone levels. Age was inversely related to both plasma testosterone levels and severity of ovarian dysfunction. Acne appeared later in patients with regular cycles and lower testosterone levels. The highest plasma testosterone levels and most severe ovarian dysfunction were most common in the teenage group.

Results of this study suggest that acne may be associated not only with a hyperandrogenic state, but also with ovarian dysfunction, and emphasize the need for careful investigation of androgen levels and ovarian function in women with acne as the chief complaint.

Reduced Sex Hormone Binding Globulin and Derived Free Testosterone Levels in Women With Severe Acne. Although acne is a well-known feature of hyperandrogenism, there are conflicting reports of normal and reduced circulating levels of sex hormone-binding globulin (SHBG) in this condition. Daphne M. Lawrence, M. Katz, T. W. E. Robinson, Maureen C. Newman, H. H. G. McGarrigle, Marcia Shaw, and Gillian C. L. Lachelin (London) measured plasma concentrations of testosterone, "derived" free testosterone, and SHBG in 47 women with moderate to severe acne. Twenty-three of these women had associated hirsutism or irregular menstrual cycles, or both. Fifteen asymptomatic, regularly menstruating women served as controls. All of the women were clinically euthyroid, and none was using oral contraceptives.

In the 24 women with acne alone, the mean plasma testosterone concentration (1.5 ± 0.3 nmole/L) was significantly higher ($P < .01$) than that in controls (1.1 ± 0.35 nmole/L). Testosterone concentrations were above the normal range (0.5–1.7 nmole/L) in 7 of these patients. In women with acne and associated hirsutism or irregular menstrual cycles, or both the mean plasma testosterone concentration (2.1 ± 0.6 nmole/L) was significantly higher than that in controls ($P < .001$) and that in women with acne alone ($P < .001$). Fifteen of these patients had plasma testosterone concentrations above the normal ranges. Mean SHBG concentrations in women with acne alone (48 ± 24 nmole/L) and in those with associated hirsutism or irregular menstrual cycles, or both (39 ± 18 nmole/L), were both significantly lower ($P < .001$) than that in controls (70 ± 19 nmole/L). The SHBG

Clin. Endocrinol. (Oxf.) 15:87–91, July 1981.

values were below the lower limit of normal in 13 of the women with acne alone and in 14 with acne and associated hirsutism or menstrual disturbances, or both. However, the difference between SHBG concentrations in the two groups of women with acne was not significant. No correlation was observed between testosterone concentrations and SHBG values. Mean free testosterone concentrations derived from SHBG and testosterone concentrations ranged from 6 to 21 pmole/L (mean, 13 ± 4 pmole/L) in control subjects, from 9 to 30 pmole/L (mean, 21 ± 6 pmole/L) in patients with acne alone, and from 15 to 50 pmole/L (mean, 31 ± 10 pmole/L) in patients with acne and associated hirsutism or menstrual disturbances, or both. Ten of the women with acne alone and 20 of those with associated hirsutism or menstrual disturbances or both, had free testosterone concentrations above the normal range.

The results show that depressed SHBG concentrations and elevated levels of derived free testosterone are frequently found in women with severe acne and that this may be a significant factor in the etiology or perpetuation of this condition, or both.

Cyproteronacetate in the Management of Severe Acne in Males. R. H. Cormane and H. L. M. van der Meeren (Univ. of Amsterdam) report the results of an investigation of the antiandrogen cyproteronacetate (CPA, 25 mg given orally once daily for at least 3 months) in the management of severe acne vulgaris in 11 men, aged 17–34 years, who did not react satisfactorily or at all to available therapy.

Marked improvement was noted in most instances. All patients responded substantially. The average improvement amounted to 1.9 grades. Side effects were minimal. Two patients perceived slight impairment of libido; 2 developed slight gynecomastia. Therapy was continued in 1 of the later patients without causing progression of the gynecomastia. No patient showed any weight gain. Routine laboratory investigations revealed no abnormalities.

High doses (100–300 mg) of CPA may cause a decrease in libido, sexual potency, and sperm count and mobility. Lower doses also may cause oligospermia. Patients given a daily dose of 5 or 10 mg of CPA had significantly decreased sperm counts but not to infertile levels. Bone marrow toxicity was not encountered. Even high doses do not influence the hypothalamic-hypophyseal-adrenal cortical axis; only if high doses are given in precocious puberty and endocrinologic disturbances are deviations in cortisol metabolism occasionally seen. The treatment is not advised in patients with severe liver dysfunctions, although in various studies effects on liver and kidney functions were not seen.

This study shows that CPA, 25 mg/day given orally, is effective in the control of recalcitrant acne in male subjects. The therapy is not recommended for minor forms of acne. The only indications are (1)

Arch. Dermatol. Res. 271:183–187, September 1981.

when acne is resistant to therapy or (2) when currently available therapy is contraindicated.

Oral Vitamin A in Acne Vulgaris. Generally, oral vitamin A therapy is not considered to be useful in the treatment of acne vulgaris. Albert M. Kligman, Otto H. Mills, Jr., James J. Leyden, Paul R. Gross, Herbert B. Allen, and Robert I. Rudolph (Univ. of Pennsylvania, Philadelphia) evaluated the effectiveness and toxicity of oral vitamin A (retinol) therapy in the treatment of acne vulgaris. Three groups of patients with serious, long-standing inflammatory acne were studied: 80 men and 56 women received 300,000 units of retinol daily for 3–4 months; 20 men received 300,000 units/day for 12 weeks; and 10 men received 300,000 units/day for the first week, 400,000 units/day for the second week, and then 500,000 units/day for 10 weeks.

Overall, about 50% of the patients showed an excellent response to treatment and 40% had a good response at the end of 3–4 months. Women appeared to respond better as none had a fair or poor response and a greater percentage had excellent results. Sebum production in women decreased by about 30% by 10 weeks. After 1 month, resolution was more rapid, with most of the pustules eliminated within 2 months. Deeper nodules were resorbed, for the most part, by 3–4 months. Back lesions were more resistant to treatment than facial lesions. In general, best results were seen in patients with many pustules and papules. Of the 20 men who received 300,000 units/day, only 4 had an excellent response, whereas 5 of the 10 men who received 500,000 units/day for 10 weeks showed an excellent response and 5 had a good response. Once treatment was stopped, most patients showed a partial relapse within 3–6 weeks. Toxicity was slight and was primarily limited to the skin (xerosis) and mucous membranes (cheilitis). Headache and minor nosebleed, both of which were well tolerated, were reported by some patients. There was no correlation between serum vitamin A levels and the therapeutic response and toxicity.

It is concluded that retinol has a definite place in the treatment of serious inflammatory acne. It is emphasized that a water-dispersed retinol emulsion was used. Guidelines for the administration of retinol are summarized.

▶ [By the time this volume of the YEAR BOOK is published, 13-*cis*-retinoic acid may be available for the treatment of severe acne. If not, megadose vitamin A is a reasonable alternative. Our results have not been as impressive overall as those of Kligman et al., but we have had some notable successes.—R.L.D.] ◀

Oral Zinc Sulfate Therapy in Acne Vulgaris: Double-Blind Trial. The exact mode of action of zinc is unknown. It plays a part in many enzyme activities and in epithelialization. It appears to be necessary in various stages of metabolism of vitamin A; a rise in vitamin A concentration has been reported to follow zinc therapy. K. C.

Int. J. Dermatol. 20:278–285, May 1981.
Acta Derm. Venereol. (Stockh.) 60:337–340, 1980.

Verma, A. S. Saini, and S. K. Dhamija compared the effects of zinc sulfate and lactose placebo in a double-blind trial in 56 patients with acne vulgaris and measured serum vitamin A concentrations. Twenty-nine patients received 600 mg of zinc sulfate per day orally and 27 patients took placebo.

Patients on placebo showed no improvement after 6 weeks; the condition in 11 was aggravated. After 6 weeks 15 patients on zinc showed some improvement, and after 12 weeks 17 (58%) showed further improvement. There was a statistically significant decrease in the number of infiltrates, papules, and cysts and a decrease in facial oiliness and associated seborrhea, but there was little effect on pustular lesions. Four patients taking zinc had nausea; in 1, treatment was discontinued because of vomiting. After 6 weeks the serum vitamin A concentrations in the zinc group rose from $20.93 \pm 4.65\mu g/100$ ml to $24.36 \pm 5.02\ \mu g/100$ ml, and at the end of the trial to $31.12 \pm 5.8\ \mu g/100$ ml ($P < .01$). The increase in vitamin A concentration was greater in the 17 patients who showed significant clinical improvement. No significant change was found in the placebo group.

Zinc is involved to some extent in acne.

▶ [There are almost as many negative trials of zinc in acne as there are positive ones. This study raises the possibility not only of differences in dietary zinc explaining the discrepancies, but differences in dietary vitamin A. One might postulate that zinc most easily would be shown to be active in acne patients whose diet is deficient in zinc, vitamin A, or both.—L.C.L.] ◀

13-*Cis*-Retinoic Acid and Acne. Acne severity and seborrhea are correlated closely, and drugs that reduce the sebum excretion rate improve the disease. Recently, an oral derivative of vitamin A, 13-*cis*-retinoic acid, reportedly improved acne in 14 severely affected patients. In 4 of these, measurements of the surface lipid content suggested substantial reduction of the sebaceous gland contribution. H. Jones, D. Blanc, and W. J. Cunliffe (Leeds, England) used 13-*cis*-retinoic acid to treat 10 patients, with beneficial effects resulting.

TECHNIQUE.—Of the 10 patients, 8 (aged 18–32 years) had severe acne unresponsive to long-term and varied antibiotic treatment. Two patients had only mild acne, but 1 (aged 49) had devastating hidradenitis suppurativa requiring a colostomy, and the other (aged 41) had widespread steatocystoma multiplex. These 2 patients were included because of the extent of their disorders and because of similarities in the pathogenesis of acne, hidradenitis suppurativa, and steatocystoma multiplex. To acquire adequate control data, all treatment was stopped for at least 6 weeks. Four patients received 0.1 mg of 13-*cis*-retinoic acid per kg and 6 patients 0.5–1.0 mg/kg. No other treatment was given. Patients were seen before treatment and at regular intervals during it.

There was a 75% reduction in the sebum excretion rate at 4 weeks that was maintained throughout the rest of the study. Clinical improvement was slower but equally dramatic. At 4 weeks, the acne

---

Lancet 2:1048–1049, Nov. 15, 1980.

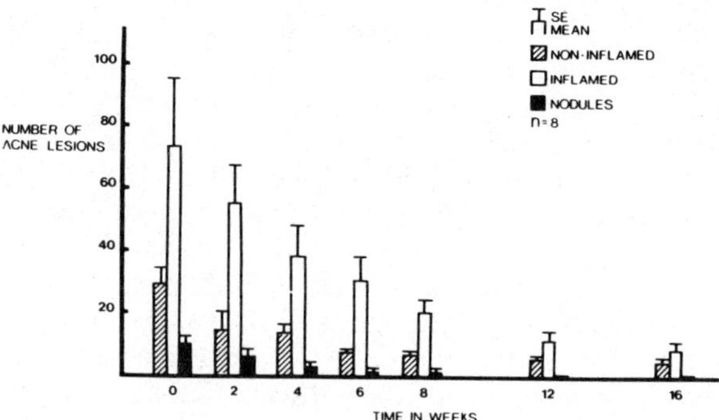

Fig 4.—Number of acne lesions occurring during treatment in all patients. (Courtesy of Jones, H., et al.: Lancet 2:1048–1049, Nov. 15, 1980.)

grade had improved by 30%, and by 16 weeks there was an 80% improvement in overall grade as well as an 80% reduction in noninflamed lesions, a 90% reduction in small inflamed lesions, and a 90% reduction in deep inflamed lesions (Fig 4).

The patients with hidradenitis suppurativa and steatocystoma multiplex did not improve, although sebum production decreased. There was a dose-response relationship: patients receiving the high dose had a greater reduction in the sebum excretion rate, although the clinical response, when expressed as a percentage change, was the same.

Clinical side effects were dose related, the most common being facial dermatitis, xerosis, and cheilitis. The most serious side effect was arthralgia, which occurred in 1 patient; the dosage of 13-*cis*-retinoic acid was reduced and the acne continued to improve, with no increase in the sebum excretion rate. Abnormalities in laboratory findings were minimal, transient, and dose related.

▶ [Treatment of severe acne is always difficult, but 13-*cis*-retinoic acid may be of considerable help. Previous reports have indicated that this drug, administered orally, produced prolonged remissions of cystic and conglobate acne (*N. Engl. J. Med.* 300:329, 1979). This article by Jones et al. again reports good results in cases of acne of such severity that most other treatments have been ineffective. At the moment, one would have to reserve use of this drug only for treatment-resistant patients. A single case report of a treatment-resistant patient tells of good results with danazol, a drug that, like the oral contraceptives, reduces testosterone levels by suppressing gonadotropins (*Cutis* 26:393, 1980). More experience with this approach will be needed before it can be considered a possible alternative.—L.E.H.] ◀

Reduction of Bacterial Skin Flora During Oral Treatment of Severe Acne With 13-*cis*-Retinoic Acid. Clinical trials of a promising new compound for the oral treatment of acne and other dermatologic disorders, 13-*cis*-retinoic acid (Ro 4-3780), are in progress. Ar-

Arch. Dermatol. Res. 270:179–183, April 1981.

thur Weissmann, Annemarie Wagner, and Gerd Plewig (Univ. of Munich) evaluated oral 13-*cis*-retinoic acid therapy in 5 randomly selected patients with severe acne unresponsive to previous treatment. No additional systemic or topical treatment was given during the trial. The effects of treatment on the bacterial flora of the skin were investigated, and a minimal inhibitory concentration (MIC) assay was used to evaluate a possible antibacterial effect of the agent in vitro.

All 5 patients responded well to the treatment, with no apparent side effects other than slight dryness of the skin and mucous membranes. The density of propionibacteria decreased steadily during treatment, the difference reaching significance after 12 weeks. Similar changes were noted for aerobic cocci on the forehead, but not on the back. The decrease in bacteria was not related to the initial dose of 13-*cis*-retinoic acid and did not correlate with clinical improvement. No inhibition of bacterial growth by 13-*cis*-retinoic acid was apparent in vitro when the growth of staphylococci and propionibacteria was assessed.

Since no in vitro antibacterial activity of 13-*cis*-retinoic acid was found in this study, the marked decrease in bacterial counts noted in vivo is attributed to changes in the bacterial habitat. A reduction in skin lipid excretion by 13-*cis*-retinoic acid could cause suppression of the bacterial flora. It remains unclear whether the change in skin bacteria is merely secondary to marked suppression of sebum excretion or whether it contributes to clinical improvement. In addition, 13-*cis*-retinoic acid shrinks the follicular infundibula, providing less space for bacterial lacunae, the predominant niche for colonization by propionibacteria.

Inhibitory Effects of 13-*cis*-Retinoic Acid on Human Sebaceous Glands. Michael Landthaler, Johann Kummermehr, Annemarie Wagner, and Gerd Plewig (Univ. of Munich) studied the effects of 13-*cis*-retinoic acid on sebaceous glands in 18 males. Studies were done by histologic, planimetric, and autoradiographic means. A dose of 1–2 mg/kg of body weight was given daily for 12 weeks.

Histologically and planimetrically, a 50% decrease in the size of sebaceous glands was observed after 3–4 weeks of treatment and a cumulative dose of about 3 gm. With higher doses and after 12 weeks of treatment, a reduction of up to 90% of pretreatment values was seen.

Additionally, in the sebaceous acini of sebaceous follicles, the ratio of the so-called differentiating cell pool (basement membrane-bound germinative cells and lipid cells [sebocytes], which contain lipid droplets in their cytoplasm) vs. the so-called undifferentiating cell pool (sebocytes that rarely produce lipid droplets at the light microscopic level and that form a spongiform skeleton throughout the sebaceous gland) changed from 2:1 to 1:7, probably indicating a disturbance of differentiation (lipid production) of sebocytes. The increase in undif-

Arch. Dermatol. Res. 269:279–309, December 1980.

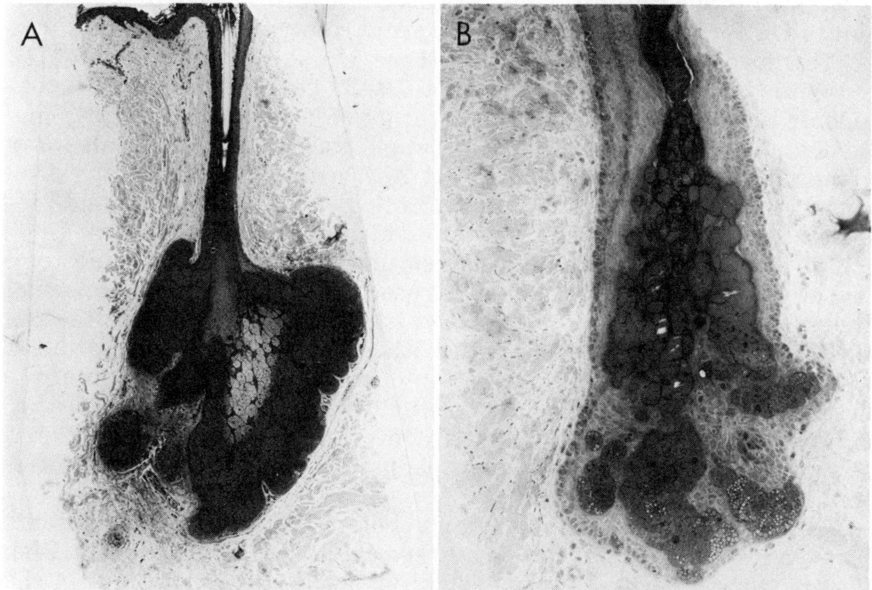

Fig 5.—13-*cis*-Retinoic acid inhibits sebocytes. **A,** before therapy. Large sebaceous follicle with abundant sebocytes in sebaceous acini. **B,** after 5 weeks of treatment with 1 mg/kg of body weight daily. Note replacement of sebaceous gland periphery by undifferentiating cells (higher magnification) and regression of sebum-producing sebocytes. (Courtesy of Landthaler, M., et al.: Arch. Dermatol. Res. 269:279–309, 1980.)

ferentiated cells could be observed histologically after only 1 week of treatment.

Histologically, the large sebaceous lobules seemed to collapse. The boundaries of the acini were replaced completely by small undifferentiating cells. Differentiating sebocytes were found only in the center of the acini, close to the sebaceous duct (Fig 5). In extreme cases, formerly large sebaceous follicles were reduced to a wicklike structure consisting of only the pilary unit. The space of the sebaceous follicles was replaced by a perifollicular fibrosis with many fibroblasts. The lower dose of 1 mg/kg of body weight also led to a marked reduction in sebaceous lobules; there seemed to be a slower and less intensive reduction with the 1-mg dose as opposed to the 2-mg dose.

The labeling index of sebocytes also regressed significantly under therapy with 13-*cis*-retinoic acid. Clinically, the patients have been in remission for up to 1 year without recurrence of seborrhea or acne.

▶ [These studies demonstrate the profound involution of sebaceous glands induced by 13-*cis*-retinoic acid. This phenomenon is probably responsible for the long remissions observed after discontinuation of treatment. It is unlikely, however, that sebaceous gland involution explains the initial resolution of severe nodulocystic acne. Within a nodule, sebaceous glands have either been destroyed by the inflammation or have dedifferentiated completely. Therefore, the initial response to 13-*cis*-retinoic acid must depend on suppression of inflammation or modulation of the reparative process.—R.L.D.] ◀

Risk Factors Promote Elevations of Serum Lipids in Acne Patients Under Oral 13-*cis*-Retinoic Acid (Isotretinoin). H. Gollnick, D. Tsambaos, and C. E. Orfanos (Free Univ. of Berlin) treated 10 patients (9 men and 1 woman, aged 19–29 years) afflicted with conglobate acne with 13-*cis*-retinoic acid given orally (Ro 4-3780, 1 mg/kg/day). After completion of a 12-week treatment, 5 patients were given a further course of therapy at 20% of the initial dose; the drug was discontinued in the other 5 patients. Serum triglyceride and cholesterol levels were measured before, during, and after therapy.

Two patients revealed abnormal serum triglyceride and cholesterol levels; triglycerides alone were increased in 1 patient and abnormal cholesterol values alone were found in 3 others. The highest serum lipid values occurred between the 8th and 12th week of treatment. These changes reversed on cessation of treatment or reduction of the dose. In some instances, values returned to normal despite further administration of the initial dose. Only in 2 patients did abnormal triglyceride and cholesterol levels persist for more than 2 weeks after treatment was discontinued.

The mean serum triglyceride and cholesterol values of all patients rose during therapy but did not exceed the upper normal limits. Risk factors such as alcohol abuse, smoking, obesity, hyperlipemia in the family history, or pretreatment values in the upper normal range were present in all patients who had significant elevations of serum lipids during treatment. Only 1 of 4 patients who revealed no elevation of serum lipids during treatment with oral 13-*cis*-retinoic acid was an alcoholic and a heavy smoker, but he claimed to have reduced alcohol consumption during therapy.

Evidence suggests that the influence of 13-*cis*-retinoic acid on serum lipids is dose-related. Individual risk factors most likely promote serum lipid abnormalities during 13-*cis*-retinoic acid treatment, and these factors should be considered in patients to be so treated. The lipid-modulating effects of oral 13-*cis*-retinoic acid cannot be regarded as specific for acne or any other disease.

▶ [Two facts emerge from this study: (1) Even short-term administration of 13-*cis*-retinoic acid in low dosage produces reversible changes in levels of serum lipids. (2) The presence of obesity, alcohol abuse, or smoking in a genetically predisposed person significantly increases the risk of these changes. Fortunately, the duration of treatment of cystic acne is brief, so even a fat patient who smokes and drinks will probably not suffer significant harm from therapy. However, when 13-*cis*-retinoic acid (Accutane) becomes readily available, it undoubtedly will be used for diseases other than severe acne. Careful patient selection and frequent monitoring will be necessary to avoid serious side effects.—R.L.D.] ◀

Topical Erythromycin Solution in Acne: Results of Multiclinic Trial are reported by Richard L. Dobson and Burton S. Belknap (SUNY at Buffalo). A total of 253 patients, who were treated in a double-blind manner by 11 investigators, received either erythromycin solution or vehicle alone. All patients had at least 10 papules or

Arch. Dermatol. Res. 271:189–196, September 1981.
J. Am. Acad. Dermatol. 3:478–482, November 1980.

pustules, 1 or more comedones, and not more than 5 nodulocystic lesions. Medications were applied twice daily for 12 weeks. Patients had not received antiacne therapy for at least 2 weeks before the study.

Significantly more vehicle-treated patients withdrew from the study because of lack of improvement or worsening of acne. Analysis of patients who completed at least 4 weeks in the study showed a significant reduction in all lesion types combined in both groups. This was not unexpected, because some components of the vehicle such as alcohol and Laureth-4 may have some value in acne therapy. Erythromycin-treated patients showed a significantly greater reduction in papules and pustules and in total lesions. Comedones also were reduced more in the erythromycin-treated group, but the difference was not significant. Overall results were better in the erythromycin-treated group after 4, 8, and 12 weeks of therapy. One patient had an urticarial type reaction 2 days after the start of erythromycin therapy, which cleared fully 6 days after treatment was discontinued.

These findings indicate significant benefit from topical erythromycin compared with its vehicle in the treatment of inflammatory lesions of acne vulgaris. No serious adverse effects were encountered in this study.

▶ [The authors have done themselves (and erythromycin) a disservice by their statistical analysis. They started with a total of 253 patients and ended with 199. Of the "lost sheep," 30 were "administrative" losses and deserved to be ignored, but 24 did not. Of the latter group, only 2 erythromycin-treated patients dropped out because of failure to improve, or actual worsening. But 19 did so for these same reasons in the placebo group. That is one hell of a difference, friends, and failure to count these in means that the results with the drug were even better than reported.—L.C.L.] ◀

Topical Clindamycin Therapy for Acne Vulgaris: A Cooperative Clinical Study. Larry E. Becker, Paul R. Bergstresser, David A. Whiting, William E. Clendenning, Richard L. Dobson, William P. Jordan, Edward Abell, Lloyd A. LeZotte, Peter E. Pochi, Jerome L. Shupack, Robert B. Sigafoes, Richard B. Stoughton, and John J. Voorhees report the results of an 8-week double-blind study conducted at 11 centers to compare 1% clindamycin hydrochloride, 1% clindamycin phosphate, and a hydroalcoholic vehicle in the treatment of moderate to severe acne vulgaris. Patients aged 12–30 years with 12–70 inflammatory papules on the face were included in the trial. Pregnant women were excluded. The 413 patients applied medications morning and night after washing with a nonmedicated soap.

A total of 358 patients completed the study. Overall pustule counts were low but the mean count was significantly lower in the patients treated with clindamycin phosphate than in the placebo group. Papule counts were lower in both clindamycin-treated groups than in the placebo group at the eighth week. Local side effects were comparable in all groups, and were mild. Twelve clindamycin-treated patients and 2 placebo patients reported diarrhea. No treatment resulted in abnormalities in posttreatment laboratory tests.

Arch. Dermatol. 117:482–485, August 1981.

Topical clindamycin is superior to a hydroalcoholic vehicle in the treatment of acne vulgaris. Significant reductions in pustule and papule counts were found in this study, and more clindamycin-treated patients than placebo patients considered themselves improved.

Topical Clindamycin Treatment of Acne: Clinical, Surface Lipid Composition, and Quantitative Surface Microbiology Response. Topical clindamycin is clinically effective in the treatment of acne vulgaris. Robert J. Thomsen, Anna Stranieri, Dianne Knutson, and John S. Strauss (Univ. of Iowa) studied the effects of topical 1% clindamycin hydrochloride hydrate in a hydroalcoholic vehicle on changes in free fatty acids in the skin surface lipids and in bacterial counts in the skin in 14 patients. Nine patients were treated with active clindamycin solution and 5 with the vehicle alone. The groups had similar degrees of initial severity and duration of acne. Two patients were taking oral contraceptives. Topical solution was applied twice daily.

Significant improvement in lesion counts was observed in the study group but not in the control group; however, only 3 patients had significant improvement. Three study patients and 1 control reported marked subjective improvement. Peeling, erythema, and burning or itching were more frequent in study patients but occurred in both groups. There were no systemic complications and no significant laboratory abnormalities. The percentage of free fatty acids was reduced by two thirds in the study group within 2 weeks and by nearly 90% after 8 weeks of treatment. The change did not correlate directly with clinical response. There were no significant changes in total numbers of organisms recovered by the surface collection technique.

The concentration of free fatty acids in the skin surface lipids is reduced significantly by topical clindamycin therapy. Clinical improvement may occur without a change in the surface microbial flora. Topical clindamycin is effective in treating inflammatory acne. The clinical response was not impressive in the present series but 8 weeks probably is an insufficient period in which to judge clinical response accurately.

▶ [Clindamycin lotion has been used widely for the treatment of acne, so the clinical experience must be better than the short-term experience reported in this article. Although the usual rationale for such treatment is thought to be due to the antibacterial effect of the drug, this study suggests that reduction of the concentration of fatty acids in skin surface lipids may contribute to the therapeutic benefit.—L.E.H.] ◀

Topical Tetracycline Hydrochloride Versus Topical Clindamycin Phosphate in the Treatment of Acne: A Comparative Study. Topical antibiotic therapy now is widely used for acne vulgaris. R. Steven Padilla, Jack M. McCabe, and Larry E. Becker (Albuquerque, N.M.) compared topical tetracycline and clindamycin therapy in 52 subjects aged 18–30 years who had 12–70 inflammatory papules or pustules on the face. None had more than 6 inflam-

Arch. Dermatol. 116:1031–1034, September 1980.
Int. J. Dermatol. 20:445–448, July-Aug. 1981.

matory nodules more than 5 mm in size. Subjects were randomly assigned to treatment with 2.2% tetracycline hydrochloride solution or 1% clindamycin phosphate solution. Medications were applied twice daily to the affected area.

Twenty-two patients treated with clindamycin and 27 treated with tetracycline completed the study. Twenty patients using clindamycin and 14 using tetracycline had a good to fair response, with a 34%–100% reduction in lesion counts. The results with clindamycin were significantly better. Only a few subjects in each group had side effects. Two patients treated with clindamycin had diarrhea, but this resolved during continued treatment in both cases.

Clindamycin phosphate was significantly more effective than tetracycline hydrochloride in reducing lesion counts in these patients with acne. No significant differences in local side effects were noted. Oral clindamycin therapy has been related to pseudomembranous colitis, but only 2 of the present patients had diarrhea, and this was attributed to viral gastroenteritis or food intolerance. Some patients using tetracycline were concerned over yellowish skin staining.

Prospective Study on Safety of Long-term Tetracycline Therapy for Acne. To assess the safety of long-term tetracycline therapy for acne, Gordon C. Sauer (Kansas City, Mo.) conducted a series of automated, multiple-analysis, blood chemistry studies (SMA 12) and blood cell counts in a prospective study of 75 patients who received low-dose tetracycline therapy for more than 1 year. All but 3 patients had acne vulgaris. Although most patients received 250 mg of tetracycline hydrochloride twice a day, 20 were treated with a daily dose of 750–1,000 mg and 1 patient received 1,500 mg/day.

All of the patients but 7 had repeated test results within normal limits. One patient, a 15-year-old girl, had a total serum bilirubin level of 1.1 mg/100 ml on the preliminary test and 1.2 mg/100 ml on the repeated test; this finding is usually associated with Gilbert's disease. A 16-year-old boy had an alkaline phosphatase level of 305 mU/ml, compared with an age-adjusted, normal high level of 272 mU/ml. A third patient, a 53-year-old man who had been treated for more than 1 year for acne rosacea, had a serum glutamic oxaloacetic transaminase level of 105 mU/ml on the preliminary test and 125 mU/ml on the repeated test. This patient also had a history of excessive alcohol intake for more than 20 years. A 15-year-old boy had a lactic dehydrogenase level of 260 mU/ml on the repeated test, compared with a normal maximum level of 221 mU/ml. Neutrophilia of 83 and 85, respectively, was present in 2 patients, and 1 patient had an eosinophilia in three tests.

The results of this prospective study corroborate the accumulating evidence that only rarely does long-term, low-dose tetracycline therapy cause serious side effects.

▶ [Sauer (*Arch. Dermatol.* 112:1603, 1976) previously reported a retrospective study of 325 patients who had received tetracycline therapy for 3 or more years. The results

Cutis 27:492–493, May 1981.

were similar to those found in the present prospective study. These data indicate that long-term low-dose tetracycline therapy, as used in dermatologic practice, is remarkably safe. They also suggest that ordering blood counts and chemistries, unless specifically indicated, is a waste of time and money.—R.L.D.] ◄

Benzoyl Peroxide: Percutaneous Penetration and Metabolic Disposition. Benzoyl peroxide, a commonly used antiacne agent, is a potent antibacterial; it is thought to penetrate into the follicles to eradicate *Propionibacterium acnes,* and is also recommended for use in other dermatoses. Sergio Nacht, David Yeung, Joseph N. Beasley, Jr., Mark D. Anjo, and Howard I. Maibach assessed the transepidermal penetration and metabolic disposition of ^{14}C-benzoyl peroxide in vitro (excised human skin) and in vivo (rhesus monkey).

In vitro, benzoyl peroxide penetrated into the skin unchanged, through the stratum corneum or follicular openings, or both, and diffused into the epidermis and dermis, where it was converted to benzoic acid. Most (95.3%) of the benzoyl peroxide originally applied topically was recovered unchanged from the skin surface at the end of 8 hours.

In vivo, benzoic acid was recovered from urine in amounts equivalent to 45% and 98% of the radiolabel following, respectively, topical and intramuscular administration of small amounts of ^{14}C-benzoyl peroxide. Three minor, as yet unidentified metabolites were found after topical, but not after intramuscular, administration; these accounted for less than 5% of the ^{14}C label in urine.

It was concluded that benzoyl peroxide penetrates as such into the skin layers and is converted therein to benzoic acid, which is absorbed into the systemic circulation by diffusing into the blood vessels of the dermis. Delayed excretion of the radiolabel after topical application, as compared with intramuscular injection, might be attributed to the longer lag time required for percutaneous absorption. Renal clearance of the metabolite is sufficiently rapid as to preclude its hepatic conjugation with glycine, since following topical administration to monkeys, no hippuric acid was found in the urine, as could have been expected had a significant amount of benzoic acid passed through the liver (as would occur following oral administration).

Calculations indicate that even under unrealistic conditions of excessive topical application, the systemic absorption of benzoyl peroxide (or of its metabolite, benzoate) cannot be greater than 500 mg/day, an amount easily handled metabolically by the mammalian organism. Thus, topical applications of benzoyl peroxide can be expected to be free of toxic systemic effects.

► [These results corroborate clinical experience. The long-term use of topical benzoyl peroxide even on extensive areas has not been associated with systemic toxicity.—R.L.D.] ◄

Skin Tumor-Promoting Activity of Benzoyl Peroxide, a Widely Used Free Radical-Generating Compound. Skin tumors can be induced in mice by a variety of chemical carcinogens and by

J. Am. Acad. Dermatol. 4:31–37, January 1981.
Science 213:1023–1025, Aug. 28, 1981.

ultraviolet light. Benzoyl peroxide is a widely used free radical-generating compound. It is an additive in cosmetics and pharmaceuticals, including those used in treatment of acne. T. J. Slaga, A. J. P. Klein-Szanto, L. L. Triplett, L. P. Yotti (Oak Ridge, Tenn. Natl. Lab.), and J. E. Trosko (Michigan State Univ.) evaluated benzoyl peroxide as a skin tumor promoter when applied topically to mice after initiation with dimethylbenzanthracene.

Benzoyl peroxide was not effective as a complete carcinogen, even in a dosage of 40 mg twice weekly for 1 year. When it was applied topically twice weekly after initiation of tumors, however, it was an effective promoter with a reasonable dose-response curve. As little as 1 mg, given twice weekly, produced a significant number of papillomas and carcinomas. The tumor response appeared to plateau at a dosage of 20 mg. Benzoyl peroxide also increased the tumor response in a dose-dependent manner when given simultaneously with 12-O-tetradecaroyl phorbol-13-acetate (TPA), a known promoter. Application of benzoyl peroxide led to epidermal hyperplasia and morphological changes similar to those caused by TPA.

Free radicals play an important role in the carcinogenic effects of irradiation and chemicals. If chemical carcinogens act through initiation and promotion, the initiation phase could involve a critical interaction of electrophilic forms of carcinogens with some cellular nucleophile. The generation of free radicals in the promotion phase could lead directly or indirectly to membrane peroxidation. Caution is indicated in the use of benzoyl peroxide and other free radical-generating compounds.

▶ [Lest we dermatologists and our patients become alarmed at this report, the facts contained therein need reiteration. (1) Benzoyl peroxide is noncarcinogenic. (2) Enormous amounts of benzoyl peroxide were applied to mice twice weekly for 1 year to demonstrate its ability to promote carcinogenesis. (3) No parallel studies were conducted with a known potent promotor such as phorbol ester to determine the relative activity of benzoyl peroxide. In this study, 40 mg of benzoyl peroxide was applied weekly. This is equivalent to the application in man of 40 gm weekly or about thirty 1-oz tubes of 5% benzoyl peroxide weekly. In addition, the strain of mice used was selected because of its ability to develop skin cancer after a single exposure to a carcinogen. Therefore, it goes beyond the bounds of reason to consider that the results of this study have any applicability to patients with acne.—R.L.D.] ◀

Skin Testing to Detect Penicillin Allergy. About one third of patients hospitalized in the United States receive antibiotic therapy, and most receive β-lactam antibiotics. Simple avoidance of these agents in patients reporting symptoms of previous allergy does not solve the problem of patients sensitized by their last exposure. Timothy J. Sullivan, H. James Wedner, Gerald S. Shatz, Lewis D. Yecies, and Charles W. Parker examined the predictive value of skin testing in 740 patients studied between 1970 and 1979, when tests were made available on a 24-hour basis at the Washington University Medical Center. Patients were tested sequentially with progressively concentrated preparations of penicilloyl-poly-L-lysine (PPL), penicil-

Allergy Clin. Immunol. 68:171–180, September 1981.

lin G (Pen G), and penicilloic acid (PA). Concentrated reagents were given percutaneously and then intradermally.

About 95% of the patients tested had a history of apparent allergic reaction to β-lactam antibiotics, and 63% were skin test positive. The rates of positivity were 93% on testing 7 to 12 months after previous reactions and 22% after 10 years or longer. Patients under age 30 more often had positive skin tests. Testing with PPL was most productive. Test-positive patients often reacted to skin testing with other β-lactam antibiotics such as ampicillin and cephalothin. No serious allergic reactions resulted from skin testing. None of 83 skin test-negative patients had acute allergic reactions to β-lactam antibiotics. Two had mild urticaria after a few days of treatment.

Testing with PPL, Pen G, and PA is a rapid, effective, and safe means of identifying patients at risk of allergic reactions to penicillin. Only the lack of a commercial source of PA prevents widespread application of this or related approaches to protecting patients from allergic reactions to β-lactam drugs and permitting their use in patients no longer allergic to them. At present, the predictive value of skin testing is uncertain if a significant period elapses before treatment is begun.

▶ [It should be noted that a systemic allergic reaction occurred in 4 of the patients tested. Because of this, the authors advocate a "progressive concentration technique" in which patients are initially tested with highly diluted antigen (1:10,000). If negative, the concentration can be increased at intervals. Given the number of β-lactam antibiotics available and the rate of introduction of new ones, what now is needed is a commercial source of specific antigens so that the possibility of sensitivity to each can be determined reliably.—R.L.D.] ◀

Topical Antibiotics and Minor Skin Trauma. James J. Leyden and Marion B. Sulzberger review the use of topical antibiotics in minor skin trauma.

Numerous early studies of various types of wounds indicated that application of appropriate antibiotics reduces the risk of infection. However, only recently have double-blind, controlled studies demonstrated that application of a combination of neomycin, bacitracin, and polymyxin reduces the incidence of staphylococcal and streptococcal infection occurring in minor skin wounds. Leyden and Kligman developed a model in which informed volunteers were wounded either with a scratch injury or with an abrasion. Six abrasions on each of 10 persons were inoculated with 1×10^5 *Staphylococcus aureus* organisms and 6 scarified areas on each of another 10 persons were inoculated with 1×10^7 *Streptococcus pyogenes* organisms. The inoculated sites were covered with an impermeable dressing for 6 hours to allow the microorganisms to become established. Each site was then treated with precisely 0.1 ml of either an ointment containing a combination of neomycin, bacitracin, and polymyxin, or a blank ointment vehicle. After 24 hours, quantitative bacteriologic cultures were obtained. Both neomycin and bacitracin proved to be highly effective in preventing infection by both *S. aureus* and *S. pyogenes*.

Am. Fam. Physician 23:121–125, January 1981.

Concerns have been expressed about absorption with resulting systemic toxicity, about the emergence of resistant strains of the microorganisms, and about the possible finding of a high incidence of allergic contact dermatitis occurring from the use of these antibiotics. With regard to the first concern, systemic side effects of nephrotoxicity, ototoxicity, and neurotoxicity have not been observed after topical use except in cases of improper massive exposure to the drugs. With regard to the possible emergence of resistant strains, this has occurred only in "closed populations," e.g., patients confined to long-stay hospitals. With regard to the development of contact dermatitis, two recent independent, well-controlled studies found that allergic sensitization to neomycin is rare and is extremely unlikely to develop when drug applications are made only occasionally to small areas of the skin for the prevention of infection in minor skin wounds.

▶ [Many of us who use such topical antibiotics for minor skin wounds are gratified to see that their use has some rationale, even in the absence of a clearly established infection.—L.E.H.] ◀

Local Treatment of Hypertrophic Scars and Keloids With Topical Retinoic Acid. Many treatments advocated for keloids have failed to give convincing results. Retinoic acid reduces normal tonofilament and keratohyalin synthesis and leads to increased production of mucoid substances and an increased epidermal cell growth rate. Cormane suggested that the inhibitory effect of retinoic acid on DNA synthesis might be useful in treatment of excessively growing scar tissues. A. M. P. Janssen de Limpens (The Hague) conducted a clinical trial of 0.05% retinoic acid as a topical treatment in 28 patients with keloids and hypertrophic scars. Solution was applied to the scars twice daily, or once a day if the surrounding skin became irritated. Nearly all patients were younger than age 36 years; most were female.

Retinoic acid application led to subjective improvement in 79% of the 21 evaluable patients. Objective assessment indicated good to fair results in 77%. Two patients developed slight atrophy at the site of scarring. One patient previously treated in many ways for extensive scarring over most of the trunk is now free from pain for the first time in years. Some patients noticed a slight decrease in hyperpigmentation of the scar.

Favorable results were obtained with topical retinoic acid applications in nearly 80% of these patients with keloids and hypertrophic scars. Two of 3 patients with intractable keloids failed to respond to retinoic acid, but 1 showed marked improvement.

▶ [This is almost too good to be true. Over the years, many remedies for keloids have been introduced, but most have been found wanting. The failures have included hyaluronidase, formalin, nitrogen mustard, tetrahydroxyquinone, and N-acetylhydroxyproline, to name only a few. Radiation seems to be useful only if applied within the day after surgery. Up until now, the least objectionable and most effective treatment has been locally injected triamcinolone. Included in this reported Dutch series were

Br. J. Dermatol. 103:319–323, September 1980.

3 patients who had proved refractory to everything else; 1 responded to retinoic acid with marked improvement. We look forward to further experience.—L.C.L.] ◄

Recurrent Urticaria: Clinical Investigation of 330 Patients.
Lennart Juhlin (Univ. Hosp., Uppsala, Sweden) used a questionnaire for 330 consecutive patients with recurrent urticaria of 3 months' to 40 years' duration seen from 1972–1978 to determine possibly relevant factors in their personal histories.

Fifty men and 50 women had urticaria only. The remainder had both urticaria and angioedema; most of these patients were women aged 24–38. Diurnal variation in urticarial attacks was reported by 53% of the patients, with most of the attacks occurring in the evening or at night. More than 33% had a history of rhinitis, asthma, or atopic dermititis. Nasal polyps, migraine, and arthralgia were present in 6%–7% of the patients, and severe psychiatric problems were reported by 16%. Abdominal disorders, primarily gastritis, were mentioned by 44%. Thirty-two percent of the patients had a history of side effects from drugs, with penicillin and aspirin most commonly reported. Food was indicated as a factor worsening the wheals by 30% of the patients; drinks were noted by 18%. Fruits, vegetables, and nuts were mentioned most often. Although all patients with physical urticaria were excluded from this series, physical factors such as exercise were reported by 20% of the patients to worsen the urticaria. Approximately 33% of the patients had one or more positive reactions to provocation tests with various food additives such as azo dyes, benzoates, butylated hydroxytoluene (BHT), butylated hydroxyanisole (BHA) sorbic acid, quinoline yellow, carotene, canthaxanthine, annatto, and nitrite; another one-third had negative reactions; and the results were equivocal in the rest. Routine laboratory studies and x-ray films of sinuses or teeth were of little value in the absence of signs or a history of other diseases. In 24% of the patients, the fibrin microclot test, an indicator of the presence of circulating endotoxins, was positive.

► [In dealing with a patient with recurrent urticaria, the question always arises as to how extensive an evaluation is indicated. Most large published series seem to agree on only one fact—in the majority of cases (90% or more), no causative factor can be detected. In this regard, this report differs in that provocative tests with various food additives were positive in one third of the patients. Whether this is generally true or depends on a highly selected patient population is unknown. This matter is of more than academic interest, since Juhlin's provocative testing requires more than 2 weeks' hospitalization. Until his results can be confirmed, most dermatologists would probably prefer to recommend an elimination diet in selected cases. However, experience has shown that this approach is usually ineffective, perhaps because of the presence of substances chemically related to food additives within "natural" foods.—R.L.D.] ◄

Localized and Systemic Hypersensitivity Reactions to Human Seminal Fluid. I. Leonard Bernstein, Bruce E. Englander, Joan S.

Br. J. Dermatol. 104:369–381, April 1981.
Ann. Intern. Med. 94(Pt. 1):459–465, April 1981.

Gallagher, Paul Nathan, and Zvi H. Marcus (Univ. of Cincinnati) studied 4 women who had severe postcoital reactions. Life-threatening systemic symptoms experienced by patients 1 and 2 required prompt treatment with epinephrine. Patient 1 had her initial anaphylactic episode 6 weeks after delivery of a normal baby and 10 weeks after the last coitus during pregnancy. Patient 2 developed anaphylactic symptoms after her first sexual intercourse. Patients 3 and 4 complained only of local symptoms (burning pain, erythema, and edema of genital tissues) lasting 24–48 hours after unprotected ejaculation. These symptoms began 4 weeks after the first intercourse in patient 3 and at the first intercourse in patient 4. All patients except patient 4 had family histories of atopy and personal allergic diatheses.

Reaginic humoral antibodies to human seminal plasma were present in the 2 women with systemic reactions. In 1 patient, IgE antibodies were demonstrated by direct skin tests, leukocyte histamine release, passive transfer to a nonallergic human recipient, the radioallergosorbent test, inhibition of the radioallergosorbent test, and neutralization of passive transfer antibodies. A similar mechanism was established in the other patient by direct skin tests and antigen-induced leukocyte histamine release. Pooled seminal plasma gave as potent skin test and passive cutaneous anaphylaxis results as did seminal plasma derived from each patient's sexual partner. Sephadex G-100 fraction 2, derived from human seminal plasma, showed greater reaginic activity than the other chromatographic fractions.

The 2 patients with histories of localized reactions did not develop humoral antibodies but did show evidence of cell-mediated immunity to seminal fluid antigens. One of these patients also had significant titers of IgM and IgG sperm agglutinating antibodies to seminal plasma.

Histocompatibility leukocyte antigen (HLA) typing of all patients and their sexual partners showed a marked degree of shared histocompatibility locus antigens in members of each of two couples.

Both localized and systemic responses to seminal fluid were eliminated by abstinence or use of condoms. The 2 patients with localized reactions in this study have been observed for more than 3 years without signs of systemic symptoms.

Prior exposure to cross-reacting antigens may provide the sensitizing stimulus accounting for reactions to seminal fluid on first sexual intercourse. Possibly, HLA sharing in sexual partners could predispose women to subsequent development of localized or systemic reactions to components of seminal fluid. The presence of specific spermatozoal IgE antibodies in one of the patients with immediate hypersensitivity symptoms may be the first recorded instance of sperm antigens being identified as anaphylactogenic.

▶ [It must be extremely deflating to the male ego to learn that his lover's facial flush was not due to passion but, rather, to histamine release!—R.L.D.] ◀

Histiocytosis X. Histiocytosis X comprises a highly variable spectrum of disease ranging from benign localized to lethal disseminated forms. Even though oral manifestations may be the first or only sign of disease, such lesions have not been emphasized adequately. Richard Fitzpatrick, Marvin J. Rapaport, and Douglas G. Silva reviewed the cutaneous and oral findings in 59 patients with histologically confirmed histiocytosis X seen during a 20-year period at the University of California, Los Angeles, Medical Center and report a new case demonstrating oral involvement.

Woman, 19, presented with a 1-year history of chronic inflammation and ulceration of the right side of the lower gingiva and chronic vulvovaginal ulcerations. Examination revealed clear drainage from both external auditory canals with moderate inflammation of both canals. There was inflammation, superficial ulcerating and granulomatous lesions of and adjacent to the lower gingiva. Looseness of the lower right molars and tenderness of the right mandible were observed. Laboratory findings consistent with diabetes insipidus were obtained. Dental roentgenograms revealed several osteolytic lesions. Electron microscopic examination of biopsy material from the oral lesions showed subepidermal edema and a cellular infiltrate containing numerous plasma cells and an admixture of histiocytes and lymphocytes. Lymphocytes, histiocytes, and eosinophils extensively infiltrated the deeper dermis. The histiocytes contained numerous free polyribosomes and a small amount of endoplasmic reticulum. Langerhans-type granules were not present. Based on the presence of typical mucosal lesions with a heavy histiocytic infiltrate, diabetes insipidus, and bone abnormalities, a diagnosis of histiocytosis X was made.

Of the 59 patients previously described with confirmed histiocytosis X, 21 had benign localized disease. Thirty-eight patients with multisystem disease were classified as having either chronic progressive or acute disseminated histiocytosis X. Cutaneous lesions were present in 76% of the patients (table) and oral lesions were present in 42%.

CUTANEOUS LESIONS OF HISTIOCYTOSIS X

Lesions	No. of Patients (%)		
	With Acute Disseminated Disease	With Chronic Progressive Disease	Total
Total	19	19	38
Skin	16 (100)	13 (100)	29 (100)
Papular scaling	15 (94)	12 (92)	27 (93)
Petechiae and purpura	11 (69)	1 (8)	12 (41)
Granulomatous ulcers	4 (25)	6 (46)	10 (39)
Vesicles and bullae	4 (25)	1 (8)	5 (17)
Nodules	1 (6)	3 (23)	4 (14)
Xanthomatous lesions	1 (6)	1 (6)	2 (7)
Bronzing	2 (13)	0 (0)	2 (7)

Arch. Dermatol. 117:253–257, May 1981.

In 19 patients with chronic progressive disease, the oral lesions usually were characterized by mandibular and/or maxillary bone lesions, subsequent loss of teeth, inflammatory necrosis and ulceration of the gingivae, and nonhealing extraction sites. In the acute disseminated group, the oral lesions were similar to the cutaneous lesions, with petechiae and purpura, vesicles, and necrosis of the palate and gingiva. Oral lesions were the initial complaint in 13% of all patients and were the only manifestation of the disease in 5%.

The correct diagnosis of histiocytosis X is often delayed when oral lesions are prominent because of such misdiagnoses as aphthous stomatitis, herpetic stomatitis, Vincent's infection, and other chronic inflammatory conditions, while jaw lesions may be misdiagnosed as cysts, osteomyelitis, and various malignant tumors. If such conditions do not respond to appropriate therapy, histiocytosis X should be considered in the differential diagnosis.

Histiocytosis X—An Immune Deficiency Disease? Studies on Antibody-Dependent Monocyte-Mediated Cytotoxicity. Because histiocytosis X (HX) cells share many features with epidermal Langerhans cells, it has been suggested that HX is a pathologic proliferation of Langerhans cells. Knud Kragballe, Hugh Zachariae, Troels Herlin, and Jørgen Jensen (Aarhus, Denmark) examined monocyte and neutrophil function in terms of antibody-dependent cell-mediated cytotoxicity (ADCC) in 6 children with HX, all of whom were in clinical remission. Only 1 child was receiving immunosuppressive therapy at the time of the study. Thirteen children of similar age served as control subjects. Antibody-dependent cell-mediated cytotoxicity was assayed using human type B Rh-negative red blood cells as target cells and hyperimmune human anti-B serum as a source of anti-target cell antibody. Fresh serum from HX patients was examined for ability to inhibit cytotoxicity of normal monocytes as was monocyte binding of IgG-coated erythrocytes.

All patients studied had become ill before age 15 months; most had had involvement of two or more organ systems. Four patients had received systemic therapy, only 1 in the past year. Monocyte-mediated cytotoxicity was reduced in all patients at various target cell-to-monocyte ratios and different periods of incubation. Neutrophil cytotoxicity was normal in 5 of the 6 HX patients studied. The proportion of monocytes that formed rosettes with IgG-coated erythrocytes did not differ from that in control subjects. Serums from the HX patients did not affect the cytotoxicity of normal monocytes. The patients had normal monocyte nuclear morphological features and cytoplasmic esterase activity.

Monocytes from children with HX in clinical remission exhibit decreased cytotoxicity. The findings suggest that HX is a disorder of the mononuclear phagocyte system and indicate a persisting functional abnormality in this cell line. An intracellular defect probably under-

Br. J. Dermatol. 105:13–18, July 1981.

lies the decreased monocyte cytotoxicity in HX. These findings support the view that HX is an immune deficiency disease.

▶ [The term "histiocytosis X" embraces three distinct conditions: Letterer-Siwe disease, eosinophilic granuloma, and Hand-Schüller-Christian disease. Ultrastructural studies have demonstrated the essential unity of these conditions as a proliferation of histiocytic cells. The abnormal cells in histiocytosis X are considered to belong to the mononuclear phagocyte system on the basis of their enzyme histochemical characteristics, properties of glass adherence and phagocytosis, and the presence of complement and receptors for the Fe fragment of IgG on cell surfaces. The results of this study by Kragballe et al. confirm abnormalities of the mononuclear phagocyte system in histiocytosis X and indicate a persistent functional abnormality in this cell line. Because most of the patients described had Letterer-Siwe disease, the results cannot be extrapolated to all persons affected with histiocytosis X. Impaired monocyte function is not necessarily associated with a bad prognosis, as suggested by the benign course of the disease in the study patients. The provocative suggestion that histiocytosis X may be an inflammatory rather than neoplastic disorder requires further investigation.—R.L.D.] ◀

Psoriasis and Its Treatment. Although psoriasis might seem to be a harmless condition, the cosmetic problem is of great importance to the patient. R. H. Champion (Cambridge, England) discusses some of the new work on the complex etiology of the disease and, in particular, the numerous treatments for more severe cases.

Central to understanding psoriasis and its treatment is the too rapid turnover of cells in the epidermis, particularly in lesions but to some extent in the clinically normal skin of psoriatics. The undisputed cause of this rapid turnover is a genetic factor with HLA associations. Changes in cyclic adenosine monophosphate and cyclic guanosine monophosphate have claimed attention for many years, but more recently there has been interest in polyamines such as putrescine and spermidine. Migration of polymorphonuclears into the skin is a cardinal feature of psoriasis. Immunologic changes also may be shown. The severity and clinical course of psoriasis are enormously variable, from occasional insignificant scaling on knees to a continual life-ruining generalized cutaneous disorder. Long-term treatment must be based on an assessment of how the disease is likely to behave with or without treatment.

For most patients, topical treatment is most logical and safe. Topical corticosteroids are prescribed—and overprescribed—for psoriasis in enormous quantities. Stronger steroids are more effective but more likely to produce atrophy and systemic absorption. The sunburn wavelengths of ultraviolet radiation (UV-B) have been used to treat psoriasis for many decades. Also, recent treatment with psoralens and ultraviolet A (PUVA) has stimulated interest in the photobiology of the skin. Serious reservations about the long-term safety of PUVA still exist, however. Powerful systemic drugs, especially corticosteroids, can control psoriasis, but because of their hazards they can only be recommended for extremely severe cases. Other systemic compounds used to treat this condition are methotrexate, hydroxyurea, razoxane, and the oral retinoids.

Br. Med. J. 282:343–346, Jan. 31, 1981.

Most patients with psoriasis are best treated with topical remedies, aided perhaps by natural sunlight or UV-B. Such topical treatments can be intermittent or on a long-term basis. Results with long-term topical steroids may be disappointing. For really severe cases, PUVA is recommended, especially for patients older than age 50. The choice of other drugs currently might be, in order of preference, methotrexate, hydroxyurea, and razoxane, although the oral retinoids may be high on the list.

▶ [Psoriasis is another disfiguring skin disease that like acne, can be difficult to treat. This article is a timely review of current methods of management. One is always interested in new approaches.

Colchicine, a microtubule disruptive agent that inhibits chemotactic migration of neutrophils, was tried as a treatment for psoriasis based on histologic evidence of infiltration of the epidermis by neutrophils in psoriatic patients. A dose of 0.02 mg/kg/day for 2 to 4 months resulted in complete clearing or marked improvement in 8 of 9 patients in whom thin plaques or thin papules were the predominant lesions. Five other patients with extensive chronic stable plaque-type psoriasis were given colchicine orally immediately after complete clearing of their skin lesions with Goeckerman's method or with methotrexate. Four of them remained free of significant skin disease during the succeeding 8 to 9 months. A considerable improvement in joint pains was noted in each of the 8 patients who suffered from arthralgias. Thus, 12 of 22 patients obtained some evidence of benefit from this treatment (*Acta Derm. Venereol.* (Stockh.) 90:515–520, 1980). As is usual with new treatments, we await the experience of others.—L.E.H.] ◀

Age Influences the Clinical and Serologic Expression of Systemic Lupus Erythematosus.

H. Alexander Wilson, Maurice E. Hamilton, Daniel A. Spyker, Carolyn M. Brunner, William M. O'Brien, John S. Davis, IV, and John B. Winfield compared the clinical and serologic characteristics of 17 patients with onset of systemic lupus erythematosus (SLE) after age 50 with those of 49 younger patients. All patients were followed prospectively for a mean of 47 months.

On initial evaluation, the older group had a lower incidence of fever, malar rash, and renal disease. Arthritis, pleuropericarditis, Raynaud's phenomenon, and muscle pain or weakness were prominent findings. Arthritis and pleuropericarditis were the most troublesome manifestations in 71% of older patients versus 28% of younger patients. Nephritis was the most troublesome manifestation in 38% of younger patients but in only 6% of older patients. During follow-up, the most significant difference between groups was a decreased incidence of nephritis in older patients. Analysis of renal disease by decade indicated that the decline in nephritis was related linearly to age. Subcutaneous nodules, most often transient, were more common in the older group.

There were longer periods of remission with increasing age. The severity of renal disease, as indicated by both the incidence and the duration of nephrotic-range proteinuria and a rise in creatinine concentration above 1.5 mg/dl, diminished with age.

Hypocomplementemia, antidouble-stranded DNA antibodies, and

Arthritis Rheum. 24:1230–1235, October 1981.

C1q precipitins occurred less frequently in older patients, and rheumatoid factor was more often present than in younger patients. Persistent rheumatoid factor positivity, encountered in 8 patients with disease onset in the fourth decade or later, was associated with chronic arthritis independent of age. Cryoglobulins, found in 80% of patients, were not age related. Younger patients tended to exhibit an inverse relationship between total hemolytic complement values and the presence of cryoglobulins; no such association was evident in patients over age 50. By multivariable regression analysis, neither single serologic indices nor combinations thereof eliminated the predictive value of age in the occurrence of nephritis.

Regression analysis suggested linear change in disease expression with age rather than distinct age-related subgroups. Among older patients, clinical and serologic patterns closely resembled those of patients with procainamide-induced lupus erythematosus. Distinction among rheumatoid arthritis, polymyalgia rheumatica, and SLE may be difficult in elderly patients.

▶ [Baker et al. (*Am. J. Med.* 66:727, 1979) previously examined the clinical manifestations of 31 patients with onset of SLE in the sixth decade or later. Pleuritis and pericarditis were the most common presenting signs. Although pulmonary abnormalities occurred more often than in patients presenting at an earlier age, Raynaud's phenomenon, lymphadenopathy, neuropsychiatric disease, alopecia, and rash were observed less frequently. Because only about 10% to 15% of all lupus cases fall into this late-onset group, such an atypical presentation may lead to a delay in diagnosis. Conservative treatment generally is indicated for these older patients, who usually have relatively benign disease; moreover, the incidence of steroid complications is increased in elderly patients.—R.L.D.] ◀

Systemic Lupus Erythematosus in Childhood. F. Caeiro, F. M. C. Michielson, R. Bernstein, G. R. V. Hughes, and Barbara M. Ansell reviewed the findings in 42 patients who developed systemic lupus erythematosus (SLE) at age 16 years or younger. Cases of drug-induced lupus and mixed connective tissue disease were excluded. The follow-up period after onset of illness ranged from 7 months to 28 years, the mean duration being 8.1 years. The 37 girls and 5 boys had a mean age at onset of disease of 12.3 years and a mean age at diagnosis of 13.5 years.

The most common presenting features were arthritis, arthralgias, rash, and fever. All patients eventually had polyarthritis or arthralgias, and 4 had deforming arthritis. Six children had proximal muscle weakness. All but 10 patients had a rash, usually the typical "butterfly" rash. Photosensitivity was found in 12 cases. More than half the patients had alopecia. Eight children had oral ulcers. Thirteen had Raynaud's phenomenon. Various forms of vasculitis were present in 23 cases. Purpura was present in 7 cases; in 3, it was associated with thrombocytopenia. Three patients had discoid lesions. Pleurisy or pleural effusion was found in nearly one third of the cases. Ten had pericarditis. Renal involvement was diagnosed in 20 cases. Eleven patients had neurologic manifestations, the most common being

---

Ann. Rheum. Dis. 40:325–331, August 1981.

grand mal seizures. Twelve patients had psychiatric manifestations, most often severe psychoneurosis and psychosis. Four patients presented with hemolytic anemia. All patients had an elevated sedimentation rate at the time of diagnosis. The lupus erythematosus cell test was positive in more than two thirds of patients tested.

All but 2 patients received steroid therapy; 9 received hydroxychloroquine. Immunosuppressive drugs were given to 15 patients. Six (14.2%) patients died, all within the first six years of illness. Three patients died of infection associated with active SLE and steroid therapy; 2 died of renal failure. At present, 4 of 36 patients are in remission without medication, and 15 are doing well on small doses of steroids. Five patients have been lost to follow-up.

The pattern and prognosis of SLE in childhood are similar to those in adults. In this series, all patients without nephritis lived at least 10 years after diagnosis. The possibility of SLE should be considered in any adolescent, particularly a girl, with polyarthritis.

▶ [As in adult SLE, the prognosis in childhood SLE depends on the development of nephritis.—R.L.D.] ◀

Mixed Connective Tissue Disease: Follow-up Study of 12 Patients With Special Reference to Cold Sensitivity and Skin Manifestations. Eija A. Johansson, Kirsti-Maria Niemi, Allan Lassus, and Marianne Gripenberg (Helsinki) describe 12 patients with an overlap syndrome compatible with mixed connective tissue disease (MCTD). Mean age of the patients was 29.9 (range 17–41) years at onset of disease; 8 were women. Patients were followed for an average of 7 years.

At the time of reexamination, Raynaud's phenomenon (the first clinical manifestation in 8 patients) and cold sensitivity were found in each patient; fever after exposure to cold (5 patients), peripheral vasospasms and aches (in cold), joint stiffness and tenderness (especially of hands), and early disability because of cold sensitivity (5 patients) were other important symptoms. Small, painful ulcerations often developed on the fingertips; gangrene occurred in 1 patient. Two patients had migraine-type headaches thought to be precipitated by exposure to cold. Muscle tenderness or weakness occurred in all but 2 female patients.

Eleven patients had swollen hands or some degree of sclerodactyly. Scaling erythematous or violaceous plaques over the extensor surfaces, especially over the hand joints, were found in 6 patients; 3 patients also had the violaceous rash over the eyelids. The conspicuous histologic feature in sclerodermatous skin was mucoid degeneration of endothelial cells in dermal capillaries and small vessels, without acid mucopolysaccharides in the vessel wall. The immunofluorescence band test was positive for IgM in 3 patients on uninvolved sun-protected skin. Immunoglobulin M was detected along the basement membrane in lesional skin from 6 patients; IgG was found in 1 case. Nuclear staining in epidermis was noted in 5 specimens.

Acta Derm. Venereol. (Stockh.) 61:225–231, 1981.

A speckled pattern of antinuclear antibodies was seen in 10 patients; 1 patient (with myasthenia gravis and cold hemagglutinin syndrome) had a nucleolar pattern; the other patient had a homogeneous fluorescence pattern. Antiribonucleoprotein antibodies were demonstrated in 6 patients and anti-Sm antibodies in 1. Patients with negative findings were clinically in remission after having received corticosteroid therapy for several years. Two patients had anti-DNA antibodies; 4 had anti-ssDNA antibodies. Two female patients had thyroiditis with high serum titers of antithyroid antibodies.

There is no outstanding skin marker typical of the MCTD syndrome. In this series it was difficult to estimate the value of corticosteroid treatment. In many cases the patient's general condition improved, but in contrast to previous findings, there was little effect on the scleroderma-like skin changes or other skin manifestations, Raynaud's phenomenon, or other symptoms induced or aggravated by cold. Esophageal and pulmonary changes were probably too advanced to respond. In northern countries, MCTD must be considered a serious illness.

▶ [In a follow-up report on the original 25 patients with MCTD, Nimelstein et al. (*Medicine (Baltimore)* 59:239, 1980) found that the inflammatory manifestations, such as arthritis, serositis, fever, and myositis, became less frequent and, when present, less severe as time progressed. These signs appeared to respond to corticosteroid treatment. Sclerodermatous manifestations, such as sclerodactyly and esophageal abnormalities, were more persistent and often unresponsive to treatment. Renal disease remained infrequent. It is possible that those patients who have persistent, corticosteroid-resistant disease with prominent sclerodermatous changes actually have true scleroderma.—R.L.D.] ◀

Does Peutz-Jeghers Syndrome Predispose to Gastrointestinal Malignancy? A Later Look. Several reports have suggested an association between intestinal carcinoma and the Peutz-Jeghers syndrome, and decreased survival has been reported among patients with this syndrome. Dimitrios A. Linos, Roger R. Dozois, David C. Dahlin, and Lloyd G. Bartholomew (Mayo Clinic and Found.) reviewed the findings in 48 patients seen with Peutz-Jeghers syndrome between 1935 and 1979. A definite diagnosis was made in 21 patients who had the complete expression of the syndrome, with mucocutaneous pigmentation and documented hamartomatous polyps.

Eleven of the 21 definitely affected patients had a family history of intestinal polyposis and mucocutaneous pigmentation. Thirteen patients had extensive, diffuse polyposis involving the stomach, duodenum, and small and large bowel. Over 80% of patients had recurrent abdominal pain from obstruction and rectal bleeding. During a median follow-up of 33 years, 6 of the 21 patients developed carcinoma. One of 15 other patients with mucocutaneous pigmentation alone developed carcinoma. Three of 7 patients with mucocutaneous pigmentation and adenomatous or hyperplastic polyps developed carcinomas. None of 5 patients without pigmentation from whom hamar-

Arch. Surg. 116:1182–1184, September 1981.

tomatous polyps had been removed from the small bowel developed cancer during follow-up.

Survival of patients with Peutz-Jeghers syndrome appears to be similar to that in the general population. There was only one possible instance of intestinal cancer arising from a hamartomatous polyp in this series. The premalignant potential of the polyps in Peutz-Jeghers syndrome, at least in the small bowel, is doubtful; a conservative surgical approach is warranted. Careful assessment of the stomach and bowel is necessary, however, because adenomatous polyps may be present, and malignancies are commonly found at these sites.

▶ [Despite scattered reports to the contrary, the polyps of Peutz-Jeghers syndrome appear to be benign, with no malignant predisposition. Because the gastrointestinal tract of affected patients is studded with hamartomatous polyps, an increased incidence of carcinoma (especially of the small bowel) presumably would be obvious if the lesions were indeed premalignant.—R.L.D.] ◀

Photobiologic Evaluation of Tanning Booths is reported by D. S. Nachtwey and R. D. Rundel (Natl. Aeronautics and Space Admin., Houston). The use of tanning booths as a substitute for natural sunlight is becoming increasingly popular. The operators generally claim that the booths simulate sunlight and therefore pose no more long-term risks than sunlight itself. Measurements were made in a custom-built tanning booth in a salon representative of such installations. Two 72 in. fluorescent sunlamps were mounted vertically in each corner, and the walls and door were covered with metallized wallpaper. Extreme anisotropy of the radiation field was observed, apparently due to a lack of sufficient ultraviolet reflectivity of the inner wall covering and lack of uniformity of the individual lamps. A highly uneven tan would result unless the user was in the exact center of the booth and rotated uniformly. At shorter wavelengths (less than 305 nm) the output of the lamps was significantly greater than the sun's.

Delayed tanning without burning is the goal of tanning booths, but some sunburn damage nearly always accompanies the induction of such a tan. The exposures necessary for greater degrees of erythema, and presumably darker tanning, cannot be readily determined. An ultraviolet radiation meter should be used by tanning salon operators to test for anisotropy and determine appropriate exposure times as lamp output declines. The use of simple, inexpensive ultraviolet radiation meters, however, can lead to serious overexposure. Since the ultraviolet radiation inside a tanning booth has a greater proportion of short wavelengths than natural sunlight, the amount of skin cancer-inducing radiation received may be twice that received for a natural suntan. One way to ameliorate this problem would be to use cellulose acetate filters, which block the shorter wavelengths. Even when equipped with such filters, however, tanning booths cause more DNA damage per minimal erythema dose than does sunlight.

▶ [Nachtwey and Rundel have calculated that 26 times as much DNA-damaging ultraviolet radiation is admitted from the fluorescent sunlamp as by the sun at 30 de-

Science 211:405–407, Jan. 23, 1981.

grees north latitude. Since the action spectrum for cutaneous carcinogenesis likely correlates with the DNA-damaging spectrum, there is significantly more DNA-damaging radiation reaching target tissue from the fluorescent sunlamps as from the sun at 30 degrees north latitude. Thus, it appears that exposure to ultraviolet radiation in suntanning booths is more carcinogenic than equivalent amounts of sunlight.—R.L.D.] ◄

Suntan Salons and the American Skin. John H. Epstein (Univ. of California, San Francisco) estimates that between 1,000 and 2,000 suntan salons are operating in the United States. Two types of salons are popular. Most commonly a fluorescent UVB (ultraviolet rays between 280 and 320 nm) light source is used. Such rays are responsible for the acute cellular injury and erythema called "sunburn," and, at least under experimental conditions, are the most carcinogenic. If the skin absorbs enough UVB energy to produce or maintain a tan, or both, enough energy has been absorbed to cause cellular damage, whether there is visible erythema or not. Acute keratitis or kerato-conjunctivitis occurs readily without appropriate protection; goggles that eliminate ultraviolet radiation but transmit visible rays should be worn. A shut-off switch should be available to the user and to an attendant who should closely supervise the units. Acute hazards from the machine itself include electric injury caused by faulty wiring and lacerations if the subject falls against the glass tubes. These can be prevented by appropriate electric installation, the use of handles by which subjects may steady themselves, and protective covers over the tubes.

The UVA (long-wave ultraviolet light, rays between 320 and 400 nm) units are found primarily in Europe. The hazards of such radiation are not fully understood. Long-wave ultraviolet light is responsible for the vast majority of exogenous photosensitivity reactions, augments the acute injury caused by the UVB rays, causes dermal blood vessel damage, and can produce lenticular injury. It appears that UVA causes less epidermal damage than UVB, but has a greater effect on the dermis.

Tanning for cosmetic purposes is not innocuous. Suntan salons supply the means for maintaining consistent cellular damage and potentially hastening the end-state of chronic actinic degeneration. Suntan salons employ no medically trained personnel to identify individuals at high risk for photodamage.

Human Sunburn Reaction: Histologic and Biochemical Studies. Barbara A. Gilchrest, Nicholas A. Soter, Jeffrey S. Stoff, and Martin C. Mihm, Jr. (Boston) investigated the ultraviolet-induced erythema reaction in 4 fair-skinned, healthy Caucasians aged 20–25, who had skin type II. Suction blister aspirates were analyzed for histamine and prostaglandin E_2 (PGE_2) content, and Epon-embedded skin biopsy sections 1μ thick from control and irradiated skin were analyzed at intervals for 72 hours after exposure to a Hanovia lamp (set at a 3 minimal erythema dose).

South. Med. J. 74:837–840, July 1981.
J. Am. Acad. Dermatol. 5:411–422, October 1981.

Major histologic changes in the epidermis included dyskeratotic and vacuolated keratinocytes (sunburn cells) and disappearance of Langerhans cells. Sunburn cells were recognized as early as 30 minutes after irradiation and were most numerous 24 hours afterward. Severely altered keratinocytes were found throughout the epidermis, but were most numerous in the lower half above the basal layer. By 72 hours, severely altered keratinocytes were principally confined to the most superficial layers, constituting a parakeratotic stratum corneum. In 2 instances, Langerhans cells were seen in apposition to severely damaged keratinocytes. The Langerhans cells identified in later sections were frequently vacuolated, as were the adjacent keratinocytes.

Melanocytes also were frequently vacuolated, swollen, and pale at 30 minutes and 1 hour after irradiation. As early as 4 hours, but more frequently at 72 hours, very large mononuclear cells with hyperchromatic nuclei, presumed to be melanocytes, were found along the basement membrane.

In the dermis the major changes were vascular, involving both the superficial and deep plexuses. Endothelial cell enlargement was first apparent within 30 minutes of irradiation, peaked at 24 hours, and persisted throughout the 72-hour study period. In 4-hour and especially 24-hour specimens, many venules and capillaries were partially occluded by endothelial cells protruding into the lumen. Minimal focal hemorrhage was noted at 24 hours.

Mast cell degranulation and perivenular edema, apparent at 1 hour, were striking at the onset of erythema 3–4 hours after irradiation and correlated with a marked reduction in the number of identifiable mast cells. Edema was absent and mast cells were again normal in number and granule content at 24 hours, when erythema peaked. By 72 hours, erythema had disappeared in individuals and was minimal in the fourth.

Dilated lymphatics containing flocculent proteinaceous-like material were visible focally in all specimens except controls. Macrophages containing melanin were observed frequently in all postirradiation specimens.

Histamine levels rose approximately fourfold above control values immediately after the onset of erythema and returned to baseline within 24 hours. The PGE_2 levels were statistically elevated even before onset of erythema, reaching about 150% of the control value at 24 hours.

These data provide the first evidence that histamine may mediate the early phase of the human sunburn reaction. Because histamine levels return to normal before peak erythema is attained, and because histamine effects are evanescent, other mediators must be responsible for the later phases.

▶ [Using Epon-embedded sections 1 μ thick, definite but subtle changes were noted in endothelial cells and keratinocytes as early as 30 minutes after ultraviolet light (UV) exposure; these increased progressively over the subsequent 24 hours. The appearance of damaged keratinocytes (sunburn cells) in the lower epidermis preceded their appearance in the upper half of the epidermis, suggesting an increased UV sensitivity of suprabasal cells. Two components of the vascular reaction to broad-spectrum UV irradiation were also documented in this study. One is characterized by the mast cell degranulation and striking perivenular edema; this coincides with the onset of erythema. Later, a more protracted reaction characterized by endothelial cell alteration and compaction of the venular bed with erythrocytes is observed; this is most severe at the time of peak erythema but extends from the latent period before the development of erythema for at least 72 hours.—R.L.D.] ◄

Additional Reading

Elias, P. M., and Williams, M. L.: Retinoids, cancer, and the skin. *Arch. Dermatol.* 117:160, 1981.

Kaplan, A. P., et al.: Exercise-induced anaphylaxis as a manifestation of cholinergic urticaria. *J. Allergy Clin. Immunol.* 68:319, 1981.

Kaplan, A. P., et al.: Idiopathic cold urticaria: In vitro demonstration of histamine release upon challenge of skin biopsies. *N. Engl. J. Med.* 305:1074, 1981.

McKenzie, M. W., et al.: Topical clindamycin formulations for the treatment of acne vulgaris. *Arch. Dermatol.* 117:630, 1981.

Monroe, E. W., et al.: Combined H_1 and H_2 antihistamine therapy in chronic urticaria. *Arch. Dermatol.* 117:404, 1981.

Trentham, D. E., et al.: Autoimmunity to collagen: A shared feature of psoriatic and rheumatoid arthritis. *Arthritis Rheum.* 24:1363, 1981.

Tsokos, G. C., et al.: Muscle involvement in systemic lupus erythematosus. *J.A.M.A.* 246:766, 1981.

Udassin, R., et al.: Cholinergic urticaria. *Arch. Intern. Med.* 141:1029, 1981.

Wenk, R. E., et al.: Tetracycline-associated fatty liver of pregnancy, including possible pregnancy risk after chronic dermatologic use of tetracycline. *J. Reprod. Med.* 26:135, 1981.

Cardiology

"The denunciation of the young is a necessary part of the hygiene of older people and greatly assists the circulation of their blood."—LO-GAN PEARSALL SMITH

The circulation of blood through organs and vessels in the adolescent—not the adult—is the purpose of this section. Obviously clinicians must be concerned with the cardiovascular system in all age groups, but in recent years increased attention has been focused on such "hot" items as hypertension and mitral valve prolapse in the adolescent. The possible association of mitral valve prolapse and hyperthyroidism is discussed in the article by Channick et al. Mitral prolapse is also seen in other organic pathological states such as Ehlers-Danlos syndrome and von Willebrand's disease. Diagnosis of mitral valve prolapse either clinically or by utilization of cardiovascular techniques is an important consideration for the administration of prophylactic antibiotics to prevent endocarditis.

Aortic stenosis in young patients may not be detected by usual methods (radiography, vectrocardiography, resting ECG). Whitmer and associates report on exercise testing in children (adolescents) before and after surgical treatment for aortic stenosis and suggest the use of exercise testing to quantify the degree of aortic stenosis, making it easy to follow up patients after surgery.

Specific cardiomyopathies and arrhythmias are other topics treated in this section, and three excellent articles on hypertension in the adolescent are included in the reading list.

Observer Variation in the Angiocardiographic Diagnosis of Mitral Valve Prolapse. Angiocardiograms often have been taken as the absolute standard for the diagnosis of mitral valve prolapse. Jerry D. Kennett, Philip F. Rust, Richard H. Martin, Brent M. Parker, and Linley E. Watson (Univ. of Missouri, Columbia) assessed the reliability of the angiocardiographic diagnosis of mitral valve prolapse by estimating the degree of agreement between observers using a defined set of diagnostic criteria. Sixty adequate left ventriculograms showing no valvular heart disease other than possible mitral valve prolapse were reviewed twice, independently, by 3 experienced angiocardiographers.

At the first review, 34 studies were considered positive for mitral valve prolapse by all 3 observers, and 8 were unanimously considered negative or equivocal. No significant difference was found between the readers in the likelihood of interpreting an angiogram as being

Chest 79:146–150, February 1981.

positive. Agreement was considerably greater than expected from chance. At the second review, 38 studies were considered positive by all observers, and 5, negative. Agreement was comparable to that observed in the first review of the ventriculograms. Intraobserver agreement was about equal to interobserver agreement.

Considerable variability was noted among different observers in this study in the angiocardiographic diagnosis of mitral valve prolapse. Agreement between observers and within observers ranged from 60% to 80%. There was little difference between agreement in determining that a ventriculogram is positive or negative for prolapse and that in selecting the specific prolapsed scallop or scallops. There is considerably more disagreement when positivity, negativity, and all subcategories of positive are considered simultaneously. Until a quantitative method is validated adequately, variability should preclude placing absolute reliance on angiocardiographic appearances as the sole or ultimate criteria for the diagnosis of mitral valve prolapse.

▶ [This is an interesting observation on the angiographic diagnosis of mitral valve prolapse. Although it is not unexpected, differences in interpretation of the echocardiographic diagnosis of mitral valve prolapse can and have taken place. The stethoscope is still the superior tool for diagnosing mitral valve prolapse, although at times the telltale auscultatory findings of a click, murmurs, or both might be absent; however, if we remember to have a high index of suspicion and specifically search for these findings with our stethoscope listening to the heart with the patient in the supine, left lateral, sitting, standing, and squatting positions, the diagnosis generally can be made. Another reason that the diagnosis of mitral valve prolapse might be missed with the stethoscope is that some patients have the findings only on inspiration, or only on expiration.—W.P.H.] ◀

Hyperthyroidism and Mitral Valve Prolapse. Mitral valve prolapse is a common disorder, apparently associated with heritable connective tissue disorders in some instances. Adrenergic tone may be elevated in symptomatic patients, and a high frequency of prolapse has been noted in thyrotoxic patients, in whom adrenergic tone is increased. Bertram J. Channick, E. Victor Adlin, Allan D. Marks, Barry S. Denenberg, Michael T. McDonough, C. Simon Chakko, and James F. Spann (Temple Univ.) sought mitral valve prolapse in 40 patients with confirmed hyperthyroidism, 9 of whom were hyperthyroid at the time of study. Twelve patients had received radioiodine, 14 had undergone subtotal thyroidectomy, and 5 had entered longterm remission after antithyroid drug therapy alone. The average interval from treatment of hyperthyroidism to the study was 7.2 years. Sixteen patients were receiving thyroid hormone at the time of study. Sixteen of 40 control patients also were taking thyroid hormone.

Mitral valve prolapse was diagnosed in 43% of the study group and 18% of control subjects, for a risk ratio of about 3.5. A significant difference remained when the patient with multinodular toxic goiter was excluded. The prevalence of mitral prolapse was not influenced by the presence of hyperthyroidism at the time of study or the current use of thyroid hormone. Seven hyperthyroid patients with mitral pro-

N. Engl. J. Med. 305:497–500, Aug. 27, 1981.

lapse had documented arrhythmias at a time when they were euthyroid. One hyperthyroid patient with mitral prolapse had subacute bacterial endocarditis 6 years after the successful treatment of Graves' disease.

Possible explanations for an association of mitral valve prolapse and hyperthyroidism include a genetic basis for both conditions; a common autoimmune basis; and increased adrenergic cardiac stimulation in hyperthyroidism. Palpitations, tachycardia, and other arrhythmias with nervousness and anxiety may be manifestations of mitral prolapse as well as of hyperthyroidism. Mitral prolapse should be sought in patients with a history of hyperthyroidism in order to provide antibiotic prophylaxis in conjunction with dental or surgical procedures.

▶ [Mitral valve prolapse is a fascinating condition. In the 1981 YEAR BOOK OF MEDICINE (p. 347), endocrine abnormalities, including elevated levels of 24-hour urinary epinephrine and norepinephrine excretion, were described. Here, its association with hyperthyroidism is noted.—E.B.] ◀

Von Willebrand Syndromes and Mitral Valve Prolapse: Linked Mesenchymal Dysplasias. Nancy J. Pickering, Jerome I. Brody and Michael J. Barrett (Med. College of Pennsylvania, Philadelphia) suspected an increased incidence of mitral valve prolapse in patients with von Willebrand's syndromes because these conditions are a form of mesenchymal dysplasia. Two-dimensional echocardiography was performed in 13 women and 2 men with von Willebrand's syndrome. Abnormal bleeding occurred in all patients but 1. Five patients had nasal and cutaneous telangiectases. The results of blood clotting studies confirmed the heterogeneity of von Willebrand's syndromes. Echocardiography also was performed in 30 healthy age- and sex-matched subjects with no history or symptoms of cardiac disease.

Mitral valve prolapse was identified in 9 of the 15 patients with von Willebrand's syndrome and in 4 of the 30 control subjects (60% versus 13.3%), a significant difference. Two of the study patients with mitral valve prolapse reported chest pain, dyspnea, or palpitations. Eight of the 9 patients had a typical systolic click and murmur. Neither the bleeding history nor the results of coagulation assays distinguished between patients with and those without mitral valve prolapse.

Mitral valve prolapse was found in more than half of the patients in this study with von Willebrand's syndrome, suggesting a relationship analogous to that among the recognized inherited abnormalities of collagen, bleeding phenomena, and cardiac lesions. The synthesis of certain coagulation factors and the normal formation of cardiovascular mesenchyma may be connected at a molecular level. It is possible that the misarrangement of polymeric factor VIII in von Willebrand's syndromes, myxomatous degeneration, and collagen-bundle disorganization in the prolapsed mitral valve, and the structural inadequacy of blood vessels in the heritable connective tissue disorders

N. Engl. J. Med. 305:131–134, July 16, 1981.

share a common pathogenesis. Von Willebrand's syndrome may explain the occurrence of cerebral embolism in mitral valve prolapse. The use of cryoprecipitate preoperatively and the administration of prophylactic antibiotics to prevent endocarditis should be evaluated in all patients.

▶ [This interesting study was based on the hypothesis that the von Willebrand syndromes are a form of mesenchymal dysplasia and that the telangiectasias, angiodysplasias, and skeletal distortions that have been described in such patients represent genetically determined defects complementary to the defect in the ability to produce factor VIII-related antigen and factor VIII- ristocetin-aggregating factor. The data presented have clinical implications for patients with von Willebrand's syndrome. They suggest that a routine search should be conducted for mitral valve prolapse in patients with a von Willebrand syndrome.—M.J.C.] ◀

Exercise Testing in Children Before and After Surgical Treatment of Aortic Stenosis. The risk and conditions under which cardiac catheterization is done make it impractical for serial investigations in the young, but significant or progressive aortic stenosis (AS) may escape detection during evaluations including radiography, vectorcardiography, and resting ECG. Exercise-induced ST depression is related to the resting gradient of left ventricular (LV) to aortic peak systolic pressure in children with AS. Preliminary studies suggest that cardiovascular adaptation to exercise shows the severity of AS and degree of recovery after surgery.

Jeffrey T. Whitmer, Frederick W. James, Samuel Kaplan, David C. Schwartz, and Mary Jo Sandker Knight (New York) studied 23 children with valvar or discrete subvalvar aortic stenosis who underwent controlled progressive bicycle exercise testing within 6 months before and 3–30 months after surgery for LV outflow tract (LVOT) obstruction. Patients were divided into 3 groups according to the preoperative resting peak systolic pressure gradient between LV and aorta: 30–69 mm Hg (group A), 70–99 mm Hg (group B), and ≥100 mm Hg (group C). Preoperatively, 19 of 23 patients (83%) showed significant ST depression (≥1.0 mm) during exercise, whereas only 7 (30%) had abnormal ST depression at rest. Postoperatively, mean exercise-induced ST depression regressed to less than 1 mm in all 3 groups. In the total population, the frequency of ST depression greater than 1 mm was significantly reduced after surgery and mean total work and peak exercise systolic blood pressure were significantly increased within 12 months after surgery. Total work increased significantly in group B within 12 months and in group C within 13–24 months after surgery, but remained unchanged in group A. Peak exercise heart rates were similar before and after surgery in each group. Peak exercise systolic pressures increased after surgery in all 3 groups, but the mean differences were statistically significant only in group C patients tested 13–24 months after surgery.

Exercise testing can be used to quantify the degree of AS, making it possible to identify patients with LVOT obstruction, to follow up

Circulation 63:254–263, February 1981.

patients with mild AS, and to follow up patients after surgical relief of LVOT obstruction. The persistence of the preoperative exercise profile or lack of a significant change toward normal after surgery suggests significant residual obstruction, cardiovascular dysfunction, an associated lesion, or a combination of the above.

The Natural History of Idiopathic Dilated Cardiomyopathy. Valentin Fuster, Bernard J. Gersh, Emilio R. Giuliani, Abdul J. Tajik, Robert O. Brandenburg, and Robert L. Frye (Mayo Clinic) conducted a 6- to 20-year follow-up of 104 patients seen in 1960–1973 with a diagnosis of idiopathic dilated cardiomyopathy. The 64 men and 40 women had a median age of 49 years at the time of diagnosis. The median follow-up was 11 years. Median time between initial clinical manifestations and diagnosis was 1.3 years. The most common presenting features were x-ray evidence of cardiomegaly, ECG abnormality, usually left ventricular conduction delay, and symptoms of heart failure. Nineteen patients had 23 episodes of systemic embolism while not receiving anticoagulant therapy, but there were no such episodes during anticoagulant therapy. At the time of diagnosis, 78% of patients had a left ventricular (LV) end-diastolic pressure above 15 mm Hg, and 62% had a cardiac index below 2.5 L/min/sq m.

At the time of the last follow-up, 77% of the patients had died, most within the first 2 years. Only 3 surviving patients had deteriorated subjectively; most patients had a normal or decreased heart size. Deaths were related to older age, a higher cardiothoracic ratio, a lower cardiac index, and an increased LV end-diastolic pressure. Half the patients had such risk factors as excessive alcohol consumption, a severe influenza-like syndrome, and a history of rheumatic fever without apparent cardiac valve involvement. These factors had no apparent prognostic significance.

Idiopathic dilated cardiomyopathy probably is the result of several factors, including alcohol ingestion and viral infections, acting together in susceptible persons. Age, the cardiothoracic ratio, and the cardiac index are highly predictive of the clinical course. Anticoagulant therapy probably should be prescribed unless contraindicated to prevent systemic embolism. Future studies of dilated cardiomyopathy should include investigation of risk factors and serial myocardial biopsies.

▶ [Since 1950, we have evaluated more than 600 patients with cardiomyopathy of the dilated type, and therefore have a long follow-up on many. These patients reflect a spectrum of findings, including severity of involvement. We have observed a number of patients who survived 10 years or longer (Segal et al.: *Curr. Probl. Cardiol.* 3:1 September 1978). Six hundred patients have been referred for evaluation because of suspected cardiomyopathy since 1961. One hundred and fifteen patients were followed-up for a minimum of 5 years or until death. The median follow-up period was 8 years and the longest was 25 years. Thirty-nine patients were observed for more than 10 years, and 6 for more than 20 years. We would like to reiterate the fact that, as the authors of the preceding article discussed, thromboembolism is a more common complication of dilated cardiomyopathy than has been realized heretofore. An-

Am. J. Cardiol. 47:525–531, March 1981.

ticoagulant therapy, unless there is some contraindication, appears justified in patients with chronic heart failure who have the dilated type of cardiomyopathy. What is necessary and worth reemphasis is the importance of early suspicion, early diagnosis, and early treatment, which can enable some patients to reverse a downhill course and achieve only a mild degree of involvement or, in some cases, even complete recovery. Unfortunately, however, by the time most patients are first seen for evaluation, they have had their disease for a longer time.—W.P.H.] ◀

Prognosis in Hypertrophic Cardiomyopathy: Role of Age and Clinical, Electrocardiographic, and Hemodynamic Features. William McKenna, John Deanfield, Azhar Faruqui, Diane England, Celia Oakley, and John Goodwin (London) reviewed the clinical course of 254 patients with hypertrophic cardiomyopathy who were followed up for 1–23 years (mean, 6 years). In most cases the diagnosis was established by left ventricular angiography. Mean age at diagnosis was 34 years.

There was a total of 58 deaths, 6 from cardiac failure and 32 occurring suddenly and unexpectedly. Nine deaths were related to cardiac surgery. One fourth of the patients who died suddenly or with heart failure had a family history of hypertrophic cardiomyopathy and sudden death, compared with 12% of surviving patients. The ECG was not prognostically useful, and no hemodynamic findings were associated with death. Sudden death was predicted by an age of 14 or under and syncope at diagnosis, a family history of cardiomyopathy and sudden death, and severe dyspnea at last follow-up. Nine of 33 patients having myotomy-myomectomy or mitral valve replacement, or both, died perioperatively, and 6 others died after 1–20 years. With improved symptomatic treatment in recent years, proportionately fewer patients have been operated on, and these have been severely symptomatic with a poor response to medical management.

Sudden death is the most common mode of death in patients with hypertrophic cardiomyopathy. A poor prognosis is better predicted by the history at the time of diagnosis and by changes in symptoms during follow-up than by any ECG or hemodynamic measures. The detection and effective treatment of arrhythmia may improve the prognosis of patients with hypertrophic cardiomyopathy. The value of amiodarone and similar antiarrhythmic agents is being examined presently.

Amiodarone in Treatment of Cardiac Arrhythmias in Children: 135 Cases. According to Philippe Coumel (Paris) and Jean Fidelle (Les Loges-en-Joses, France), because of the many different types of arrhythmias, some of which are refractory and peculiar to children, and because of the limitations of therapeutic choice due to greater drug toxicity, amiodarone is a considerable asset in the pediatric age group.

They report their experience with 80 boys and 55 girls (mean age, 10.2 years) who were treated and followed during 1971–1979, who

Am. J. Cardiol. 47:532–538, March 1981.
Am. Heart J. 100:1063–1069, December 1980.

had predominantly atrial (69%) and postoperative (61%) arrhythmias. These were accompanied by clinical cardiac failure in 27%; and by isolated radiologic cardiomegaly in 40%, and were well tolerated hemodynamically in only 33%. In 46% the arrhythmias had lasted more than 2 months, and in 55% they were resistant to the usual pediatric drugs such as digitalis, disopyramide, beta blockers, atropine, and verapamil. Initial treatment was a daily oral dose of 800 mg of amiodarone adjusted to surface area. This was maintained for an average of 2 weeks, then was reduced by half, and finally was given only 5 days each week. Most patients were also given digitalis therapy.

Results were considered good when stable sinus rhythm was reestablished, average when the cardiac rate was reduced but the arrhythmia was not perfectly controlled on the ECG, and poor when treatment was clinically and electrocardiographically ineffective. Results were good in 81 patients (60%), average in 44 (33%), and poor in only 10 (7%). Cause of the arrhythmia, mechanism, localization, and resistance to other antiarrhythmics do not affect drug efficacy; longer duration of the arrhythmia (more than 2 months) resulted in lower effectiveness ($P<.10$). Delay before response to treatment was evaluated in 91 patients and was 1–16 days, with a mean of 4.1 days. The delay before relapse after interruption of treatment was assessed in 34 patients with serious, chronic and recurring arrhythmias. Mean delay was 3.3 weeks; in 24 patients, the interval before relapse was 2 weeks or less. Both duration of treatment and the child's age affected the delay. Amiodarone cured or improved 6 of 10 patients with arrhythmias in this series and improved the tolerance of the dysrhythmias in 3 of 4 of remaining children. The drug is metabolized more rapidly in children.

The overall effectiveness of amiodarone should not cause it to replace other antiarrhythmics; its problems of tolerance and thyroid toxicity prevent its use as an initial simple therapeutic approach. However, the younger the child and the more recent the arrhythmia, the more likely oral amiodarone is to terminate reciprocal junctional paroxysmal tachycardia, atrial tachycardia, or ventricular tachycardia, while avoiding the dangers of other antiarrhythmics. The authors believe that the patients with poor myocardial performance also tolerate the drug well. Long-range therapy does not have to be maintained except in special resistant life or death childhood arrhythmias.

▶ [Amiodarone is another "miracle drug" not released by the FDA. Adult experience in selected institutions in the United States is favorable, Pediatric experience is nonexistent.—A.S.N.] ◀

Lyme Carditis: Cardiac Abnormalities of Lyme Disease. Lyme disease, thought to be transmitted by the tick *Ixodes dammini,* consists of erythema chronicum migrans followed by neurologic, cardiac, and/or joint involvement. Allen C. Steere, William P. Batsford, Marc

Ann. Intern. Med. 93:8–16, July 1980.

Weinberg, Jonathan Alexander, Harvey J. Berger, Steven Wolfson, and Stephen E. Malawista (Yale Univ.) report data on 20 patients with cardiac abnormalities of Lyme disease. All patients but 1 were diagnosed by the occurrence of erythema chronicum migrans. The 16 male and 4 female patients were aged 6–58 years. In 18 cases the illness began in the summer. The initial associated signs and symptoms sometimes suggested aseptic meningitis. Features of heart disease appeared a median of 21 days after the onset of the skin lesion. Fifteen patients still had skin lesions when heart disease was present, and 7 had meningoencephalitis. Thirteen patients had joint involvement.

The most common cardiac abnormality was fluctuating atrioventricular (AV) block, but 13 patients had more diffuse cardiac involvement. Ten patients had high-degree AV block. Ten patients had diffuse T wave flattening or inversions. One patient presented in atrial fibrillation. Four patients had a mildly reduced left ventricular (LV) ejection fraction. Eighteen patients had an elevated erythrocyte sedimentation rate, 14 had an elevated serum IgM level, and 13 had cryoglobulins containing IgM and sometimes IgG. Nine patients received prednisone in daily doses of 40–60 mg. With this drug there was a decrease in degree of AV block within 24–48 hours and usually complete resolution within 1–2 weeks. Aspirin was followed by improvement in some cases. Eight patients received penicillin for erythema chronicum migrans.

Although the most common cardiac abnormality was fluctuating AV block, Lyme disease was recognized primarily by extracardiac findings in these patients. Circulating immune complexes may play a pathogenetic role in Lyme disease, but the presence of cryoglobulins does not correlate well with cardiac involvement. Patients with high-degree AV block or first-degree block and a PR interval longer than 0.3 second should be hospitalized. Patients with heart block may be treated initially with a temporary pacemaker and aspirin, but prednisone is given if meningoencephalitis is present, complete AV block lasts more than 1 week, or the cardiac status deteriorates and cardiomegaly is present.

▶ [Lyme disease generally is diagnosed by the occurrence of erythema chronicum migrans (ECM). A red macular papule expands to form a large annular lesion, usually with a bright red outer border and partial central clearing. In another study presented by these authors (Steere, A.C., et al.: *Ann. Intern. Med.* 93:1, 1980), evidence was presented that ECM should be treated with oral penicillin G, 250,000 units a day, or tetracycline, 250 mg four times a day for 7 to 10 days. However, there is no evidence that this method of therapy affects Lyme carditis.

For an excellent brief summary on Lyme disease, see *Morbidity and Mortality Weekly Report* (30:49, 1981). Lyme disease, an illness of uncertain cause, is manifested typically by ECM and by recurrent bouts of arthralgia and arthritis. Most cases begin in June, July, or August. It is more common in male subjects, and most cases have been reported in Connecticut, along the Atlantic seaboard and across the upper northern half of Wisconsin and southeastern Minnesota. It is thought to be part of a disease process caused by a penicillin-sensitive infectious agent transmitted by *Ixodes* ticks. In a minority of cases there are neurologic manifestations, such as aseptic meningitis, encephalitis, and cranial or spinal neuropathies. No specific diagnostic tests or examinations are available to establish the diagnosis.—E.B.] ◄

Idiopathic Recurrent Sustained Ventricular Tachycardia in Children and Adolescents. Ventricular tachycardia is an uncommon arrhythmia in children. Victoria L. Vetter, Mark E. Josephson, and Leonard N. Horowitz (Philadelphia) used programmed electric stimulation and catheter endocardial mapping to study the electrophysiologic characteristics and mechanisms of recurrent sustained ventricular tachycardia (VT) in 7 pediatric patients. The age at diagnosis ranged from 5 to 18 years and the age at electrophysiologic study ranged from 7 to 22 years. Each patient had had at least four spontaneous episodes of VT prior to the study. None of the patients had abnormal hemodynamics at the time of catheterization and angiography; one patient had anomalous takeoff of the right coronary artery from the left coronary cusp.

Atrionodal-bundle and His-ventricular intervals were obtained in 5 subjects. The cycle length of spontaneous episodes ranged from 330 to 480 msec (mean, 410 ± 54), and all patients showed atrioventricular dissociation during VT. In the basal stage, VT could be initiated reproducibly in 2 patients, 1 by rapid ventricular pacing and the other by single ventricular stimuli and rapid ventricular pacing. In 1 patient, VT could be initiated by single ventricular premature stimulus only after the administration of lidocaine. In the other 4 patients, VT could not be initiated by any of the various methods used. In 1 patient, VT could be terminated reproducibly in the basal state by a single ventricular premature stimulus or rapid ventricular pacing. In another patient, VT could be terminated by single ventricular premature polarization only after the administration of lidocaine. In a third patient, VT could be terminated intermittently in the basal state but at other times required the administration of phenytoin for reproducible termination. In the other 4 patients, VT could not be terminated by electric stimulation either before or after drug administration. Electric stimulation not only did not terminate VT in these patients but also reset it. In 5 patients, atrial pacing resulted in ventricular capture, converting the QRS complex to a supraventricular configuration without terminating VT. The QRS configuration was right bundle-branch block (RBBB) in 3 patients and left bundle-branch block (LBBB) in 4 (Fig 6). The site of origin of VT was the right ventricular outflow tract in the 4 patients with LBBB configuration. In the 3 patients with RBBB configuration, the sites of origin were the inferobasal wall of the left ventricle, the mid right ventricular septum, and the mid left ventricular septum, respectively.

The results show that in 4/7 patients the VT had an automatic rather than a reentrant mechanism and originated more frequently in the right than in the left ventricle; this contrasts with the adult experience, in which 90% fulfilled the criteria for reentrant mecha-

Am. J. Cardiol. 47:315–322, February 1981.

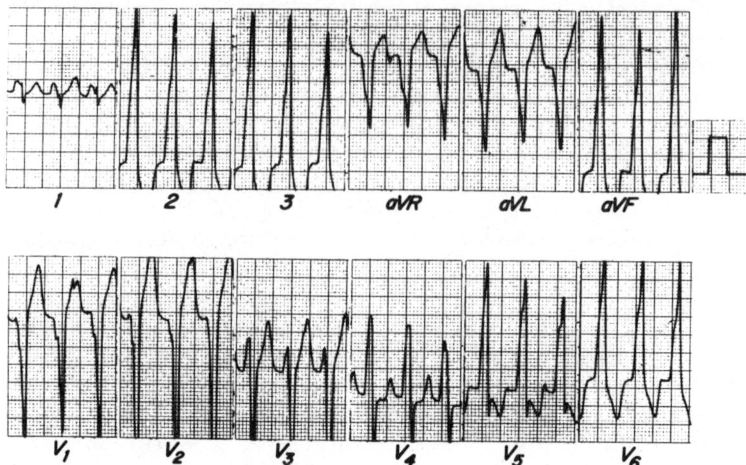

Fig 6.—Patient 5. Electrogram during ventricular tachycardia. It is typical of the ventricular tachycardias with a LBBB configuration observed in this group of patients. The right precordial leads show an rS or QS pattern, and the limb leads show an inferior axis with all monophasic R waves in leads II, III, and a VF. (Courtesy of Vetter, V. L., et al.: Am J. Cardiol. 47:315–322, February 1981.)

nism. Also, in contrast to adults with ventricular tachycardia, none of these patients was proved to have structural heart disease. On the basis of these two features, electrophysiologic studies seem less useful in the management of these children than in adults.

Ventricular Tachycardia in Children is discussed by Albert P. Rocchini, Patrick O. Chun, and MacDonald Dick to assess factors that are important in determining the prognosis of children with this arrhythmia. Records of 38 children who had ventricular tachycardia were reviewed. Patients were aged 1–20 years, and follow-up ranged from 0.5 to 12 years. Patients were classified according to presence or absence of known structural heart disease. Among the 21 with structural heart disease were 5 with mitral valve prolapse, 4 with repaired tetralogy of Fallot, 3 with myocarditis, 3 with prolonged Q-T syndrome, and 6 with other lesions. In 17, there was no known heart disease. Ventricular tachycardia was diagnosed at a mean of 9.8 years in patients with and at a mean of 11.5 years in those without underlying disease. There were three deaths among patients with organic disease and none among those without. Catheterization was done in 19 patients with and 5 patients without underlying heart disease; left ventricular abnormalities were present in 8 of the patients with and none of the patients without heart disease. Seventeen of the 21 patients with known heart disease were symptomatic, with cardiac arrest occurring in 5, syncope in 5, and dizziness in 7. Only 6 of the patients without heart disease had symptoms, including syncope (3)

Am. J. Cardiol. 47:1091–1097, May 1981.

and dizziness (3) each in 3 ($P<.01$). All symptomatic patients had rates of more than 150 beats per minute, whereas all but 1 of the asymptomatic patients had rates of less than 150 beats per minute ($P<.01$). Graded treadmill exercise testing was done in 21 patients. Exercise increased the degree of ventricular arrhythmia in 8 of the 11 symptomatic patients but decreased or abolished the arrhythmia in 9 of the 10 asymptomatic patients ($P<.01$).

Antiarrhythmic therapy was given to 28 of the 38. Effectiveness was assessed with both 24-hour Holter monitoring and graded treadmill exercise testing. Therapy effectively abolished ventricular tachycardia and greatly decreased the number of premature ventricular complexes in symptomatic patients, but was less effective in the asymptomatic patients. The presence of underlying heart disease, rate of the ventricular tachycardia, and results of graded treadmill exercise tests are useful in predicting prognosis. Antiarrhythmic therapy is suggested only for patients who are symptomatic or those with tachycardia rates exceeding 150 beats per minute or with exacerbation of tachycardia on exercise. Propranolol seemed to be effective in management of arrhythmias associated with mitral valve prolapse, and a combination of this drug with phenytoin abolished the ventricular tachycardia associated with prolonged QT. Phenytoin alone was helpful in controlling the postoperative arrhythmias of patients with tetralogy of Fallot.

► [The two preceding articles are very interesting in that they discuss a real therapeutic dilemma, ventricular tachycardia in children. In contrast to adults, particularly those with coronary heart disease, asymptomatic ventricular tachycardia in children without heart disease is a benign condition, and needs neither electrophysiologic studies nor pharmacologic suppression. Ventricular tachycardia in children with structural heart disease, congenital or rheumatic, on the other hand, may be life-threatening and demand vigorous drug therapy. Patients with aortic valve disease and ventricular ectopy should be considered candidates for aortic valve surgery.— A.S.N.] ◄

Additional Reading

Abinader, E. G., and Oliven, A.: The effect of congesting cuffs on echo- and phonocardiographic findings in mitral valve prolapse. *Chest* 80:197, 1981.

Beasley, B., and Kerber, R.: Does mitral prolapse occur in mitral stenosis? Echocardiographic-angiographic observations. *Chest* 80:56, 1981.

Bisset, G. S., III, et al.: Clinical spectrum and long-term follow-up of isolated mitral valve prolapse in 119 children. *Circulation* 62:423, 1980.

Dungan, W. T., et al.: Arrhythmogenic right ventricular dysplasia: A cause of ventricular tachycardia in children with apparently normal hearts. *Am. Heart J.* 102:745, 1981.

Ellison, R. C., et al.: Obesity, sodium intake, and blood pressure in adolescents. *Hypertension* 2(Suppl. I):I–78, 1980.

Falkner, B., et al.: Cardiovascular characteristics in adolescents who develop essential hypertension. *Hypertension* 3:521, 1981.

Fiddler, G. I., and Scott, O.: Heart murmurs audible across the room in children with mitral valve prolapse. *Br. Heart J.* 44:201, 1980.

Fuchs, R. M., and Achuff, S. C.: Auscultatory findings of mitral prolapse mimicking aortic stenosis and regurgitation. *Am. Heart J.* 101:351, 1981.

Hanson, M. R., et al.: Brain events associated with mitral valve prolapse. *Stroke* 11:499, 1980.

Jaffe, A. S., et al.: Mitral valve prolapse: A consistent manifestation of type IV Ehlers-Danlos syndrome: The pathogenetic role of abnormal production of type III collagen. *Circulation* 64:121, 1981.

Lichstein, E.: Site of origin of ventricular premature beats in patients with mitral valve prolapse. *Am. Heart J.* 100:450, 1980.

Maron, B. J., et al.: Prognostic significance of 24-hour ambulatory electrocardiographic monitoring in patients with hypertrophic cardiomyopathy: A prospective study. *Am. J. Cardiol.* 48:252, 1981.

Oliven, A., and Abinader, E.: Postural-related supraventricular tachyarrhythmia in the mitral valve prolapse syndrome. *Am. Heart J.* 102:130, 1981.

Rice, G. P. A., et al.: Mitral valve prolapse: A cause of stroke in children? *Dev. Med. Child. Neurol.* 23:352, 1981.

Walsh, P. N., et al.: Platelets, thromboembolism, and mitral valve prolapse. *Circulation* 63:552, 1981.

Weber, K. T., et al.: Amrinone and exercise performance in patients with chronic heart failure. *Am. J. Cardiol.* 48:164, 1981.

Wei, J. Y., and Fortuin, N. J.: Diastolic sounds and murmurs associated with mitral valve prolapse. *Circulation* 63:559, 1981.

Woodruff, J. F.: Viral myocarditis: A review. *Am. J. Pathol.* 101:427, 1980.

Zahka, K. G., et al.: Cardiac involvement in adolescent hypertension: Echocardiographic determination of myocardial hypertrophy. *Hypertension* 3:664, 1981.

Hematology/Oncology

"To be is to do."—PLATO

Hematological problems and neoplastic diseases unfortunately comprise a large portion of the adolescent health care physician's day. Pediatric patients are living longer into the adolescent years with dreaded diseases. Therefore the clinician must not only be knowledgeable about the basic medical, surgical and chemical aspects of these diseases but also strive to better understand their psychosocial aspects. The job of caring for an adolescent or young adult with a hematologic or oncologic problem can be overwhelming, not only for the adolescent and his family but also for the health care provider. Both physician and patient can "burn out" in trying to treat this particular disease state, and therefore "to be and to do" becomes a monumental task for both.

Articles in this section deal with the latest treatment available to the adolescent cancer patient as well as specific neoplastic diseases and hematologic states. Of special interest is the article by Torti et al. on extralymphatic Hodgkin's disease. The authors note that limited (localized) extralymphatic disease carries an excellent prognosis, and with appropriate treatment success with this rare disease is possible. Results of long-term treatment of children and adolescents with Hodgkin's disease are reported by Williams and associates who point out that the chief long-term side effect of treatment has been growth retardation but that most surviving patients are leading normal productive lives.

The article on the epidemiology of testicular cancer in young adults is extremely important because of the numbers of adolescent males who present with this malignancy. Testicular cancers of germ cell origin account for at least 95% of the testicular malignancies in young adult men. When one considers that the mortality rate from testicular cancer in individuals aged 15–19 years has increased substantially, it is important that the clinician understand this condition in order to diagnose it early.

The article by Pratt et al. also deserves attention. Half the patients in this series of 31 children and adolescents with malignant melanoma died, but multiple adjunct chemotherapy may hold promise for the treatment of both adults and children with metastatic melanoma.

Management of depression in patients with advanced cancer is discussed by Goldberg. This important article emphasizes the need for concern about the total patient and emphasizes the importance of support systems. The article covers the various stages through which the individual progresses after the cancer is diagnosed. Identification and correction of the underlying medical disease without addressing the emotional and social issues is not treating the entire patient. Those individuals who work with adolescent and young adult cancer patients realize that depression is a major concern and therefore will find this article extremely helpful. In the article on cancer prevention as a realizable goal, Berenblum discusses prevention by *interfering with* as distinguished from *eliminating* the causative agent. Prevention by interference could theoretically operate at three different levels: (1) during the precarcinogenic stage; (2) during the course of carcinogenic action; and (3) during the postcarcinogenic stage. This discussion of concepts concerning the treatment of cancer in all age groups is certainly applicable to adolescents and young adults, as is the article by Cairns which discusses genetics and the origin of human cancers. Finally, the link between diet and cancer is an important consideration, and an article assessing the methodologies for studying this relationship is included in the reading list.

Use of Prognostic Factors in Improving Design and Efficiency of Clinical Trials in Childhood Leukemia: Children's Cancer Study Group Report. Denis R. Miller, Sanford Leikin, Vincent Albo, Leonard Vitale, Harland Sather, Peter Coccia, Mark Nesbit, Myron Karon, and D. Hammond note that prognostic factors are exerting an increasingly apparent and important effect on the results of comparative treatment regimens in childhood acute lymphoblastic leukemia. Between February 1975 and March 1977, 883 previously untreated children with acute lymphoblastic leukemia (ALL) were entered on a Children's Cancer Study Group protocol (CCSG 141) designed to evaluate prognostic factors that influence the rate of induction of complete remission, duration of remission, and overall survival. A second purpose was to identify subsets of patients with high

Fig 7.—Schema for CCSG 141. (Courtesy of Miller, D. R., et al.: Cancer Treat. Rep. 64:381–392, Feb.—Mar. 1980.)

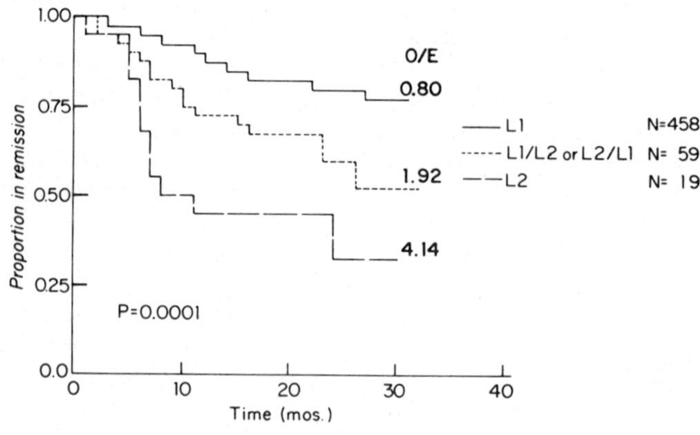

Cancer Treat. Rep. 64:381–392, Feb.–Mar. 1980.

risk of early treatment failure or with particularly favorable prognoses.

Stratification was based upon the initial white blood cell count (WBC); the schema is presented in Figure 7. Patients with initial WBC of $< 20 \times 10^9$/L were given induction therapy of prednisone (PDN), vincristine (VCR), L-asparaginase (L-ASP), cranial radiation therapy of 2400 rad plus 6 weekly injections of intrathecal methotrexate (MTX), and maintenance therapy consisting of daily 6-mercaptopurine (6MP), weekly MTX, and monthly pulses of VCR and PDN for 12 months, after which VCR and PDN were discontinued

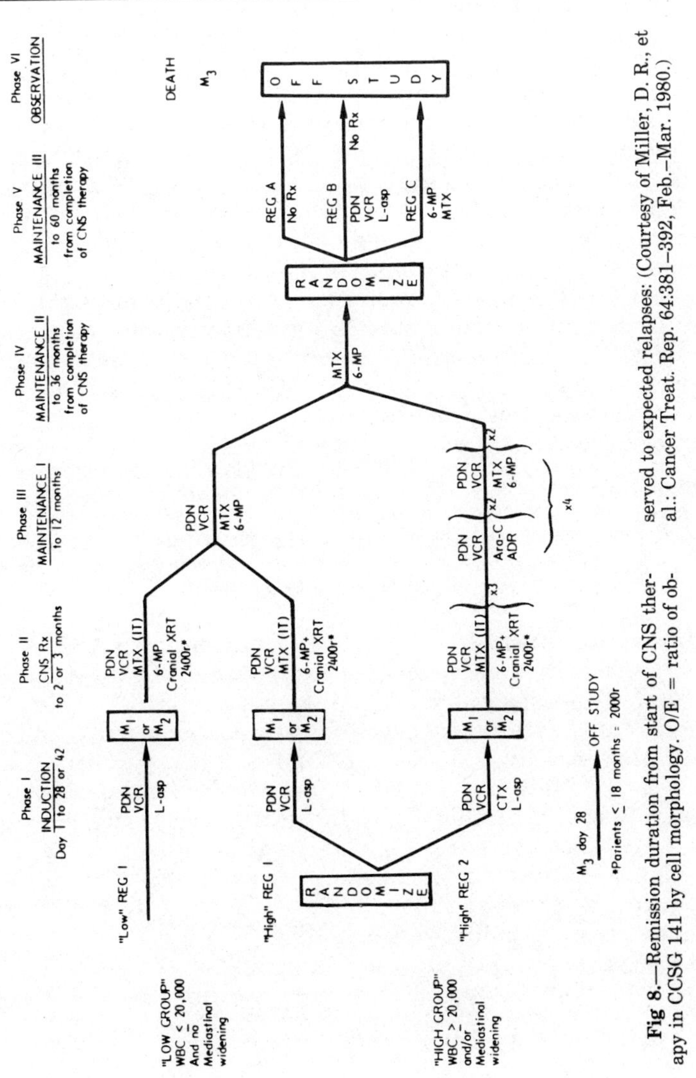

Fig 8.—Remission duration from start of CNS therapy in CCSG 141 by cell morphology. O/E = ratio of observed to expected relapses: (Courtesy of Miller, D. R., et al.: Cancer Treat. Rep. 64:381–392, Feb.–Mar. 1980.)

(regimen 1). Children with initial WBC $< 20 \times 10^9$/L were randomized to receive either regimen 1 or a more intensive program (regimen 2) consisting of PDN, VCR, L-ASP, and cyclophosphamide as induction therapy, intensive CNS prophylaxis with intrathecal MTX twice weekly, and intermittent cycles of POCA (PDN, VCR, cytosine arabinoside, and Adriamycin) or POMP (PDN, VCR, MTX, and 6MP) for 12 months. Thereafter, maintenance therapy was similar to the standard regimen.

The overall rate of complete remission (CR) was 94.2%. Key unfavorable factors predictive of remission induction were: patient age > 10 years, initial WBC $> 20 \times 10^9$/L, and decreased serum immunoglobulin levels. The following factors were associated with unfavorable prognoses leading to bone marrow relapse and death: WBC $\geq 20 \times 10^9$/L; age > 7 years; CNS leukemia at the time of diagnosis; L_2 morphology as determined by the French-American-British classification (Fig 8); hemoglobin level ≥ 11 gm/dl; decreased levels of serum immunoglobulins G, A, and M; and M_3 bone marrow status ($> 25\%$ lymphoblasts) on day 14 of induction. At the time of this report, none of the 41 patients, aged 3–7 years, who had initial WBC $< 10 \times 10^9$/L, L_1 lymphoblasts, normal levels of immunoglobulins, and M_1 bone marrow on day 14 had sustained an adverse event.

Identification of prognostic factors should permit more efficient and effective design of future protocols by refining the classification of ALL, decreasing the toxic risks to patients with a better prognosis, and improving the relatively short duration of remission and survival for patients with a poor prognosis.

▶ [This study evaluates prognostic factors that influence induction rate, remission duration, and survival in patients with acute lymphoblastic leukemia, and identifies subsets of patients with a high risk of early failure. It appears to be one of the first attempts to coordinate different prognostic variables in one article. There are problems associated with the excessive use of prognostic factors without recognition of the heterogeneity of the disease; therefore, alternate attempts at generating bases for treatment purposes are important. Nevertheless, this is an important article.— R.L.C.] ◀

Treatment of Acute Myelogenous Leukemia in Children and Adults. Progress in acute myelogenous leukemia (AML) therapy during the past 2 decades has not equaled the advances attained in the management of acute lymphocytic leukemia. Howard J. Weinstein, Robert J. Mayer, David S. Rosenthal, Bruce M. Camitta, Felice S. Coral, David G. Nathan, and Emil Frei III (Boston) designed a protocol to address the problem of relapse from complete remission in AML in 83 consecutive patients younger than age 50 years. Patients in remission were treated for 14 months; early and intensification of chemotherapy, sequential drug combinations, and high-dose continuous infusions of cytarabine were included.

Of the 83 patients, 58 (70%) had a complete remission. Forty patients entered complete remission with 1 course of therapy; 18 pa-

N. Engl. J. Med. 303:473–478, Aug. 28, 1980.

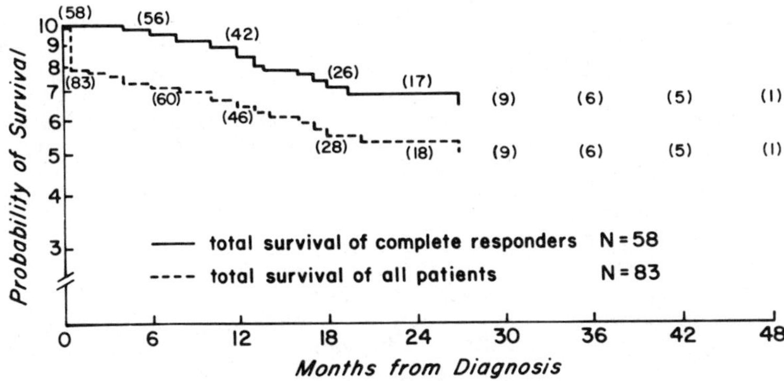

Fig 9.—Kaplan-Meier analysis of survival. Figures in parentheses refer to patients at risk during the interval. (Courtesy of Weinstein, H. J., et al.: N. Engl. J. Med. 303:473–478, Aug. 28, 1980.)

tients required 2 courses. Rates of complete remission were similar in patients aged 0–17 years and 18–50 years. Five patients were younger than age 12 months at the time of diagnosis, and 4 of these had a complete remission. Of the 25 patients without complete remissions, 15 had leukemia resistant to therapy, and 10 died of infection during a period of bone marrow hypoplasia. A Kaplan-Meier analysis predicted that 49% ± 17% of patients (mean ±2 SD) who entered complete remission will remain free from disease at 2 years. Twenty-two patients completed therapy, and the median follow-up after cessation of treatment was 11 months. Only 4 of these 22 patients suffered relapse. There were 22 relapses, 2 deaths during remission, and 5 withdrawals during remission. In the age group 10–17 years, the CNS was the first site of relapse in 7 patients. Survival curves are shown in Figure 9. The projected median survival time for all patients was 27 months. The early decline in this curve is due to the 1-month median survival time of patients who did not enter complete remission. These curves suggest that more than 65% of patients with complete remission will be alive 2 years after diagnosis. Toxic manifestations were more severe during induction of remission than during intensive sequential chemotherapy. All patients had reversible alopecia. The present study suggests that AML can be controlled by chemotherapy in many patients.

▶ [Howard J. Weinstein, Assistant Professor of Pediatrics at Harvard Medical School and of Oncology at the Sidney Farber Cancer Institute, Boston, writes:

"The AML study was closed to patient entry in May 1980 and the data have been updated through July 1, 1981. A total of 61 children (aged 10–17 years) entered the study and 45 (74%) achieved complete remission. There have been a total of 18 relapses: bone marrow (9), central nervous system (8), and myeloblastoma (1). The median follow-up of children remaining in remission is 29 months. By life table analysis, the probability that a patient will remain in continuous complete remission from 2 to 5 years is 55%. Twenty-two children have completed all therapy, and the median follow-up after cessation of therapy is 1 year. Only 4 of these 22 patients have relapsed after cessation of treatment. These data continue to indicate that intensive chemotherapy in children with AML results in prolonged remissions. It is also possible to discontinue this therapy after a finite period (15 months in our study) and expect continued remissions without maintenance therapy. The only factor influencing the length of remission in our AML study was the morphological appearance of the leukemic cell. Children with acute monocytic (FAB classification M-5) leukemia have a statistically significant shorter duration of remission compared to those patients with other subtypes of AML. Because of the incidence of meningeal recurrence in this study, we are now administering prophylactic intrathecal cytosine arabinoside.

"What is the best treatment for a patient with AML in remission? Is bone marrow transplantation superior to intensive chemotherapy? Prospective controlled trials are being performed (Children's Cancer Study Group—Mark Nesbit et al.) to address this question. The early transplant data suggest long-term remission in the majority of patients given transplants during first remissions. Marrow transplantation is only applicable to a minority of patients and is of at least equal hazard with chemotherapy. Immunologic progress will certainly improve the efficacy and feasibility of marrow transplantation in AML, but we also expect continued improvement in the chemotherapy of AML."] ◄

Leukemia and Other Cancers After Radiotherapy and Chemotherapy for Hodgkin's Disease. Jean-F. Boivin (McGill Univ.) and George B. Hutchison (Harvard Univ.) reviewed data on 1,553 patients with Hodgkin's disease (HD) seen between 1940 and 1975 and analyzed follow-up findings through 1976.

Excluding basal and squamous cell carcinomas of skin, trichoepitheliomas, and in situ carcinomas of cervix uteri, 27 cancers were observed 1 year or more after the diagnosis of HD. There were 21 solid tumors and 6 cases of acute nonlymphocytic leukemia. The estimate of the relative risk (RR) of leukemia in patients treated with intensive chemotherapy was 140 relative to the general population. In the subgroup treated with both initial intensive radiotherapy and intensive chemotherapy, the RR was 270; in the subgroup not treated with initial intensive radiotherapy but exposed to both late radiotherapy and intensive chemotherapy, the RR was 250. Leukemia never followed intensive radiotherapy without chemotherapy. For second cancers other than leukemia and non-HD lymphomas, RRs were generally not significantly different from the null value one. Series of patients will have to be followed for longer intervals before more definitive statements can be made regarding second cancers other than leukemia.

The observed leukemias occurred within 4 years after chemotherapy (few person-years of experience were available 5 or more years after chemotherapy). The absence of leukemias in patients not receiving chemotherapy suggests that neither HD itself nor irradiation is a risk factor for leukemia, but that chemotherapy may be a strong risk factor. General population comparison and the Mantel-Byar estimate of RR support the general conclusion that intensive chemotherapy is a risk factor for leukemia. It is also possible that leukemia is a characteristic of progressing HD, but that risk of leukemia is reduced or abolished when the disorder is successfully controlled. Another explanation might be that an immune-deficient state leads to both progression of HD and occurrence of leukemia.

JNCI 67:751–761, October 1981.

▶ [All 6 patients with leukemia were treated with nitrogen mustard, procarbazine and prednisone. All 6 also received vincristine, vinblastine, or both; 3 patients also received other drugs, including bleomycin, Adriamycin, semustine, cyclophosphamide, or chlorambucil. Since publication of this study, 8 additional cases of leukemia have been diagnosed among the original 1,553 patients. Seven of these occurred after intensive chemotherapy. The eighth may have represented the late occurrence of leukemia in a patient treated with radiotherapy alone.—R.L.D.] ◀

Extralymphatic Hodgkin's Disease: Prognosis and Response to Therapy. Disseminated extralymphatic Hodgkin's disease has been reported to have a poor prognosis, while patients with localized extralymphatic disease have a better survival.

Frank M. Torti, Carol S. Portlock, Saul A. Rosenberg, and Henry S. Kaplan (Stanford Univ.) evaluated 318 patients with pathologic stage IA to IIIA Hodgkin's disease who entered randomized trials comparing lymphatic radiotherapy alone with radiotherapy plus 6 cy-

Fig 10.—Overall result of patient population studied. (Courtesy of Torti, F. M., et al.: Am. J. Med. 70:487–492, March 1981.)

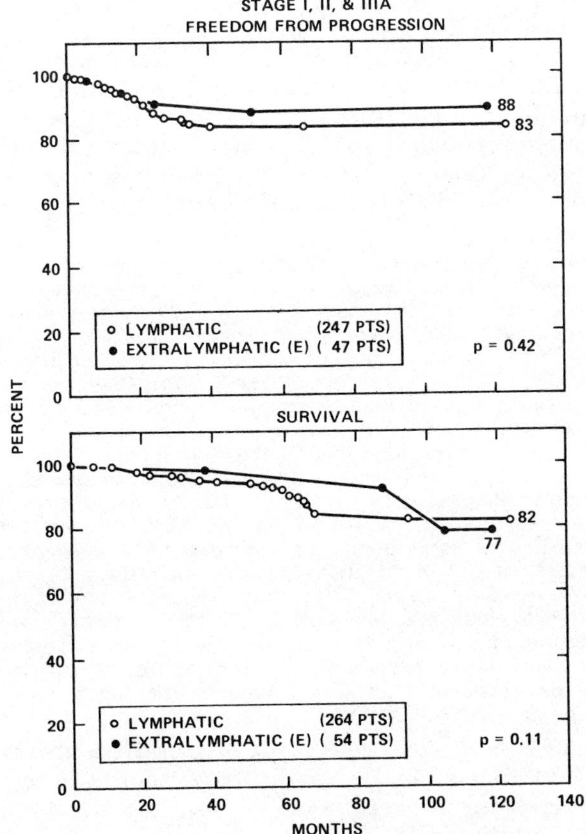

cles of adjuvant chemotherapy with MOPP (mustard, Oncovin, procarbazine, and prednisone), MOP (mustard, Oncovin, and procarbazine), or PAVe (procarbazine, alkeran, and vinblastine). Fifty-four patients had extralymphatic lesions. Pericardial disease was treated with additional radiation therapy in patients not given chemotherapy. Lung lesions in such patients were treated with a full dose of 4,400 rad. Median follow-up was 54 months.

Fourteen patients had pericardial involvement, 7 as the only extralymphatic disease. Nodular sclerosis histology predominated among patients with extralymphatic lesions; this appeared to reflect more frequent mediastinal involvement in these cases. Relapses occurred with about equal frequency within each stage in patients with extralymphatic disease (5 patients) and those without.

Survival and freedom from progressive disease were similar for patients with and those without extranodal disease (Fig 10). Three of the 54 patients with extralymphatic lesions died. Two were patients given radiotherapy alone who died of unrelated causes. The type of treatment did not significantly influence survival in patients with extralymphatic disease.

Limited extralymphatic Hodgkin's disease carries an excellent prognosis. These patients survived as well as patients with nodal disease of equivalent stage. Addition of chemotherapy to radiotherapy did not improve survival in patients with extralymphatic disease, and there appears to be no reason to add adjuvant chemotherapy to optimal radiotherapy solely because of the presence of localized extralymphatic disease.

▶ [Patients with Hodgkin's disease presenting with extralymphatic disease unassociated with detectable lymph node involvement are exceedingly rare. Overwhelmingly, the disease appears to originate in lymph nodes and usually spreads to anatomically contiguous nodes in an orderly fashion. The biologic and therapeutic significance of extralymphatic spread of Hodgkin's disease was discussed at the Ann Arbor conference in 1971 (*Cancer Res.* 31:1860, 1971). At that conference, it was a widely held clinical impression that disseminated extralymphatic disease had a poor prognosis. It also was shown that survival in patients with Hodgkin's disease was significantly better in those with localized extralymphatic disease contiguous to lymph nodes than in those with disseminated extralymphatic disease. The Ann Arbor conference thus designated local or limited extralymphatic disease (E lesions) as a substage within stage I, II, and III disease. This decision in regard to staging classification was based on the assumption that local spread to extralymphatic sites occurs by contiguity and not by hematogenous dissemination. Recently, however, a report by Levi and Wiernik (*Am. J. Med.* 63:365, 1977) suggested that prognosis in pulmonary extralymphatic Hodgkin's disease is worse than in disease with intrathoracic adenopathy but without extralymphatic spread. The present article describing a large experience at Stanford University suggests that survival of patients with localized extralymphatic disease is not significantly different from that of patients without extralymphatic spread.—M.J.C.] ◀

Long-Term Results of Treatment of Children and Adolescents With Hodgkin's Disease. Successful treatment of Hodgkin's disease has led to increasing concern over adverse late effects of treatment. Judith Wilimas, Elizabeth Thompson, and Kirby L. Smith (St. Jude

Cancer 46:2123–2125, Nov. 15, 1980.

Children's Res. Hosp., Memphis, Tenn.) report findings in a long-term follow-up of 54 patients with Hodgkin's disease, treated in 1967–1972. The median age at diagnosis was 11 years. Thirty patients had stage IIB or more advanced disease, and 7 had stage IV disease. All patients received radiotherapy and chemotherapy. Three patients have been lost to follow-up. Thirty-eight patients remain in continuous complete remission a median of 90 months after diagnosis. Nine patients have died, 4 of progressive disease, and 6 have relapsed. Two of the 6 patients with relapse have died.

Three patients died of pneumonitis early during treatment. One died with presumed pneumococcal sepsis and 1 with acute myelocytic leukemia, which developed 47 months after diagnosis. Among 40 patients younger than age 16 years when given radiotherapy, those given more than mantle therapy appeared to have a lower growth rate. One patient has significant scoliosis. None has clinical evidence of hypothyroidism. No patient has clinically apparent pulmonary dysfunction. Five women are amenorrheic. Three patients have had psychological problems requiring medical attention. At least 12 patients are employed, and 13 are still in school. One woman and 1 man have each had a normal child.

Three fourths of patients in this series remain in continuous complete remission 71–130 months after diagnosis of Hodgkin's disease. Many had advanced disease at diagnosis.

The chief long-term side effect of treatment has been growth retardation. Most surviving patients are leading normal productive lives. Attempts to reduce morbidity from treatment should not compromise present cure rates, since growth retardation represents minimal morbidity in exchange for long-term disease-free survival.

▶ [This is a useful study providing follow-up data on young patients treated for Hodgkin's disease 10 or more years ago. Several points are worth noting. First, the incidence of acute myelogenous leukemia appears to be lower than that reported in many other series of intensively treated patients. Although most of the patients in this series are beyond the median time for development of acute myeloblastic leukemia, they still remain at risk of developing this disease or another secondary neoplasm.

The reported 3% incidence of pneumococcal sepsis is somewhat lower than that described in other series, despite the fact that no patient was taking prophylactic antibiotics or had received pneumococcal vaccine.

The data presented here suggest that the most striking retardation in growth occurred in children irradiated before age 6 years and those irradiated between ages 12 and 13 years.—M.J.C.] ◀

Lymphoblastic Lymphoma in Adults: Results of a Pilot Protocol. Lymphoblastic lymphoma is a recently established subgroup of the diffuse non-Hodgkin's lymphomas that occurs primarily in adolescent boys. The disease has many similarities to T cell acute lymphocytic leukemia (ALL). Approximately 50% of the patients present with a mediastinal mass. Involvement of the bone marrow is seen at diagnosis in 25%–30% of the patients and during the course of the disease in 80%; central nervous system (CNS) relapse is common. C.

Blood 57:679–684, April 1981.

Norman Coleman, James R. Cohen, Jerome S. Burke, and Saul A. Rosenberg (Stanford Univ.) evaluated an intensive chemotherapy program in the treatment of 13 patients with histologically proved lymphoblastic lymphoma. An additional patient with T cell ALL was treated by the same protocol.

Of the 14 patients, 11 presented with mediastinal masses, 5 with bone marrow involvement, and 1 with CNS disease. The chemotherapy program consisted of induction with cyclophosphamide, adriamycin, vincristine, and prednisone (modified CHOP); consolidation and CNS prophylaxis with methotrexate intrathecally and by high-dose intravenous injection, citrovorum factor, and L-asparaginase; reinforcement with CHOP, and maintenance with 6-mercaptopurine and methotrexate. The duration of treatment was 1 year. The median age of the patients was 22 years (range 16–50 years), and the ratio of male to female patients was 2.5:1.

The clinical response was complete in all patients. A pathologic complete response was seen in all cases of bone marrow involvement. Four of the 13 patients without initial CNS disease relapsed; 3 had primary CNS relapse, and 1 had a recurrent abdominal mass. There were 5 deaths, 2 from drug toxicity, 2 from CNS relapse, and 1 from chronic myelogenous leukemia, which was diagnosed at the same time as the lymphoblastic lymphoma. Hematologic toxicity was severe, with 50% of the patients reaching a white blood count nadir of less than 100/cu mm during induction; the CNS prophylaxis phase was well tolerated. The median follow-up was 19 months, and all patients completed the planned therapy. The actuarial survival rate at 3 years was 61%, and the relapse-free survival was 56% (Fig 11).

The results of this pilot study demonstrate that an aggressive ALL-

Fig 11.—Actuarial survival and freedom from relapse in 13 of 14 patients with adult lymphoblastic lymphoma. (Courtesy of Coleman, C. N., et al.: Blood 57:679–684, April 1981.)

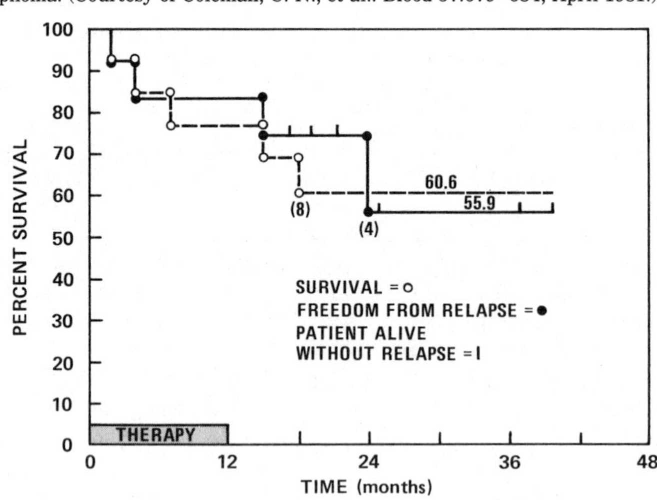

like protocol is successful in treating adult patients with lymphoblastic lymphoma and gives results similar to those achieved in the treatment of childhood lymphoblastic lymphoma.

▶ [The neoplastic cells of lymphoblastic lymphoma are morphologically similar to the blast cells of acute lymphocytic leukemia and are predominantly T cells. It is not surprising, therefore, that the disease has many similarities to T cell ALL, and many authorities consider lymphoblastic lymphoma and T cell ALL to be variants of one disease (Dow et al.: *Blood* 50:671, 1977). Before its identification as a nosologic entity distinct from other non-Hodgkin's lymphomas, lymphoblastic lymphoma often was treated by local radiation therapy or cyclic chemotherapy with cyclophosphamide, Adriamycin, vincristine, and prednisone, or by both regimens. Median survival generally was short (8–13 months). Beginning about 1977, many groups of investigators began treating patients with this disease with more aggressive protocols resembling those used in the treatment of childhood acute lymphoblastic leukemia. Central nervous system treatment was added to deal with the frequent occurrence of disease in this site.

The results of this pilot study from Stanford University are encouraging for the treatment of adult lymphoblastic lymphoma patients. It should be noted that high-dose methotrexate with citrovorum factor rescue failed to prevent CNS relapse in 3 of 13 patients and that drug toxicity led to 2 deaths. These investigators plan to modify their protocol by earlier use of CNS prophylactic therapy, which would include cranial irradiation and intrathecally administered methotrexate. They plan to avoid the use of high-dose methotrexate and to lower the dose of cyclophosphamide.—M.J.C.] ◀

Fibrolamellar Carcinoma of the Liver: A Tumor of Adolescents and Young Adults With Distinctive Clinico-pathologic Features. John R. Craig, Robert L. Peters, Hugh A. Edmondson, and Masao Omata (Univ. of Southern California, Los Angeles) report on the histopathologic features of 23 hepatocellular carcinomas that allowed recognition of a distinct clinical and pathologic variant of hepatocellular carcinoma. These features include deeply eosinophilic plump hepatocytes and abundant fibrous stroma arranged in thin parallel bands around small nests and clumps of the malignant hepatocytes (Fig 12). In addition, approximately half of the tumors had distinct tumor cells with cytoplasmic pale bodies (Fig 13). Electron microscopy revealed prominent and abundant mitochondria. Most of the tumors occurred in noncirrhotic livers and were solitary. Two tumors had prominent deep fibrous scars in their central areas causing the gross appearance to resemble focal nodular hyperplasia. The histologic features may simulate focal nodular hyperplasia, hepatocellular adenoma, metastatic islet cell carcinoma, and paraganglioma.

The distinctive clinical features are the young age of the patient (mean 26.4 years compared with 55 years for all hepatocellular carcinoma patients the authors have seen) and the tumor's equal incidence in both sexes, which differs from the usual distribution of 3.6 males to 1 female for all hepatocellular carcinomas. Major clinical symptoms included abdominal pain and malaise. None of 4 patients tested had elevated serum α-fetoprotein levels, and α_1-antitrypsin phenotypes were monozygotic in 2 patients. Eighteen patients (82%)

Cancer 46:372–379, July 15, 1980.

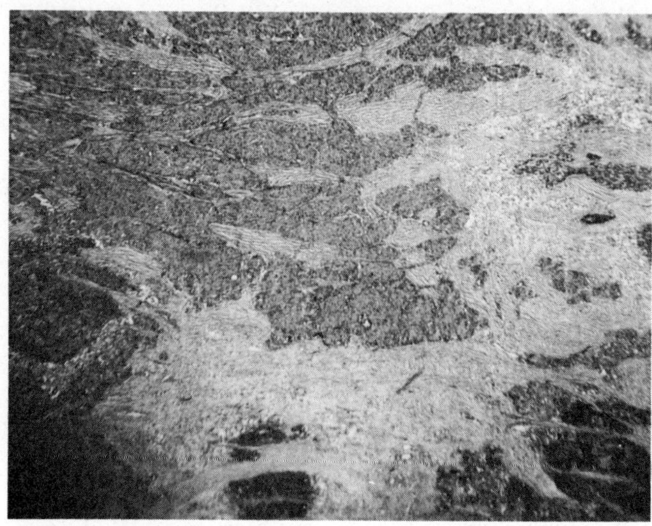

Fig 12.—Typical mixture of dense fibrous tissue in thin fibrous strands, intermingled with epithelial component. Hematoxylin-eosin; ×80. (Courtesy of J. R. Craig.)

underwent laparotomies, with surgical resections accomplished in 48%.

The long-term survival information based on 20 patients indicated an average survival of 32 months, with 3 long-term survivals at 5, 10, and 15 or more years. The longest patient survival without resection was 22 months. The sites of metastases differed from those usu-

Fig 13.—Typical cytoplasmic pale bodies in epithelial component with lamellar fibrosis at the margins of the photograph. Hematoxylin-eosin; ×250. (Courtesy of J. R. Craig.)

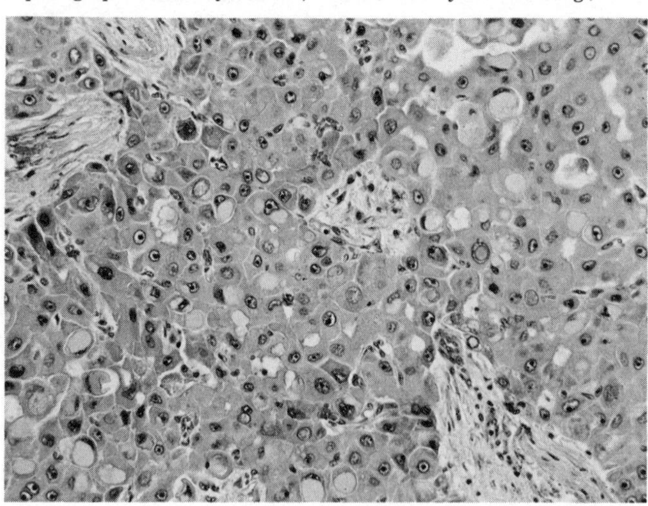

ally seen in hepatocellular carcinoma by occurring more frequently in abdominal lymph nodes and peritoneum. The carcinoma's equal incidence in both sexes and the absence of oral contraceptive therapy in most of the female patients indicate no causal relationship to oral contraceptive use. Clinical and pathologic recognition of this variant is important to encourage surgical resection and potential cure.

▶ [This is an excellent account of a variant of the usual hepatocellular tumor. Fibrolamellar carcinoma has distinctive histologic findings.—R.L.C.] ◀

Coffee and Cancer of the Pancreas. Brian MacMahon, Stella Yen, Dimitrios Trichopoulos, Kenneth Warren, and George Nardi (Harvard School of Public Health, Boston) questioned 369 patients with histologically proved cancer of the pancreas and 644 control patients about their use of tobacco, alcohol, tea, and coffee. The authors report that they found a weak positive association between pancreatic cancer and cigarette smoking, but no association with the use of cigars, pipe tobacco, alcoholic beverages, or tea. A strong association between coffee consumption and pancreatic cancer was evident in both sexes. The association was not affected by controlling for cigarette use.

For the sexes combined, there was a significant dose-response relationship ($P \cong 0.001$); after adjustment for cigarette smoking, the relative risk associated with drinking up to 2 cups of coffee per day was 1.8 (95% confidence limits, 1.0 to 3.0); the risk with 3 or more cups per day was 2.7 (1.6 to 4.7). The authors conclude that this association should be evaluated with other data; if it reflects a causal relationship between coffee drinking and pancreatic cancer, coffee use might account for many of the cases of this disease in the United States.

▶ [This article generated an enormous response in the literature and has raised a controversial issue that is yet to be resolved. The controversy concerns the possible precision of the authors' observations and further investigation will be required before these questions can be answered satisfactorily.—R.L.C.] ◀

Occult Testicular Leukemia: Testicular Biopsy at Three Years Continuous Complete Remission of Childhood Leukemia: A Southwest Oncology Group Study. F. B. Askin, V. J. Land, M. P. Sullivan, A. H. Ragab, C. P. Steuber, P. G. Dyment, J. Talbert, and T. Moore explain that with the development of effective chemotherapy for acute lymphocytic leukemia (ALL) of childhood, long-term continual complete remission (CCR) is being attained. In addition to control of the bone marrow, clinical success has been extended further by the ability to prevent central nervous system (CNS) relapse. However, extramedullary relapse in other sites remains an obstacle to cure and is all too frequently evidence of inadequate disease control despite continued bone marrow remission. Numerous reports have documented the appearance of clinically overt testicular involvement as an initial manifestation of recurring disease. The authors report

N. Engl. J. Med. 304:630–633, Mar. 12, 1981.
Cancer 47:470–475, Feb. 1, 1981.

results of the Southwest Oncology Group Pediatric Division investigation of the incidence, pathologic features, prior therapy, and sequelae of occult testicular leukemia (OTL) among 59 patients who had testicular biopsies after 3 years of CCR while receiving chemotherapy.

Between June 1977 and December 1978, OTL was discovered at 3 years of CCR from the time of diagnosis of acute lymphoblastic leukemia in 5 of 59 (8.5%) patients who underwent bilateral wedge testicular biopsy at participating Southwest Oncology Group institutions. Forty-five of the 54 patients who had normal biopsies (78% of the total group of 59) remained free of recurrent ALL at a median time of 18 months (range 13 to 23 months) since the biopsy procedure, whereas 8 relapsed for the first time (5 in the bone marrow, 1 in the sclera, 1 simultaneously in the bone marrow and testes, and 1 in the testes) at a median time of 12.5 months (range 4 to 22 months) after the normal testicular biopsy.

Each of the 5 patients whose biopsies revealed OTL received bilateral testicular radiation at a dose of 2400 rads during 2½–3 weeks and intensive systemic chemotherapy and CNS reinforcement therapy with intrathecal chemotherapy with or without cranial irradiation.

Fig 14.—Clinically occult testicular leukemic infiltrate. Low-power photomicrograph shows extensive infiltrate between the tubules. This patient was 4 years old. Hematoxylin-eosin; ×90. (Courtesy of Askin, F. B.: Cancer 47:470–473, Feb. 1, 1981.)

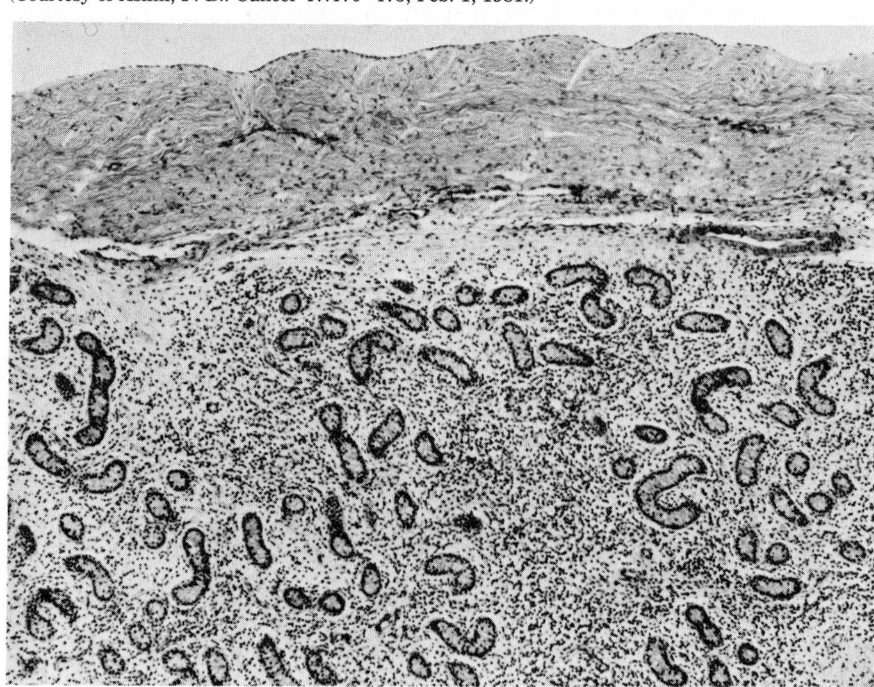

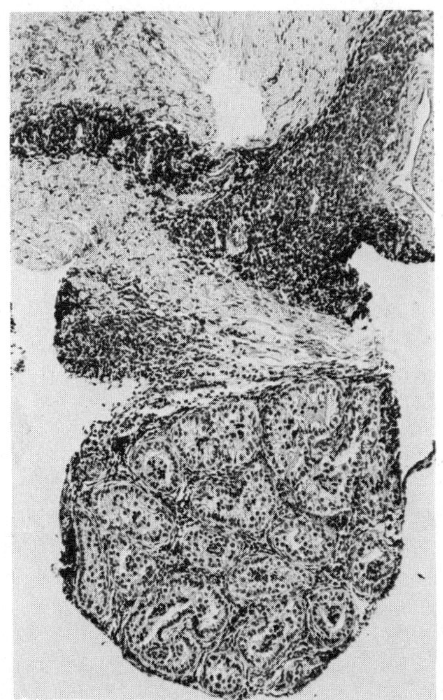

Fig 15.—In this case, the most florid infiltrate lies beneath the testicular tunic and around blood vessels. Hematoxylin-eosin; ×150. (Courtesy of Askin, F. B.: Cancer 47:470–473, Feb. 1, 1981.)

The histologic features of OTL were essentially those described in cases of overt testicular relapse. The testicular tubules were generally widely separated by dense bands of cells 7–10 μ in diameter (Figs 14 and 15). The individual cells had a small rim of cytoplasm, and the nuclei had coarse or ropey chromatin, with one or more small nucleoli. In some instances, the nuclei were markedly convoluted. In a few cases, involvement of the tunica albuginea was noted (Fig 15).

In 2 of the 4 patients who underwent bilateral biopsy, infiltrates were present in both testes. The intensity of involvement from each side of the paired organs differed markedly. Based on this investigation, the authors conclude that routine bilateral testicular biopsy at the time that treatment is discontinued is of value.

▶ [Occult testicular leukemia is being recognized with increasing frequency in patients who are seemingly free of ALL. Bilateral testicular biopsy at the time treatment is discontinued probably should be established as a routine procedure. Although the number of patients subjected to the investigation is small, the apparent absence of complications and the information it provides demands the attention of investigators participating in the care of these patients.—R.L.C.] ◀

The Epidemiology of Testicular Cancer in Young Adults. For a white male subject in the United States, the lifetime probability of testicular cancer developing is about 0.2%, compared with 3.8% for prostatic cancer. The epidemiologic features of cancers of the testis, prostate, and breast in men are compared in the table. David Schot-

Am. J. Epidemiol. 112:232–246, August 1980.

COMPARISON OF EPIDEMIOLOGIC FEATURES OF CANCER OF THE TESTIS, PROSTATE, AND BREAST IN MEN

Factor	Testis	Prostate	Breast
Magnitude (United States) (16)	About 5000 new cases/yr. About 1000 deaths/yr. 1% of cancer incidence.	64,000 new cases/yr. 21,000 deaths/yr. 17% of cancer incidence.	900 new cases/yr. 300 deaths/yr. <0.2% of cancer incidence.
Age	Bimodal age-mortality curve with a prominent peak at 25–34 and a lesser peak after 70 (white males). Third National Cancer Survey indicated testis cancer to be most frequent site during 20–34. Under age 15, germ cell tumors (yolk sac carcinoma and teratoma) comprise 65–75% of testicular tumors. Over 15, germ cell tumors comprise 95% of testicular tumors. The peak incidence period is comprised of embryonal, seminoma and teratoma cell types. Choriocarcinoma is a rare form of germ cell tumor which usually occurs in combination with other germ cell types (17–19).	Rare before 50 then increases steadily with age (20, 21).	Rates begin to rise at 45–50, and increase regularly beyond 75+ (22).
Secular trend	Between 1937–1975, overall decrease (11%) in age-adjusted mortality in US. Age-specific rates increased between 15–34 years and decreased for all age groups after 60. Between 1937 and 1969–71, incidence in whites doubled, and significant age-specific increases were observed for ages 15–44 (4).	Between the First National Cancer Survey in 1937 and the Third National Cancer Survey in 1969–71, incidence increased in blacks by 155% and in whites by 41%. Peak rates for nonwhites born from 1896–1900, with some decline among men born after 1900 (23, 24).	Stable (22, 25)
Geography	Highest age-adjusted incidence rate in Denmark and lowest for some African countries. Highest rates tend to occur for North American whites, United Kingdom and Northern European countries (10, 11).	Highest for United States blacks. At least 20-fold difference in incidence, with lowest in Japan, rare in Central and South America and parts of Africa. Western Europe more common than Eastern Europe. Japanese migrants to US have markedly higher rates than Japanese in Japan, although still less than half that of US whites (26–28).	Little international variation—lowest in Japan and Finland. Increased in Egypt, accounting for more than 6% of all cancers in men (22, 25).

112

Race, religion, socioeconomic status	Incidence and mortality about 4× higher among whites than among blacks who do not manifest early peak at 25–34. Higher incidence among men of higher social class. No consistent relationship with religion independently of social class and residence. The most extreme positive social class gradient suggested for embryonal carcinoma (29–32).	American blacks with significantly higher rates of invasive cancer than in African blacks, while rates for occult or noninvasive cancer are about equal. Low incidence for Israeli Jews and Russian-born Jews in New York City. No consistent relationship with socioeconomic status (33, 34).	Slight excess in US blacks compared to whites. Increase in European Jews. Some studies have suggested higher rates in upper social class (22, 35).
Residence	Several studies have suggested higher risks among men from rural areas, particularly for seminoma. In Denmark the opposite trend was noted for all germ cell tumors (36, 37).	Increased urban (38).	Slight urban excess (22, 35).
Marital status	No consistent significant pattern suggested. The relationship may vary by cell type and age at diagnosis (13, 32).	Mortality higher in ever married than in single persons; highest rates in widowed and divorced (20–23).	Several studies have suggested highest mortality in divorced males (22).
Family history	Isolated sibling and twin case reports. In the absence of national twin registries or population studies, concordance by cell type, laterality and age at diagnosis requires further study. Single case report of bilateral teratomas in nontwin brothers with Klinefelter syndrome (39, 40).	Fathers and brothers of patients are at increased risk (26–28).	At least 5 families reported with multiple male members (41–44).
Occupation	Higher risk in "white collar" subgroups such as "professionals" and "managers". Specific occupations have not yet been identified (45).	Cadmium production workers; rubber workers; chemists; chemical and pharmaceutical industry workers; other occupational groups cited by Third National Cancer Survey (28).	No relationships identified.
Gonadal function	Increased risk in cryptorchidism with hypospermia and abnormal androgen steroidogenesis. ? Orchitis and epididymitis (mumps, other causes) with subsequent atrophy has been suggested in clinical reports (46–49).	Prevalence of prostate cancer at autopsy diminished in patients with moderate to severe cirrhosis of liver; although prior hyperestrogenism presumed, circulating blood levels not recorded. No consistent differences in profile of urinary hormone metabolites observed in patients and controls or between normal Japanese and Americans. Normal growth and function of prostate dependent on androgen and estrogen levels in plasma and prostatic tissues (23, 28).	Increased risk with Klinefelter syndrome which is associated with hypogonadism, decreased testosterone production, decreased responsiveness to pituitary gonadotropin stimulation: ? increased risk in patients with orchitis; ? increased risk in Egyptian males as a result of bilharzial infection of liver and hyperestrogenism; ? general metabolic abnormality in estrogen steroidogenesis (41, 50–56).

COMPARISON OF EPIDEMIOLOGIC FEATURES OF CANCER OF THE TESTIS, PROSTATE, AND BREAST IN MEN—(CONTINUED)

	Testis	Prostate	Breast
Sexual activity and fertility	No primary relationship yet established (13).	Increased history of venereal disease and number of premarital and extramarital sexual partners, increased coital frequency. Studies have suggested enhanced rather than defective fertility (13, 20).	No relationship identified.
Benign precursor lesions	Gonadal dysgenesis—as in the female, more commonly associated with seminoma (dysgerminoma) or gonadoblastoma (57, 58).	Although some investigators have suggested that 43 per cent of prostatic cancer may be attributed to benign prostatic hypertrophy, a historical cohort study failed to demonstrate relationship with clinically diagnosed, invasive cancer (59–61).	No indication that gynecomastia is precancerous condition (62).
Other factors	? Inguinal hernia (80). ? Trauma—physical, sustained heat injury (63, 64). ? Prenatal estrogen administration (65). ? Congenital anomalies of genitourinary tract (66, 67).	Positive correlation between prostate cancer mortality and consumption of dietary fat, and with international variation in colon and rectum and breast cancer (women) mortality (26). Positive correlation with suspended particulate air pollutants. Herpes simplex type 2 and cytomegalovirus isolation studies have been inconclusive (68, 69).	Radiation to chest reported in several instances (41).

tenfeld et al. investigated the relationship, if any, between prenatal diethylstilbestrol (DES) exposure and testicular cancer because of a history of such exposure in several young patients with a diagnosis of testicular cancer. Review was made of data on 228 patients seen in 1965–1977 with testicular cancer. All were white and born in the United States between 1950 and 1965. A total of 193 questionnaires have been completed. Both neighborhood control subjects and hospital cases of lymphoma were used for comparison.

An undescended testis was present at birth in 11.6% of cases, 3.6% of hospital control subjects, and 4.9% of neighborhood control subjects. The risk ratio for the hospital control comparison was significant. Cancer occurred on the same side as the maldescent in 15 of 20 evaluable cases; 1 patient had bilateral cryptorchidism. Embryonal carcinoma was present alone in 5 cases and as a mixture of cell types in 14 patients with cryptorchidism. Two patients had teratocarcinoma, and 1 had seminoma. The mean age at diagnosis of testicular cancer in patients with cryptorchidism was 20 years. The use of DES and other hormones in pregnancy was higher in the mothers of patients than in the control groups, but the differences were not significant. Only 1 case of maldescent was associated with maternal use of DES.

This study failed to show that prenatal hormone exposure increases the risk of testicular cancer to a moderate or marked degree. Further study is needed to assess the potential role of oral contraceptives, which were prescribed commonly after 1960.

▶ [Testicular cancers of germ cell origin account for at least 95% of malignant neoplasms of the testis in adult men. Age-specific and age-adjusted United States mortality rates per 100,000 white male subjects for testicular cancer during the period 1936 to 1976 indicates some changing trends within specific age groups. The mortality rate for testicular cancer has shown significant increases in males aged 15–19 years (0.3 in 1936 to 0.6 in 1976), 20–24 years (1.0 to 1.6), and 25–29 years (1.3 to 1.9). After age 60, the mortality for testicular cancer shows significant declines. The group aged 15–29 years could have been exposed to DES in utero, hence the attempts of the authors in this study to show an association. The association is not present, and male offspring of DES mothers should not be alarmed by the possibility of an increased risk of testicular cancer. Also, it is important to note that in Denmark, where the rising trend to this young age group has been even more impressive with regard to testicular cancer mortality, DES use was at a minimum.

Mebust (*Cancer Control for the Professional* 8:17, 1981) provides an update on carcinoma of the testis. Some 2,500 new cases of testicular carcinoma are discovered in the United States annually. The socioeconomic impact of testicular carcinoma has been devastating because of its predilection for young men and because of its poor prognosis. In the past 10 years, significant advances in diagnosis, staging, and therapy have improved survival. Lymph node dissection has been demonstrated to be effective in controlling nonseminomatous germinal cell tumors. A 5-year survival rate after retroperitoneal node dissection is estimated at 65%, in contrast to the 5-year survival rate of 13.5% after radiation therapy. In seminomatous tumors, radiation therapy continues to be the primary means of controlling retroperitoneal metastasis. Two thousand to 3,000 rad to the retroperitoneum results in a 5-year survival of 90% to 95%. In patients with pulmonary metastasis, radiation therapy is still appropriate but the survival rate declines to 30% to 50%. Multidrug chemotherapy in conjunction with aggressive surgery provided the most significant therapeutic approach. Multidrug therapy increases survival time, and recent reports suggest we are approaching a

100% response rate using various combinations of therapeutic drugs. In summary, the prognosis in patients treated with an aggressive approach has been improved dramatically within the past 10 years.—C.E.D.] ◄

Testis Cancer Incidence: Suggestion of a World Pattern. Cancer of the testis may indicate risks to the genome besides that of malignant disease. Following detailed analyses of a pronounced increase in Denmark and its possible causes, Johannes Clemmesen (Copenhagen) studied the international distribution of the disease. Because changes in morbidity and international differences are largely determined by rates for younger men, he reviewed morbidity data for the three consecutive 5-year age groups from 25 to 39 years from a number of countries and regions with cancer registries, mainly based on the tables of "Cancer Incidence in Five Continents" (International Union Against Cancer 1966, World Health Organization IARC 1976).

Minimal incidence was reported from the small cancer registries for African Bantus, rural as well as urban. Low rates were found for American Negroes, Singapore Chinese, Malay, Israeli-born Jews, Jews born in Africa and Asia, and people in Bombay, Sao Paolo, Quebec, and Finland, increasing in approximately that order. Moderate

SELECTED TESTIS CANCER MORBIDITY RATES (UICC 1960, 1970; WHO IARC 1976)

Location	Year	Number of cases	Male population (× 100 000)	25–29 years	30–34 years	35–39 years	All ages
				\multicolumn{4}{c}{Morbidity rates per million male population}			
Bantu negroes							
Johannesburg	1953–55	2	2.6	0	0	0	3
Kyadondo	1954–60	1	1.2	0	0	0	1
Bulawayo	1968–72	0	1.1	0	0	0	0
Detroit, negroes	1969–71	8	3.6	28	0	36	7
Singapore							
Chinese	1968–72	32	7.8	0	8	29	8
Malay	1968–72	2	1.5	0	0	26	3
Bombay	1968–72	103	32.3	7	14	8	6
Japan							
Osaka	1970–71	56	38.2	6	15	17	7
Miyagi	1968–71	27	8.8	0	22	11	8
Sao Paolo	1969	32	27.9	28	18	31	11
Quebec	1969–72	173	29.9	24	32	37	14
Israeli Jews							
Native	1967–71	15	5.6	30	20	17	5
Africa-Asia born	1967–71	19	3.3	16	12	31	11
US-Europe born	1967–71	47	3.5	68	106	46	27

Int. J. Androl. (Suppl. 4):111–122, March 1981.

Finland	1966–70	132	22.5	22	26	24	12
Sweden	1959–61	290	37.3	44	70	55	26
	1966–70	535	39.5	60	57	59	27
England							
Birmingham	1960–62	152	23.5	59	32	45	22
	1968–72	351	25.3	76	71	54	28
South Metropolitan	1960–62	292	38.8	57	79	40	25
	1967–71	650	41.9	70	77	70	31
Manitoba, Canada	1969–72	57	4.9	73	54	112	29
USA							
Upstate, New York	1959–61	277	44.0	41	63	42	21
	1969–71	322	50.4	64	43	52	21
Connecticut	1960–62	93	12.7	66	46	89	24
	1968–72	203	14.7	63	66	40	28
Alameda, Calif.	1960–64	60	3.9	83	59	68	31
	1969–73	100	4.2	73	136	85	48
New Zealand							
Europeans	1962–66	183	12.1	93	84	56	33
	1968–71	182	12.9	83	88	104	35
Maori	1962–66	15	0.95	89	106	87	31
	1968–71	17	1.1	103	75	135	38
Norway	1959–61	186	17.9	66	108	85	35
	1972–76	425	19.9	102	83	105	43
Hamburg	1963–66	133	8.5	40	102	59	39
	1969–72	177	8.4	117	136	124	53
Denmark	1943–47	342	22.0	73	69	66	34
	1968–72	739	24.5	107	160	182	61

rates were reported for Israeli Jews born in Europe or the United States, non-French (non-Catholic?) Canadians, and people in Sweden and New York State, exclusive of New York City.

The United Kingdom had similar results from all its registries, and might perhaps be included in the moderate group. However, morbidity rates rose from 1960 to 1972, and age-adjusted mortality rates show a rise from 5.9 per million in 1911–1914 to 15.2 in 1967. Therefore, English data may be logically included with the high-risk groups showing a rate increase, such as those found in Connecticut, Alameda County, California, New Zealand (Europeans and Maori), Norway, Hamburg, and Denmark.

Earlier studies, most hampered by small numbers, suggest higher rates for professionals than for lower socioeconomic groups and for Protestants than for Catholics. Conflicting observations from Denmark and Norway on urban and rural morbidity have now been reconciled by mounting rates in both areas.

The findings, whose main features are shown in the table, indicate a long-term increase in morbidity from testis cancer in the industrialized world. The increase varies in pace, as illustrated by the data from upstate New York and Alameda County, California. It seems to have reached its peak in Denmark, Hamburg, and Norway and is becoming apparent in England, whereas Finland shows no increase. The increase will facilitate analysis of possible causes.

The steep increase with age beginning at puberty may well be due to the proliferative qualities of cells attained at that age. However, the possibility that prenatal causative factors are involved deserves analysis, as suggested by data from Israel.

▶ [Different trends in incidence of testis cancer now seem discernible, which conforms with the observations for England reported by Joan Davies (*Lancet* 1:928–931, 1981).—R.L.C.] ◀

Ewing's Sarcoma: Ten-Year Experience With Adjuvant Chemotherapy. Gerald Rosen, Brenda Caparros, Anita Nirenberg, Ralph C. Marcove, Andrew G. Huvos, Cynthia Kosloff, Joseph Lane, and M. Lois Murphy (Meml. Sloan-Kettering Cancer Center, New York, N.Y.) describe their experience during the past decade using three different adjuvant chemotherapy protocols for the treatment of primary Ewing's sarcoma. During the first 5 years, success in increasing the disease-free survival of patients with Ewing's sarcoma was attributed to the use of Adriamycin in the T-2 chemotherapy protocol. In 1975, when it was evident that the total dose of Adriamycin received by children would have to be limited to 500 mg/sq m or less, combination chemotherapy was instituted with cyclophosphamide, Adriamycin, methotrexate, and vincristine, alternating with bleomycin, cyclophosphamide, and dactinomycin. Bio-chloroethyl nitrosourea (BCNU) in combination with cyclophosphamide was also used. Although this regimen appeared to be effective in reducing the bulk of the primary tumor prior to surgery or radiation therapy, it called for 5 consecutive days of chemotherapy in most of the cycles, and prolonged delays in the resumption of chemotherapy were attributed to the use of BCNU. The protocol was subsequently revised over the next 5 years to yield 2 days of intensive combination chemotherapy approximately every 3 weeks (Fig 16).

Patients with extremity lesions had local therapy delayed until the completion of 2 cycles of chemotherapy to reduce the bulk of the primary tumor or to allow pathologically eroded bones to heal before megavoltage radiation therapy is started. The major toxicity of the current protocol included fever and neutropenia, requiring hospitalization, that occurred in approximately one third of the patients. By careful monitoring of the patients' blood counts, keeping the hemoglobin above 10 gm/dl, and admitting any patient to the hospital who had fever and an absolute neutrophil count below 1000/cu mm, there have been no drug-related deaths or severe toxicity. The current combination chemotherapy regimen appears to be extremely effective in rapidly reducing the bulk of disease in primary tumors, and has allowed the delay of radiation therapy to axial tumors until 3 or 4 cy-

Cancer 47:2204–2213, May 1, 1981.

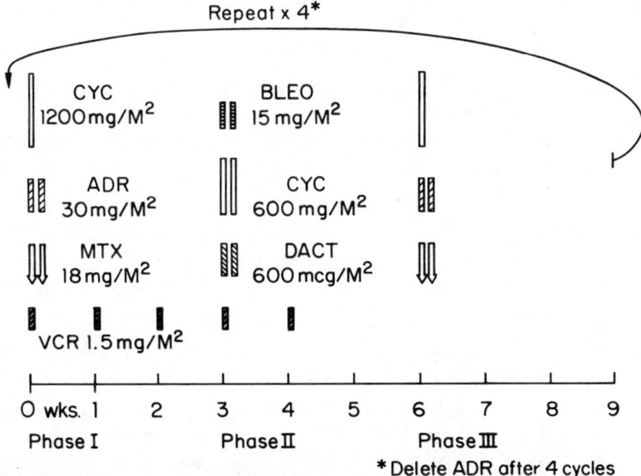

Fig 16.—The current combination chemotherapy protocol used for patients with Ewing's sarcoma and other small cell sarcomas. Careful monitoring of the patient's blood cell count 1 week after each course of chemotherapy and then every other day until the white blood cell count and platelet count have passed through their nadir has prevented severe or life-threatening toxicity among patients undergoing this aggressive chemotherapy protocol. (Courtesy of G. Rosen.)

Fig 17.—The disease-free survival of 66 patients with primary Ewing's sarcoma according to the location of the primary tumor. All patients received, in addition to local therapy, adjuvant chemotherapy with one of the three Adriamycin-containing regimens used at the Memorial Sloan-Kettering Cancer Center over the past 10 years. (Courtesy of Rosen, G., et al.: Cancer 47:2204–2213, May 1, 1981.)

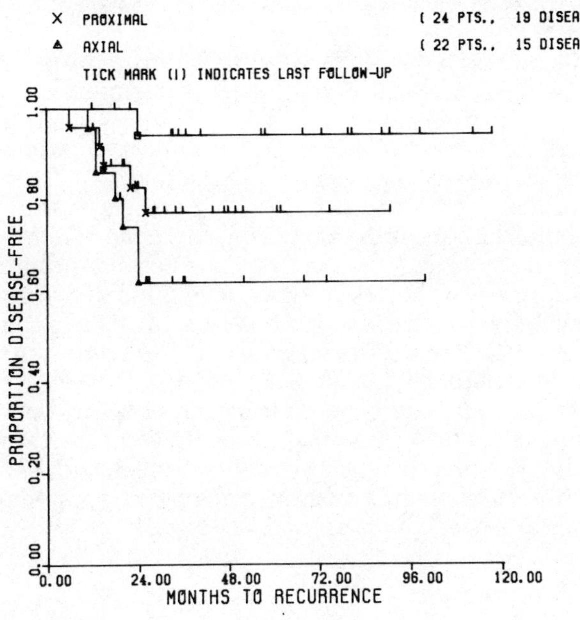

cles of chemotherapy can be administered, thereby increasing patients' tolerance for chemotherapy and requiring fewer drug dosage reductions.

Figure 17 shows the overall disease-free survivals obtained in 66 patients according to the site of the primary tumor. Of note, the only patient to relapse with a distal extremity lesion was a patient who had a local recurrence at the site of the primary tumor after administration of radiation therapy. The higher percentage of patients with pelvic or axial tumors who are disease-free survivors is attributed to the use of surgical resection of the primary tumor following preoperative chemotherapy. A major problem in the treatment of Ewing's sarcoma is still the local recurrence of primary tumors after treatment with radiation therapy. The expected local recurrence rate after radiation therapy is in the vicinity of 20% to 30%, even with the addition of aggressive combination chemotherapy and full-dose megavoltage radiation therapy. This failure rate exceeds the overall failure rate of approximately 20% with combination chemotherapy and local treatment for Ewing's sarcoma. Aggressive combination chemotherapy is extremely effective in the treatment of primary Ewing's sarcoma, and the addition of surgical resection for the primary tumor has given a disease-free survival rate of approximately 85%.

▶ [This study coordinates the results of a 10-year experience in 67 consecutive patients with primary (nonmetastatic) Ewing's sarcoma treated with adjuvant chemotherapy and radiation therapy or surgery to the primary tumor. Of significance is the incidence of local recurrence of approximately 20% and an overall disease-free survival of 76% in patients treated with radiation therapy and 85% surgery. The article emphasizes that chemotherapy should receive increasing recognition as an essential component of treatment of the primary tumor. It may cause reduction in tumor size and allow the pathologically eroding bone to heal before initiation of radiation therapy.—R.L.C.] ◀

Bone Sarcoma as a Second Malignant Neoplasm in Children: Influence of Radiation and Genetic Predisposition. Anna T. Meadows, Louise C. Strong, Frederick P. Li, Giulio J. D'Angio, Odile Schweisguth, Arnold I. Freeman, R. D. T. Jenkin, Patricia Morris-Jones, and Mark E. Nesbit, for the Late Effects Study Group report that as more children are surviving for long periods after the diagnosis and treatment of cancer in early life, attention is being drawn to a complication of cure. These survivors have second malignant neoplasms (SMN) at rates higher than age-specific incidence rates indicate they should. Important questions have been raised about the relationship between aggressive therapy (drugs and radiation) and the predisposition to develop SMN.

The Late Effects Study Group, a consortium of 13 pediatric oncologic centers, obtained information on 188 persons whose first cancers occurred in childhood and who subsequently developed SMN. Bone sarcomas were the most frequent SMN, with 34 new osteogenic sarcomas and 6 chondrosarcomas arising in the study group. Radiation

Cancer 46:2603–2606, Dec. 15, 1980.

therapy, genetic susceptibility, or both played a role in all but one of these cancers; chemotherapy with 2 alkylating agents may have been responsible for the development of an osteosarcoma outside of an irradiated field in a patient who had relapsed Hodgkin's disease. Conspicuous in this group of 40 patients were 16 patients who had bilateral retinoblastoma, a disease now believed to occur as a result of a germinal mutation (Knudson's hypothesis). Of these 16 patients, 11 developed tumors of the facial bones 3 to 14 years after irradiation, and 5 developed sarcomas of long bones without irradiation 12 to 16 years later. Seven other persons were judged to carry a predisposition to cancer because of family history (5 patients), neurofibromatosis (1 patient), or hemihypertrophy (1 patient).

Ages at diagnosis of bone sarcoma and intervals between first and second neoplasms were compared for patients with or without prior irradiation and with or without predisposing conditions. Although patients with inherited conditions had their first neoplasms diagnosed at younger ages than the other patients did (2 years vs. 8 years), only those who subsequently received radiation treatments developed bone sarcomas in the first decade of life. These patients had a significantly shorter latent period (7 years) than those with genetic disease who had not been irradiated (13 years). This observation is consistent with a two-mutation hypothesis stating that persons who inherit a tumor predisposition are further along in the neoplastic development process than those without the diathesis are. In this case, radiation, by providing the second event, shortens the time to SMN development.

Children without genetic disease who were irradiated before the age of 5 years differed from those irradiated after 8 years of age by taking longer (12 years vs. 8 years) to develop bone sarcomas. In both groups, however, bone tumors appeared during the usual second and early third decades of life. Exposure to radiation or any mutagenic event occurring at the time of increased cell division may hasten neoplastic development because it provides an additional event in cells already at greater risk for sustaining spontaneous mutations.

The study of SMN in children continues to provide clues to carcinogenic mechanisms and, in particular, to the role of heredity and therapeutic agents in the etiology of neoplasia.

▶ [This is the first attempt to document the incidence of bone sarcoma as a second malignant neoplasm in children. The authors emphasize the importance of radiation and genetic predisposition. The article may serve as a base for future investigations to determine the relationship of genetic and environmental mutagens in the etiology of primary and secondary childhood neoplasia.—R.L.C.] ◀

Current Concepts Review: Surgical Staging of Musculoskeletal Sarcoma. William F. Enneking, Suzanne S. Spanier, and Mark A. Goodman (Gainesville, Fla.) report that recent advances in diagnostic radiology, chemotherapy, radiotherapy, and reconstructive surgery have encouraged a proliferation of protocols for managing musculoskeletal sarcoma. These protocols often use adjunctive

J. Bone Joint Surg. [Am.] 62–A:1027–1030, September 1980.

chemotherapy or irradiation and, although their long-term effectiveness is unknown, offer alternatives to amputation. If sufficient data are to be accumulated for timely evaluation of clinical trials in these rare neoplasms, interinstitutional cooperation is essential. An urgent need for standard terminology defining surgical stage and surgical procedures exists.

A surgical staging system for musculoskeletal sarcoma should: (1) incorporate the most significant prognostic factors describing progressive degrees of risk, (2) define progressive stages of disease having specific implications for surgical management, (3) furnish guidelines for using adjunctive therapies, and (4) facilitate interinstitutional and interdisciplinary cooperation and data comparison.

The usual determinant of a desired surgical margin for definitive surgical treatment of a musculoskeletal sarcoma is whether the lesion tends to recur locally but has little risk of metastasis (low grade) or is an aggressive lesion with significant tendency to both local recurrence and metastasis (high grade). How a particular surgical margin is accomplished is influenced by the anatomical setting.

The three stages that relate stage of disease to surgical procedure selection and adjunctive measures are: stage I—low-grade lesions, without metastases, of any histogenesis, well to moderately differentiated, and having low mitotic rates; stage II—high-grade lesions, without metastases, of any histogenesis, poorly differentiated, and having high mitotic rates, necrosis, and vascular invasion; stage III—stage I or II lesions with regional or distant metastases.

Stages are stratified by the intracompartmental (A) or extracompartmental (B) anatomical setting of the lesion. Intracompartmental (A) lesions are confined within well-defined anatomical structures: bone, joint, or fascially defined functional muscle group compartments. Extracompartmental (B) lesions either arise or secondarily extend into extrafascial spaces or planes having no natural anatomical barriers to extension, or into another compartment. Pathologic or surgical examination of lesions has confirmed that the anatomic setting may be reliably assessed preoperatively by relevant history, physical examination, and radiographic studies.

The staging system is summarized as follows: IA—low-grade intracompartmental, IB—low-grade extracompartmental, IIA—high-grade intracompartmental, IIB—high-grade extracompartmental, and III—either grade, any anatomical setting, regional or distant metastases.

The ease with which others might use this system was assessed in a retrospective study involving the Musculoskeletal Tumor Society, whose members contributed records of 397 patients analyzed for probability of survival as a function of stage (Fig 18).

The probability of patient survival at each stage each year is different ($P < 0.01$). Stage IA and IB lesions are not statistically different, but the difference in their surgical management justifies separation.

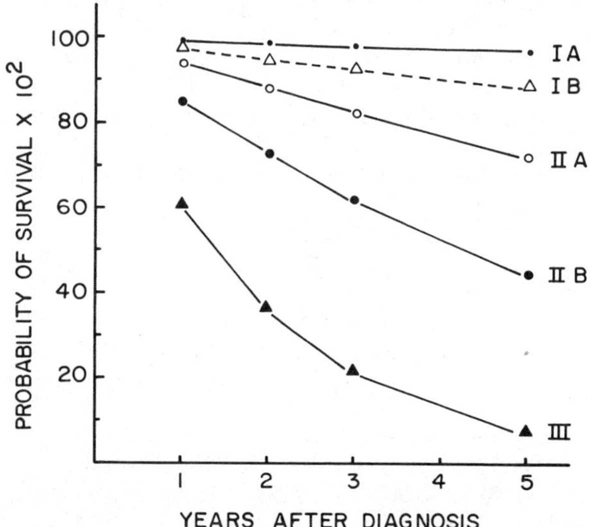

Fig 18.—The probability of survival as a function of surgical stage for 397 patients with soft tissue and bone sarcoma as a function of surgical stage. (Courtesy of W. F. Enneking.)

Stages IIA and IIB are different ($P < 0.01$). Data for bone and soft parts sarcomas analyzed separately indicate that the system works for both.

The system clearly separates patients into low- and high-risk populations. Patients with stage I lesions have low local recurrence and metastatic rates; those with stage II lesions have higher local recurrence rates and substantially higher metastatic rates. Because surgical treatment and the need for adjunctive therapy are different, the stages should be analyzed separately for evaluation of treatments.

Surgical planning is made easier by the description of progressive stages of disease having specific surgical implications. Previous work has shown that if the surgical procedure is to be definitive, a wide margin is required for stage I lesions, and a radical margin is required for stage II lesions. When a lesser margin is achieved, local recurrence rates increase substantially, and adjunctive therapies to suppress local recurrence may be indicated. For intracompartmental (A) lesions of either stage, a wide or radical margin can often be accomplished by a local procedure. Extracompartmental (B) lesions of either stage often require an ablative procedure to secure either a wide or radical margin.

▶ [One of the great advances in oncology has been functional clinical staging systems. Enneking proposes a clinically oriented system equally applicable in bone and soft tissue sarcomas of the extremities. The American Joint Committee on Cancer's staging system is a usable system once the specimen has reached the pathologist's laboratory, but this is little help to the clinician in staging and evaluating the patient's disease preoperatively.—R.L.C.] ◀

Osteofibrous Dysplasia of the Tibia and Fibula. M. Campanacci and M. Laus (Istituto Ortopedico Rizzoli, Bologna, Italy) explain that osteofibrous dysplasia of the tibia and fibula is not a well-recognized entity. The authors have seen 35 patients with the disease, 31 of whom had histologic documentation. Twenty-two comparable cases have been reported in the literature, with such diagnoses as ossifying fibroma, congenital fibrous dysplasia, and congenital fibrous defect of the tibia. The main differential diagnosis is with fibrous dysplasia and with adamantinoma of a long bone.

Twelve of the patients in this study had long-term follow-up, ranging from 5 to 20 years (average, 10 years), and some of the lesions regressed spontaneously. Osteofibrous dysplasia seldom has even a moderate tendency to progress during childhood, but it does recur frequently after curettage or subperiosteal resection. Such recurrences generally are moderately progressive or not progressive at all. Any progression of the lesion comes to an end after puberty.

Attempts at radical surgery either for the primary disease or after recurrence do not seem to be necessary. Surgery should be delayed as long as possible and should be restricted to patients who have extensive lesions. In the authors' opinion, marginal subperiosteal excision should not be attempted in patients younger than age 15 years because the lesion will likely recur. In many cases, biopsy appears unnecessary, because clinically and radiographically the lesion is so typical that the physician can be reasonably confident about the diagnosis. The occasional pathologic fracture may be treated by plaster-cast immobilization. The authors have not seen any patients with multiple fractures, and therefore doubt that surgery is ever mandatory before age 15. If a patient has repeated fractures, or if the lesion is rapidly progressive, it would be necessary to resort to wide extraperiosteal resection and massive grafting. Marginal excision is likely to be successful in patients who are older than age 15 years; however, it should not be necessary to treat the lesion then because it often is asymptomatic. The results of surgical treatment usually are good even in patients who have a recurrence, fracture, or pseudarthrosis.

▶ [The benign entity described here, also called "ossifying fibroma," has been recognized only within the past several years. The intracortical localization, osteoblastic rimming of the bone, and the fact that this lesion may regress spontaneously differentiate it from fibrous dysplasia.—R.L.C.] ◀

Radiation Therapy in the Treatment of Aggressive Fibromatoses. Harvey M. Greenberg, Robert Goebel, Ralph R. Weichselbaum, Joel S. Greenberger, John T. Chaffey, and J. Robert Cassady (Harvard Med. School, Boston) review their experience with 12 patients who had aggressive but histologically benign connective tissue tumors (9 desmoids and 3 neurofibromas) and were treated with either radiation or radiation plus surgery. Treatment planning emphasized normal tissue sparing and included individually shaped lead alloy

J. Bone Joint Surg. [Am.] 63–A:367–375, March 1981.
Int. J. Radiat. Oncol. Biol. Phys. 7:305–310, March 1981.

blocks, subcutaneous and lymphatic strip sparing in extremity lesions, extensive use of oblique and rotational fields, and a shrinking field technique in appropriate cases. Treatment breaks were initiated to alleviate either abdominal symptoms or skin reactions to therapy. Those patients who had appendicular desmoids were treated with varying fraction sizes ranging from 140 to 250 rad per day, while those with abdominal desmoids were treated with from 150 to 180 rad per day.

Long-term local control was accomplished in 8 of 9 patients with desmoid tumors and 2 of 3 with neurofibromas. In the successfully treated patients, local control was obtained with minimal long-term complications when compared with radical surgical procedures that would have been necessary for cure.

The data presented here, in conjunction with earlier published reports, suggest that megavoltage irradiation is effective in treating bulky, locally recurrent tumors and should be used in patients in whom resection is either not feasible or is disfiguring, or in those in whom the likelihood of recurrence is high. However, the relative roles of radiation and surgery need to be more clearly defined. When delivered in appropriately high dose, radiation appears capable of controlling even bulky tumors for long periods of time. In those patients in whom gross surgical removal of tumor can be achieved, but with close margins, postoperative treatment should be given, especially in those cases where local recurrence would threaten neural or vascular structures.

▶ [These lesions often grow so slowly that the 14 months indicated in this study is minimum follow-up, and even a mean of 36 months is a bit on the short side for recurrence of these tumors. Also, despite the fact that gross tumor is left behind, it sometimes does not progress over a period of time and may well become static.

The patient may develop different lesions at different sites. A biopsy specimen should be taken from each site.—R.L.C.] ◀

Malignant Melanoma in Children and Adolescents. Charles B. Pratt, Michael K. Palmer, Nicholas Thatcher, and Derek Crowther (Manchester, England) reviewed experience with 31 patients, under age 21, admitted between 1945 and 1977 for treatment of malignant melanoma. The 21 girls and 10 boys had a median age of 14 years; 16 were under age 13 at diagnosis. Fourteen patients had head and neck lesions, including 2 with choroid melanoma; 9 had trunk and 8 had extremity lesions. Twenty-five patients had clinical stage I disease at diagnosis. Four had regional node involvement and 2 had generalized melanoma. No patient had a family history of melanoma. Twelve patients had had lesions since birth.

Surgery was the primary treatment for all patients. Four patients received radiotherapy as part of initial treatment, and 4 were irradiated for painful or disfiguring metastases. Only 2 patients received chemotherapy or chemoimmunotherapy. Fifteen patients are free from apparent disease after 2 to 18 years. Overall median survival

Cancer 47:392–397, Jan. 15, 1981.

was about 8 years, but median disease-free interval was only 20 months. Stage had a highly significant influence on outcome, but survival was unrelated to anatomical site of the primary lesion or age at diagnosis. No significant trend in survival was apparent over the period of review. The extent of initial surgery did not significantly affect survival.

Half the patients in this series of children with malignant melanoma died. Multiple-agent chemotherapy may hold promise for the treatment of both adults and children with metastatic melanoma. The clinical features and level of skin infiltration must be defined in individual cases to relate the expected prognosis to the planning of definitive surgery.

Bowenoid Papules of the Penis. The designation "bowenoid papulosis" represents the histologic finding of intraepithelial carcinoma of the penis presenting clinically as benign-appearing papules.

Margot S. Peters and Harold O. Perry (Mayo Clinic and Found.) describe a case of multiple bowenoid papules of the penile shaft. A biopsy specimen of one papule showed the typical histologic pattern of squamous cell carcinoma in situ. Clinical examination showed multiple 3- to 4-mm red-brown, slightly shiny papules covered with a fine scale located on the anterior aspect of the penile shaft (Fig 19).

Because of the diverse clinical appearance of bowenoid papulosis and the morphological resemblance to such conditions as lichen planus, psoriasis, condyloma acuminatum, verrucous seborrheic keratoses, and pigmented nevi, the possibility of squamous cell carci-

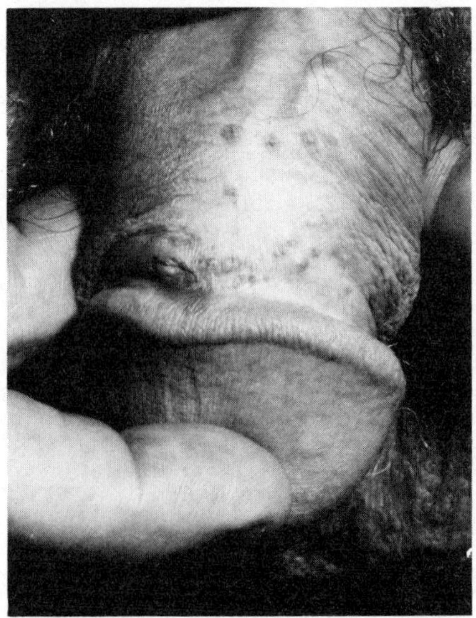

Fig 19.—Discrete, relatively uniform, grouped and isolated papules on penile shaft. (Courtesy of Peters, M. S., and Perry, H. O.: J. Urol. 126:482–484, October 1981.)

J. Urol. 126:482–484, October 1981.

noma in situ emphasizes the need for histologic examination of such lesions. The age of the patient, location of the lesion, and circumcision are factors that may modify the clinical expression of this condition. Bowenoid papulosis, pigmented penile papules with changes of carcinoma in situ, multicentric pigmented Bowen's disease, erythroplasia of Queyrat, and Bowen's disease are all current designations of different clinical expressions of intraepithelial carcinoma of the penis with the histologic pattern of squamous cell carcinoma in situ.

The risk of primary internal malignant disease developing in patients with intraepithelial carcinoma of the penis may or may not be significantly increased. Of those reported cases of penile or vulvar carcinoma in situ associated with internal malignant disease, most involve the prostate, bladder, or rectum. Carcinoma in situ of the penis has been found in or associated with genital warts. Electron microscopic studies have been negative for virus in many cases of bowenoid papulosis. However, a recent study did demonstrate viral particles in such lesions.

The natural history and prognosis of bowenoid papulosis have not yet been defined; individual case reports have illustrated different types of biologic behavior. Bowenoid papules have the potential for regression, persistence, or recurrence. Because invasive and metastatic squamous cell carcinomas have developed from lesions of Bowen's disease or erythroplasia of Queyrat, caution should be exercised with respect to bowenoid papulosis of the penis; its potential for progression to invasive carcinoma is unknown. On this basis, patients should be treated as having carcinoma in situ. Modalities suggested include simple excision, cryosurgery, and 5-fluorouracil therapy. Shave excision followed by curettage-electrodesiccation has also been recommended.

▶ [Bowenoid papulosis, which usually occurs on the shaft of the penis, has also been reported in the groin and axillae and on the labia and breasts of women. Although histologically similar to erythroplasia of Queyrat, the two conditions usually can be readily differentiated clinically. Lesions of bowenoid papulosis typically present as asymptomatic, multiple, approximately 4-mm papules on the shaft of the penis. Patients are usually young (average age, younger than 30 years) and almost all have been circumcised in infancy. The solitary lesions of erythroplasia of Queyrat, which commonly measure 10 mm in diameter or greater, occur in older persons and are often associated with pain or pruritus. The condition is not seen in persons circumcised in infancy. Many patients with bowenoid papulosis have been treated previously for a viral genital eruption, either herpes progenitalis or condyloma acuminata. Lesions of bowenoid papulosis may be clinically indistinguishable from condyloma. Many patients with a history of herpes progenitalis have received photoinactivation therapy, a procedure thought to increase oncogenic potential. Virus-like particles have been reported in bowenoid papulosis, but seem to be larger than the herpes virus. Kaufman et al. (*N. Engl. J. Med.* 305:483, 1981) recently reported the occurrence of herpesvirus-induced antigens in squamous cell carcinoma in situ of the vulva. Careful reading of the article indicates that most of their patients were, in fact, suffering from bowenoid papulosis rather than true preinvasive squamous cell carcinoma. Recognition of bowenoid papulosis as a distinct entity is necessary to avoid subjecting these patients to unnecessary radical surgery. The biologic potential of such lesions, if left untreated, remains unknown.—R.L.D.] ◀

Herpesvirus-Induced Antigens in Squamous Cell Carcinoma In Situ of the Vulva. Raymond H. Kaufman, Gordon R. Dreesman, Joyce Burek, Matti O. Korhonen, David O. Matson, Joseph L. Melnick, Kenneth L. Powell, Dorothy J. M. Purifoy, Richard J. Courtney, and Ervin Adam (The Univ. of Texas M. D. Anderson Hosp. and Tumor Inst. at Houston) note that squamous cell carcinoma in situ of the vulva is appearing with increasing frequency, particularly in women under 40 years old. It has been suggested that common pathogenic factors, possibly viral, may be associated with carcinogenesis of the vulva, cervix, and vagina, and a temporal relation between this disease and genital herpesvirus (HSVE2) infection has been noted. Recently, the authors detected an HSV2-specific DNA-binding protein in 38% of human tissues with histopathologic features of severe dysplasia or carcinoma of the cervix. In this report, they identified HSV2 DNA-binding proteins in biopsy samples from patients with carcinoma in situ of the vulva.

Tissue and serum specimens were collected from the vulvas of 19 patients. In 9 patients the biopsy revealed squamous cell carcinoma in situ; in 1 instance the biopsy revealed severe dysplasia. In another patient, a previous biopsy had revealed squamous cell carcinoma in situ, and the later biopsy revealed mild dysplasia. Four patients with condyloma acuminatum and 4 patients seen for periodic checkups had biopsy specimens taken from normal tissue and were included as controls. Sections were cut for staining with hematoxylin and eosin, and adjacent sections were cut for immunologic staining. The latter sections were stained by indirect immunoperoxidase and indirect immunofluorescence methods. The primary serums used in the staining procedures included anti-HSV2, a rabbit antiserum prepared by immunization with purified HSV2 that had been grown in rabbit kidney cells; anti-ICSP34/45 and anti-ICSP11/12, rabbit antiserums to HSV2-infected cell-specific proteins 34/35 and 11/12, respectively; anti-VP143, a rabbit antiserum to nonstructural HSV2 protein; and a normal rabbit serum obtained from a nonimmunized animal.

Antigens induced by HSV2 were found associated with squamous cell carcinoma in situ of the vulva in 9 of 10 patients. The HSV2-induced antigens are DNA-binding proteins normally present in the nuclei of infected cells, but in the neoplastic cells they were found in the cytoplasm. Whole virion structural antigens were not present, although there was serologic evidence of previous HSV2 infection in patients tested for the presence of antibodies. None of the patients with normal tissue or with condylomata acuminatum demonstrated the presence of the HSV2-induced antigens.

The observations reported here and the recent parallel rise in the prevalence of both HSV2 infections and vulvar carcinoma in situ, particularly in women under 40 years of age, suggest an undetermined association between HSV2 infection and this type of neoplasia.

N. Engl. J. Med. 305:483–488, Aug. 27, 1981.

▶ [For the past decade gynecologists have been concerned about the unexplained increase in the incidence of carcinoma in situ of the vulva, especially among young women. The authors' findings of herpes simplex virus type II in the surgical specimens of 9 of the 10 patients studied with carcinoma in situ of the vulva most likely explain not only the increased rate of this disease but also its etiology: sexual transmission of herpes type II virus.—R.L.C.] ◀

Management of Depression in the Patient With Advanced Cancer. Richard J. Goldberg (Rhode Island Hosp., Providence) points out that as medical therapies continue to lengthen survival time of patients with cancer, quality of survival and the emotional consequences of illness and its treatment become more prominent. Depression in some form is an issue that must be faced by many patients and clinicians dealing with advanced cancer and is the most frequent reason for psychiatric referral in this population. While estimates of the prevalence of depression in patients with advanced cancer vary, depending on the population studied and the criteria used to define depression, moderate to severe depressive symptoms generally occur in approximately 23% of cancer patients.

When confronted by patients with advanced cancer who are depressed, the clinician should not assume that the depression is an unavoidable outcome of the situation. Symptoms suggesting depression in these patients may result from one or more medical aspects of the disease, including metabolic encephalopathies, brain tumors, cerebral metastases, nutritional impairments, and drug effects. Also, depression is virtually impossible to evaluate in a patient with severe ongoing pain. When appropriate and adequate analgesic medication is used to treat pain in patients with advanced cancer, symptoms of depression often resolve spontaneously.

After a review of medical factors that can lead to depression, the next step is to address the major psychosocial issues commonly associated with depression in this group of patients. *Social support* is important in maintaining mental and physical health. Advanced cancer brings with it isolation, a loss of social acceptability, and a sense of abandonment—all of which can be sources of depression in the patient. Whenever possible, the physician should meet with patient and key support together in order to observe their interactions and to help facilitate better sharing and communication. As the disease progresses, there is also risk of alienation between physician and patient. Regular contact and communication of concern is a valuable positive intervention and can be a crucial element in counteracting some of the impersonality involved in the highly technical therapies offered to patients with advanced cancer.

Loss of control is a second factor that may be critical in precipitating depression. The patient should be given appropriate opportunities to exercise some form of control (i.e., choice) over his or her therapy and environment. Sharing information about diagnosis should be considered an important part of allowing the patient to share control.

JAMA 246:373–376, July 24, 1981.

Third, *loss of bodily integrity* or a body part creates grief often characterized by signs and symptoms typical of depression. The physician should not assume that each patient reacts to loss in a predictable way but should ask questions that allow the patient to reveal his or her own private issues. Regardless of whether the issue of dying is brought up directly by the patient, signs of the physician's willingness to discuss this topic are important.

In cases where the symptoms of depression are severe and do not respond to the identification and correction of underlying medical disorders or to addressing emotional and social issues, the adjunctive use of antidepressant medication may be very helpful. Positive clinical effects of tricyclic antidepressants for depression associated with advanced cancer are common, although this topic has not been critically researched yet.

▶ [The New Wave in the nascent subspecialty of oncologic psychiatry is best represented in this clearly written article, which grounds the depressive illness of cancer patients in the neuraxis rather than the imagination. The article's message is well put: Depression in cancer patients is not only an autonomous medical illness, but also a symptom that requires exhaustive differential diagnosis, for it is often secondary to other organic brain disorders.—R.L.C.] ◀

Cancer Prevention as a Realizable Goal. Isaac Berenblum (Weizmann Inst. of Science, Rehovot, Israel) points out that opinions about the scope of cancer prevention in man have changed greatly over the years. It was originally thought of in a very limited sense: avoid contact with specific occupational carcinogens. Subsequently, this was extended to avoidance of all kinds of environmental factors suspected of inducing or facilitating human cancer development. More recently, the possibilities of *interfering* with the carcinogenic process have been studied, as distinct from *eliminating* the causative agents. The aim of the author was to analyze, based on contemporary knowledge of carcinogenesis mechanisms, the ways such interference could operate. A blueprint for more effective cancer prevention in man could thus be developed.

Prevention by interference could theoretically operate at three different levels: (1) during the precarcinogenic stage; (2) during the course of carcinogenic action; and (3) during the postcarcinogenic stage.

Examples of prevention during the *pre*carcinogenic stage include (1) interfering with nitrosamine formation in vivo, e.g., by vitamin C; (2) encouraging metabolic detoxification of precursor carcinogens, rather than allowing their conversion to ultimate carcinogens; and (3) stimulating the body's defenses against carcinogenic action.

Interference *during* carcinogenic action has to be considered separately. In the primary, initiating phase of carcinogenesis, the repair of gene mutations is to be encouraged. In the promoting phase, the process may be blocked at various stages of the long latent period.

Interference during the *post*carcinogenic phase may appear to be a

Cancer 47:2346–2348, May 15, 1981.

contradiction in terms. In fact, early detection of established neoplasia, followed by appropriate therapy, is in a sense prevention, since the condition is prevented from reaching a stage no longer curable.

Of the various postulated methods of interference, that related to the promoting phase undoubtedly holds the best prospects. The current intensive studies of mechanisms of tumor promotion are likely to provide clear leads to rational methods of cancer prevention. These would replace haphazard attempts based on trial and error.

▶ [The author believes 70% to 90% of cancers are influenced by the environment. He proposes directing cancer prevention at three levels and believes that by manipulation of the enzymatic detoxification processes, cancer will be controlled.—R.L.C.] ◀

The Origin of Human Cancers. John Cairns (Imperial Cancer Res. Fund, London) notes that different human populations tend to suffer from different kinds of cancer: the inhabitants of third world countries have an excess of liver cancer, those of Western nations have an excess of cancer of the breast and colon, the Japanese have an excess of stomach cancer, etc. Most of this variation must be due to varied diets, customs, and environment rather than to differences in genetic constitution, because nations have been observed to undergo changes in cancer incidence from one generation to the next and migrant populations tend to take on the pattern of cancer that is characteristic of their new homes. Cancer is therefore thought to be a preventable disease.

In the Western world the two most common cancers are cancer of the skin and the lung, and each of these happens to be so strongly dependent on a single factor (that is, sunlight and smoking, respectively) that their cause could be identified without the need for any understanding of the underlying mechanism of carcinogenesis. The preventable causes of the other common cancers are less clear-cut. Eventually the techniques of nucleic acid chemistry should allow all the differences in nucleotide sequence and gene expression that distinguish a cancer cell from its normal counterpart to be itemized, and perhaps at that point the steps involved in carcinogenesis will cease to be in doubt. But until then, one must be content with circumstantial evidence. This review discusses the evidence and makes certain deductions about the molecular biology of human cancer.

In the last decade, the routes leading to genetic diversity have become much better understood. Diffusion of heritable information is now known to occur not only by "legitimate" recombination between homologous regions of different genomes, but also by "illegitimate" recombination between largely nonhomologous regions (which can be in different parts of the genome or even in different individuals). The second of these processes is equivalent to a chromosomal rearrangement and allows the shuffling of certain modules of information ("transposons") so that new combinations of genes can be tested for

Nature 289:353–357, Jan. 29, 1981.

survival advantage. The process depends on the presence of certain short sequences in the DNA that are the substrates for various recombinational enzymes ("transposases") and it represents a much more drastic form of genetic variation than localized changes in base sequence because it can alter the expression of whole regions of the genome.

The author believes that the steps leading to human cancer are likely to be genetic transpositions. It is therefore important to find out what classes of external agents or features of cellular behavior raise the frequency of such transpositions. Interestingly, conventional mutagens often appear to have no effect. Indeed, it was the inability of any mutagen to raise the spontaneous reversion rate of certain forward mutations in *Escherichia coli* that initially marked out these mutations as being unusual and eventually led to the discovery that they were due to the movement of insertion sequences; similarly, the movement of certain transposable elements in yeast has been found to occur "spontaneously" but does not appear to be strongly catalyzed by any of the common mutagens. However, rates of transposition can be influenced by external factors. For example, transpositions are only a minor cause of mutation in rapidly multiplying bacteria, but they are a major source of forward mutations in stationary cultures; the growth of *Drosophila* cells in vitro leads to the proliferation of certain repetitive sequences; the frequency of the transpositions that produce variegation in *Drosophila* and in *Antirrhinum* petals is inversely related to temperature; and the integration of a tumor virus can be associated with transpositions in the neighboring host DNA. Lastly, many mutagens are known to cause sister chromatid exchanges and other chromosomal interactions in mammalian cells, although it is not always clear to what extent these gross changes are functionally equivalent to genetic transpositions.

The assay of mutagens using bacterial tester strains has been one of the most fruitful practical results of molecular genetics. Its success stems from the fact that the chemistry of DNA is the same for all forms of life and so the chemistry of mutagenesis (and of repair) also tends to be the same. The molecular biology of transposition promises to be more idiosyncratic. However, it is still too early for there to have been much systematic molecular biologic investigation of the factors that trigger transpositions, either in prokaryotes or in eukaryotes. The rate of movement of most transposons will have been subject to evolutionary pressures, and many transposons will therefore have acquired their own individual controls. Thus, it may not be a simple matter to devise a general assay for the factors that drive carcinogenic transpositions.

▶ [The author presents and discusses evidence that suggests that many, possibly most, human cancers are not caused by conventional mutagens but are rather the consequence of gene transposition. He contends that local changes in DNA sequence, produced by conventional mutagens, make only a minor contribution to our national cancer death rate. This is a provocative but, as yet, less than compelling argument.—R.L.C.] ◀

Additional Reading

Bagley, F. H., et al.: Changes in clinical presentation and management of malignant melanoma. *Cancer* 47:2126, 1981.

Batata, M. A., et al.: Testicular cancer in cryptorchids. *Cancer* 49:1023, 1982.

Beitner, H., et al.: Further evidence for increased light sensitivity in patients with malignant melanoma. *Br. J. Dermatol.* 104:289, 1981.

Berek, J. S., et al.: Laparoscopy for second-look evaluation in ovarian cancer. *Obstet. Gynecol.* 58:192, 1981.

Bernstein, I. L., and Sigmundi, R. A.: Tumor anorexia: A learned food aversion? *Science* 209:416, 1980.

Broadbent, V. A., et al.: Medulloblastoma in children: Long-term results of treatment. *Cancer* 48:26, 1981.

Chow, C. W., et al.: Malignant carcinoid tumors in children. *Cancer* 49:802, 1982.

D'Angio, G. J., et al.: Treatment of Wilms' tumor: Results of the second national Wilms' tumor study. *Cancer* 47:2302, 1981.

Feibleman, C. E., et al.: Melanomas of the palm, sole, and nailbed: Clinicopathologic study. *Cancer* 46:2492, 1980.

Graham, S.: Diet and cancer. *Am. J. Epidemiol.* 112:247, 1980.

Lynch, H. T., et al.: The cancer family syndrome: Rare cutaneous phenotypic linkage of Torre's syndrome. *Arch. Intern. Med.* 141:607, 1981.

Melicow, M. M.: Tumors of the testis: In the forefront of oncology—Review and preview. *Urology* 17:54, 1981.

Mora, R. G., and Burris, R.: Cancer of the skin in blacks: Review of 128 patients with basal cell carcinoma. *Cancer* 47:1436, 1981.

Mora, R. G., and Perniciaro, C.: Cancer of the skin in blacks: I. Review of 163 black patients with cutaneous squamous cell carcinoma. *J. Am. Acad. Dermatol.* 5:535, 1981.

Nakayama, H.: Clinical and histologic studies of the classification and the natural course of the strawberry mark. *J. Dermatol. (Tokyo)* 8:277, 1981.

Pendergrass, T. W., and Davis, S.: Incidence of retinoblastoma in the United States. *Arch. Ophthalmol.* 98:1204, 1980.

Pollard, H. H., Chairman, Cancer of the Pancreas Task Force: Staging of Cancer of the pancreas. *Cancer* 47(Suppl.):1631, 1981.

Pratt, C. B., et al.: Malignant melanoma in children and adolescents. *Cancer* 47:392, 1981.

Rickard, K. A., et al.: Effectiveness of enteral and parenteral nutrition in the nutritional management of children with Wilms' tumors. *Am. J. Clin. Nutr.* 33:2622, 1980.

Saemundsen, A. K., et al.: Epstein-Barr virus-carrying lymphoma in a patient with ataxia-telangiectasia. *Br. Med. J.* 282:425, 1981.

Endocrinology, Metabolism and Nutrition

"Dear Dr. Shearin:
Thank you for coming to our school and telling us about the human
body. I thought it was very interesting how the penis grows. I knew
some stuff about the body. Now I know a lot of stuff about it. Thanks
to you.
Your friend John."—(Letter from a 12-year-old biologically mature
male after a human development lecture)

Passing through puberty is exciting and confusing at times for both
doctor and patient. The adolescent is experiencing the changes, and
the doctor is trying to explain all of the biological events. Endocrine
research in this area is still in its infancy. The endocrine and metabolic aspects of adolescent health are still a challenging area in adolescent medicine. The papers offered in this section constitute only
a minimal portion of the voluminous literature that is available
today.

Articles on diabetes are plentiful in this section, either as abstracts
or as references. One of particular interest deals with limited joint
mobility in childhood diabetes mellitus and increased risk for microvascular disease. Rosenbloom et al. attempted to substantiate a relationship between these two factors, and their results strongly suggest
that limited joint mobility is an early sign of microvascular complications in the diabetic patient.

It is difficult indeed to appreciate all of the endocrine and metabolic
aspects of anorexia nervosa. The several articles on anorexia nervosa
in this section indicate the importance of understanding this condition endocrinologically and metabolically. The article on abnormal
gastric emptying in primary anorexia nervosa suggests the presence
of a hypothalamic disorder. The discussion of neurochemical abnormalities in anorexia nervosa by Gwirtsman and Gerner also emphasizes that this condition is a form of hypothalamic disturbance. In the
article on continuous infusion of lutenizing hormone releasing hormone (LHRH) in patients with anorexia nervosa, the authors note
that plasma luteinizing hormone (LH) value and LH response to
LHRH are depressed in patients with anorexia nervosa at low body
weight but increase as weight is regained. All these articles should
be required reading for the clinician working with anorexia nervosa.
Papers discussing psychologic aspects are included under Mental
Health.

Limited Joint Mobility in Childhood Diabetes Mellitus Indicates Increased Risk for Microvascular Disease. Restricted mobility of small and large joints has been observed, along with thick, tight, waxy skin and impaired growth, in adolescents with long-standing diabetes. Arlan L. Rosenbloom, Janet H. Silverstain, Dennis C. Lezotte, Kathryn Richardson, and Martha McCallum (Univ. of Florida, Gainesville) attempted to substantiate a relationship between limited joint mobility and early microvascular complications in a series of 309 diabetics aged 1–28 years. Joint mobility was assessed by the patient attempting to approximate the palmar surfaces of the interphalangeal joints of the hands tightly, with the fingers fanned, as shown in Figure 20.

Limited joint mobility was found in 92 patients (30%). It was not associated with sex, daily insulin dosage, diabetes control, or the most recent hemoglobin A_1 level. One third of the patients with joint limitation had thick, tight, waxy skin that could not be tented. In 5 cases microvascular signs developed at the same time as joint limitation, whereas in the other patients microvascular complications developed after a mean of 2.7 years. The frequency and severity of microvascular complications both increased with the degree of joint limitation after $4^{1}/_{2}$ years of diabetes. The risk of developing microvascular com-

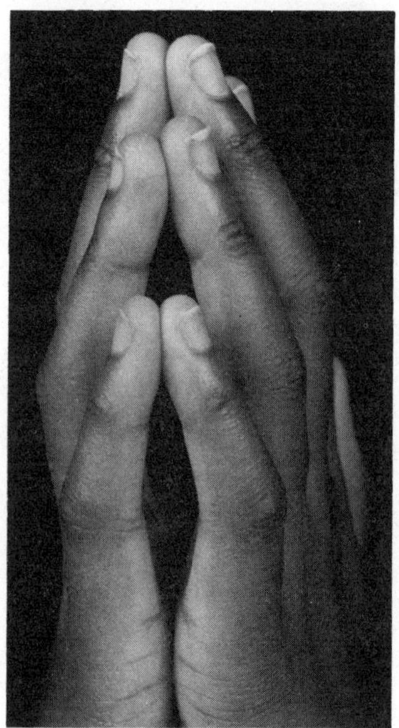

Fig 20.—Attempted approximation of palmar surfaces of proximal and distal interphalangeal joints. Inability to approximate palmar surfaces demonstrates limited mobility of all joints. (Courtesy of Rosenbloom, A. L., et al.: N. Engl. J. Med. 305:191–194, July 23, 1981.)

N. Engl. J. Med. 305:191–194, July 23, 1981.

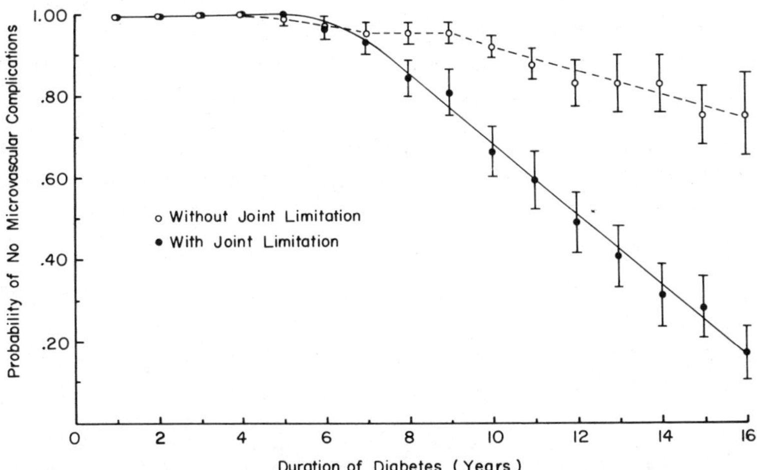

Fig 21.—Life-table analysis of risk for development of microvascular complications. Limits shown are standard errors for each estimate; doubling the standard error of the estimate gives the 95% confidence limits of the estimate. (Courtesy of Rosenbloom, A. L., et al.: N. Engl. J. Med. 305:191–194, July 23, 1981.)

plications is related to both joint limitation and the duration of diabetes in Figure 21.

Limited joint mobility is found in a population of diabetics at particular risk of development of early microvascular complications. Recognition of this relationship will permit the more selective use of newer techniques for long-term physiologic control of diabetes, to determine whether such control can delay or prevent the development of microvascular disease.

► [This is an interesting observation. I would be inclined to believe that the limited joint mobility and tight skin are a result of microvascular disease that has not yet manifested itself in the more usual locations.—W.G.R.] ◄

Physical Symptoms Related to Blood Glucose in Insulin-Dependent Diabetics. Diabetes is an example of a disease state in which physical symptoms do not prompt the patient to take corrective action, and in which neither the patient nor physician can determine which symptoms are indicative of pathologic features. James W. Pennebaker, Daniel J. Cox, Linda Gonder-Frederick, M. G. Wunsch, W. S. Evans, and Stephen Pohl (Univ. of Virginia) carried out a within-subject correlational procedure in which 30 hospitalized insulin-dependent diabetics completed a symptom checklist just before the blood glucose level was measured several times a day for 6–10 days, and simple correlations were computed for each symptom and the blood glucose level. The mean age was 32 years. Eleven patients had adult-onset diabetes. The mean duration of diabetes was 13.7 years. The

Psychosom. Med. 43:489–500, December 1981.

mean blood glucose level during the study was 150.9 mg/dl. The mean level of hemoglobin A_1 at the outset was 10.7.

Most subjects had several symptoms that were closely correlated with glucose fluctuations. The symptoms that correlated with glucose levels differed from one subject to another. Symptom-glucose correlations were reliable and were not related to sex, age, duration of diabetes, or other individual difference variables. Among the symptoms that correlated most closely with blood glucose levels were tremor; light-headedness; dryness of the nose, eyes, or mouth; hunger; a sweet taste; and weakness.

In most insulin-dependent diabetics, certain symptoms are reliably correlated with fluctuations in blood glucose levels. The covarying sensations differ considerably from one patient to another. Studies are under way to determine whether the symptom-blood glucose relationships are consistent over time and setting in larger patient groups, and whether informing patients of their covarying symptoms will improve their ability to estimate their blood glucose levels. The within-subjects paradigm may prove useful in increasing the compliance of diabetics who must constantly monitor their glucose levels.

Colonic Dysfunction in Diabetes Mellitus. Constipation is frequent in diabetes mellitus, but its pathogenesis is poorly understood. William M. Battle, William J. Snape, Jr., Abass Alavi, Sidney Cohen, and Seth Braunstein (Univ. of Pennsylvania) performed myoelectrical and motility studies in diabetics and correlated the findings with peripheral nerve conduction, the rate of gastric emptying, and the clinical features. Studies were performed in 12 patients with insulin-dependent diabetes, aged 25–59 years, and 10 normal subjects aged 21–50 years. The patients had no history of alcoholism or pancreatic disease. All but 1 had clinical evidence of autonomic insufficiency. No patient was acutely ill at the time of study. Colonic myoelectric and motor activities were monitored for 90 minutes after ingestion of a 1,000-calorie meal. Gastric emptying was measured with the use of ^{99m}Tc-sulfur colloid in a test meal.

Diabetics had a lesser spike activity response than normal subjects after the meal. Six severely constipated patients had no postprandial colonic spike response. The pattern of gastrocolonic responses is shown in Figure 22. Gastric emptying of the liquid test meal was reduced in the diabetics, but 3 patients had adequate gastric emptying. Five diabetics had simultaneous abnormalities in gastric emptying and in the colonic spike response. There was no correlation between peripheral nerve conduction velocities and either the colonic spike response or gastric emptying. Neostigmine (0.5 mg, intramuscularly) or metoclopramide (20 mg, intravenously) stimulated colonic spike activity and increased the motility index in both diabetics and normal subjects. Colonic motility increased in diabetics after injection of 20 mg of metoclopramide, but the response to 10 mg was less marked.

Gastroenterology 79:1217–1221, December 1980.

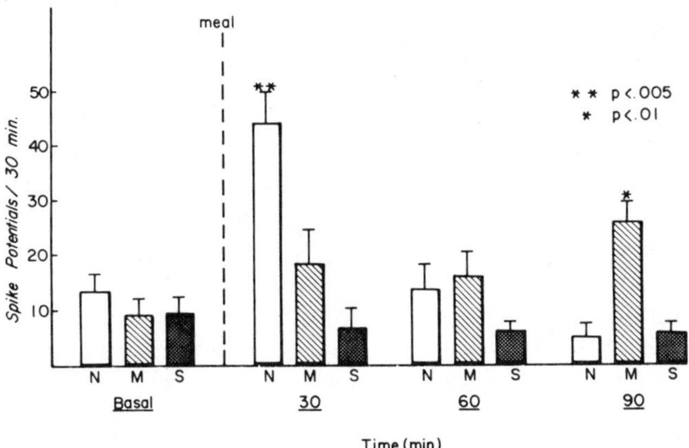

Fig 22.—Pattern of gastrocolonic response to 1,000-calorie meal in normal subjects and patients with diabetes mellitus. Spike response for basal fasting 30-minute period is compared with successive postprandial 30-minute periods: 0–30 minutes, 30–60 minutes, and 60–90 minutes. N = normal, M = mild constipation, and S = severe constipation. (Courtesy of Battle, W. M., et al.: Gastroenterology 79:1217–1221, December 1980.)

Diabetics with severe constipation have a totally absent gastrocolonic response to feeding, indicating that increased postprandial colonic motility may be physiologically important for a normal bowel movement. The abnormal colonic motility in diabetics presumably is related to autonomic neuropathy of the gastrointestinal tract. Metoclopramide stimulates colonic myoelectric and motor activity in a dose-related manner, and several of the present patients noted a significant improvement in constipation while taking metaclopramide for the treatment of diabetic gastropathy.

Prepubertal Endogenous Major Depressives Hyposecrete Growth Hormone in Response to Insulin-Induced Hypoglycemia. About half of severe adult depressives exhibit growth hormone (GH) hyporesponsivity to insulin induced hypoglycemia. Such hyporesponsivity might result from a functional decrease in noradrenergic stimulation of postsynaptic receptors in certain hypothalamic paths. Joaquim Puig-Antich, Mary Ann Tabrizi, Mark Davies, Raymond Goetz, William J. Chambers, Frieda Halpern, and Edward J. Sachar (New York) hypothesized that prepubertal endogenous major depressives would hyposecrete GH in response to insulin-induced hypoglycemia. Twenty-seven drug-free children aged 6 to 12 years were tested. Ten fit Research Diagnostic Criteria for major depressive disorder of the endogenous type, 10 had nonendogenous major depressive disorder, and 7 fit DSM-III criteria for nondepressed neurotic disorder.

All subjects had glucose nadirs 50% or less of baseline. The endogenous depressives significantly hyposecreted GH during tolerance

Biol. Psychiatry 16:801–818, September 1981.

testing, compared with the other two groups. Discrimination was maximal when a cutoff value of 4 ng/ml for peak plasma GH concentration in the first 60-minute postinsulin sample was used. By this criterion, 90% of endogenous major depressives, half the nonendogenous depressives, and no neurotics hyposecreted GH. When a cutoff point of 102 ng/ml × minutes for the area under the GH curve data was used, all endogenous depressives, 40% of nonendogenous depressives, and no neurotics hyposecreted GH.

These preliminary findings strongly support the hypothesis that prepubertal endogenous major depressives hyposecrete GH in response to insulin-induced hypoglycemia. The test appears to be quite specific for prepubertal depression. The results further support the similarity between child and adult major depressive disorders. Insulin resistance, as is observed in adult depressives, has not been demonstrated conclusively in prepubertal patients.

▶ [This study is characteristic of the revived interest in the insulin tolerance test as a marker for endogenous depression. As reported in the study by Winokur et al. (see 1–12), adult depressives have diminished prolactin responses to insulin much more frequently than blunted GH responses. It would also have been interesting to examine the prolactin response in the prepubertal children with depression and neurotic disorders studied here. The implied linkage between adult and childhood depression through this neuroendocrine finding is paralleled by reports of abnormal dexamethasone suppression tests in both groups. The use of neuroendocrine testing to confirm the diagnosis in children with depressive syndromes should be approached with great caution because there are many unknown factors which influence hormone response in these procedures. Assay reliability may be a major problem.—H.Y.M.] ◀

Clinical Recognition of Juvenile Hypothyroidism in the Early Stage. Acquired juvenile hypothyroidism is among the most common endocrine diseases of childhood. The clinical manifestations of this disorder vary with the age at onset and the degree of thyroid dysfunction, and some cases may not be clinically recognized. V. Abbassi, E. Rigterink, and R. P. Cancellieri (Georgetown Univ., Washington, D.C.) reviewed the clinical manifestations of biochemically confirmed acquired hypothyroidism found in 19 of 78 children and adolescents seen in a 5-year period with goiter or abnormal thyroid function tests or both. Biochemical hypothyroidism was documented from elevated thyroid-stimulating hormone (TSH) and low thyroxine (T_4) levels in 18 cases. One patient had low T_4 and TSH levels resulting from hypopituitarism.

Eight patients had chronic lymphocytic thyroiditis. One had Down's syndrome. One patient was thought to have abnormal thyroid iodoprotein secretion, and 1 had undergone removal of a thyroglossal duct cyst that contained all his ectopic thyroid tissue. One patient had become hypothyroid after thyroidectomy for presumed Graves' disease. Age range was 4½–16 years. Presenting features are shown in Table 1; clinical findings are listed in Table 2. Fifteen patients had a goiter. Growth retardation was observed in 6 patients, including 1 with GH deficiency as well. Most patients with cutaneous changes

Clin. Pediatr. (Phila.) 19:782–786, December 1980.

TABLE 1.—SUMMARY OF PRESENTING SYMPTOMS IN
19 HYPOTHYROID PATIENTS

Symptom	Number of Patients
Overweight	9
Fatigue/Lethargy	8
Cold Intolerance	7
Poor Growth	6
Constipation	6
Headache	1
Hip Pain	1
Vaginal Bleeding	1
Asymptomatic	4

had facial puffiness. Serum T_4 level ranged from 0.3 to 4.9 µg/dl. Serum TSH concentration was increased significantly except in the patient with hypopituitarism. Triiodothyronine concentration was undetectable in the serum of 3 patients and reduced or borderline in 7. Eight of 16 patients had significant titers of antithyroid antibody.

This series included children with severe, prolonged hypothyroidism, including growth retardation, and others with hypothyroidism of apparently short duration, in whom classic symptoms and features of myxedema often were absent. The most consistent overall finding was goiter. Thyroid palpation is an important part of the routine pediatric examination, especially in girls. Replacement therapy for 6 to 12 months will normalize the size of the thyroid gland in most cases. When this occurs, treatment is stopped for 6 weeks and thyroid function is reevaluated. Replacement therapy is reinstituted if persistent hypothyroidism is evident. Questionable findings call for TRH testing or reassessment of thyroid function 4–6 weeks later.

▶ [Both Table 1 and Table 2 are valuable. Note the preponderance of goitrous hypothyroid children in this group; goiter has become the single most reliable manifes-

TABLE 2.—SUMMARY OF CLINICAL FINDINGS IN 19
HYPOTHYROID PATIENTS

Finding	Number of Patients
Goiter	15
Obesity	10
Skin Changes	10
Facial Puffiness	8
Short Stature	6
Abnormal Deep Tendon Reflexes	5
Bradycardia	4
Cretinoid Facies	2
Carotenemic Discoloration	2
No Finding*	6

*Goiter excluded.

tation of potential or existing hypothyroidism in children. The authors state, "Interestingly enough, scholastic performance of none of the children, including those with severe and prolonged hypothyroidism, had been affected." One might ask (at some risk) whether this is a reflection more of the state of these children or of the schools that they attend.

Lest you conclude that the spectrum of presentation of juvenile hypothyroidism is completely covered in this article, you should know that Riddlesberger (*Radiology* 39:77, 1981) describe 5 young girls in whom hypothyroidism was associated with cystic ovaries that improved with replacement thyroid therapy. In addition, 2 of the girls showed evidence of precocious puberty.

Is there anything new about the manifestations of hypothyroidism in adults? There is. Look ahead.—T.B.S.] ◄

Obesity and Its Role in Polycystic Ovary Syndrome. Obesity is a hallmark of the polycystic ovary syndrome, which includes the triad of obesity, hirsutism, and anovulation, and recent findings suggest that obesity may be a causative factor. Stephen R. Plymate, Bruce L. Fariss, Martin L. Bassett, and Louis Matej (Madigan Army Med. Center, Tacoma, Wash.) studied 55 consecutive patients who had been infertile for 2 years. All patients had normal husbands, no cervical or tubal problems, normal prolactin levels, and evidence of oligo-ovulation or anovulation. No patient was less than 90% of ideal body weight. Those weighing more than 145% of ideal weight and those weighing less than 120% had comparable testosterone and estradiol levels (table). Testosterone levels were high-normal or elevated. Both sex steroid-binding globulin (SSBG) and LH levels were higher in obese patients than in patients of normal weight. No differences in FSH or prolactin levels were noted. Levels of SSBG correlated with body weight.

In patients with polycystic ovary syndrome or a tendency to develop the syndrome, a decrease in the level of SSBG and an increase in that of free testosterone may contribute to the syndrome becoming manifest. The rise in the free testosterone level associated with increased body fat would increase the amount of estrone formed from peripheral conversion of testosterone, in turn increasing LH secretion and suppressing FSH secretion. Increased levels of free testosterone also may suppress follicular maturation by a direct action on the ovary. Not all obese women have the syndrome, so the change in SSBG may not be

PLASMA HORMONE MEASUREMENTS IN OBESE AND NORMAL
WEIGHT WOMEN WITH POLYCYSTIC OVARY SYNDROME*

	Obese (n = 30)	Normal wt (n = 25)	P
T (ng/ml)	0.83 ± 0.06	0.80 ± 0.05	NS
SSBG (ng DHT/ml)	7.14 ± 0.64	14.7 ± 1.09	<0.0001
LH (μIU/ml)	23.4 ± 4.3	13.8 ± 0.81	<0.05
E_2 (pg/ml)	91 ± 17	60 ± 12	NS

*Values are means ± SEM.

J. Clin. Endocrinol. Metab. 52:1246–1248, June 1981.

the primary factor, but it may be significant in patients who have another defect leading to polycystic ovary disease. Whether the problem with SSBG is a reduced response to estrogen or increased clearance is not known.

▶ [I have visited the Madigan Army Medical Center several times, so that this group of investigators are friends and, being friends, they must suffer. The patients all had "normal husbands." Really? All named Jack Spratt, no doubt.

The authors here make a reasonable guess that the reduction in sex steroid-binding globulin levels, along with the rise in the free testosterone concentrations, may be an important etiologic factor in the genesis of polycystic ovaries in these obese women. These reciprocal changes in SSBG and free testosterone levels have also been noted in women with severe acne (Lawrence et al.: *Clin. Endocrinol. (Oxf.)* 15:87, 1981); the weights of these women were not recorded.

Multiple hormonal changes are being uncovered in obese women. For instance, in contrast to the effect of feeding described in the preceding article, Cavagnini et al. (*J. Endocrinol. Invest.* 4:149, 1981) find that prolactin secretion in obese patients is impaired. It will take time to sort all of this out.—T.B.S.] ◀

Subclinical Anorexia Nervosa. There is substantial evidence that anorexia nervosa is not rare in females and that it may be increasing in prevalence. The occurrence of subclinical anorexia nervosa in individuals with serious problems of eating and weight concern has been proposed. Garner and Garfinkel described the Eating Attitudes Test (EAT) for evaluating behavior and attitudes characteristic of anorexia nervosa. E. J. Button and A. Whitehouse (Univ. of Southampton) undertook a study of "normal" subjects who scored high on the EAT. The test was administered to 446 female and 132 male students at a College of Technology and to 1 male and 13 female patients who fulfilled strict diagnostic criteria for anorexia nervosa. The patients, aged 13 to 38 years, had a mean age at onset of illness of 15 years and were a clinically heterogeneous group.

No male scored high on the EAT, but 28 female students (6.3%) scored in the "anorectic" range. Interviews with these subjects and with 28 subjects who did not score high indicated that symptoms of

PERCENTAGE OF ANORECTIC PATIENTS, HIGH-SCORING STUDENTS AND RANDOM CONTROL STUDENTS DISPLAYING SPECIFIED FEATURES OF ANOREXIA NERVOSA

	Female anorexics (N = 13)	High-scoring students (N = 28)	Control students (N = 28)
Dieting	100	100	57
Weight loss of 5 kg or more	100	71	17
Weight loss of 9 kg or more	100	39	7
Amenorrhoea (>6 months duration)	100	14	0
Self-induced vomiting	46	39	0
Overactivity	92	39	4
Subterfuges to avoid eating	62	36	0
Detailed calorie counting	54	32	0
Encouraging others to eat	77	32	0
Binging	31	18	0
Laxative abuse	46	18	0
Hoarding of food	31	7	0
Increased interest in cooking/food	77	0	0

Psychol. Med. 11:509–516, August 1981.

anorexia nervosa were common in the high-scoring group but virtually absent in the student control group (table). The two groups did not differ significantly in weight; both groups were heavier than the patients. High-scoring students, however, had had a lower minimum weight since puberty than control students.

The findings indicate that a substantial proportion of postpuberal females develop a subclinical form of anorexia nervosa. Awareness of this may lead to the eventual development of effective ways of helping these persons. There appears to be a good case for preliminary evaluation of a small-scale health education program directed primarily at female adolescents in the school context. Close cooperation between researchers and those directly concerned with adolescents in the school setting will be necessary.

▶ [There is a methodological problem here. A purist would insist that the Eating Attitudes Test must be a variable independent of the abnormal behavior noted in the table in order for it to support the conclusion that these individuals suffer from "subclinical" anorexia nervosa. If, for example, a question on the test is "Do you ever vomit?", the individual who answers "yes" would show this as a behavioral aberration as well.

Regardless, I hold the intuitive conviction that, as proposed by Fries (*Acta Psychiatr. Scand.* [*Suppl.*] 248, 1974), there is a continuum of behavior extending from the girl with normal eating habits to the patient with florid anorexia nervosa. Those who travel in middle- or upper middle-class circles cannot help observing females with ages ranging up to the fifties who are fanatic joggers or who, at mealtime, have an insatiable craving for lettuce and celery but eat very little else. One such woman of my acquaintance has succeeded in making herself amenorrheic. She is in her late thirties and is anxious enough to bear children to have taken increasingly large doses of clomiphene without effect. Intellectually, she recognizes the problem, its genesis, and its cure, but she simply cannot "gain weight."

As an incorrigible inventor of acronyms, I must say that the Eating Attitudes Test (EAT) arouses my admiration. A sample of my own creations: *TBNT*, which means "thanks, but no thanks," constructed when I was asked to become a cub scout leader; *NAAFC*, not a civil rights organization, but "nutty as a fruitcake"; and *GOYA*, not an artist, but a peremptory command to Fellows and residents when it's time for endocrine rounds: "Get off your ass."—T.B.S.] ◀

Abnormal Gastric Emptying in Primary Anorexia Nervosa. Most etiologic studies of anorexia nervosa have focused on psychosocial factors. Few studies of gastrointestinal function have been made, although patients often report early satiety, epigastric discomfort, and spontaneous vomiting. S. Holt, M. J. Ford, S. Grant, and R. C. Heading (Edinburgh) assessed the gastric emptying of solid and liquid components of a physiologic test meal in 10 female patients with primary anorexia nervosa and 12 healthy subjects, using a scintiscanning method with ^{113m}In-diethylenetriamine penta-acetic acid as a marker of the liquid phase and ^{99m}Tc-sulfur colloid as a marker of the solid phase. The meal consisted of corn flakes, sugar, and milk. The patients, aged 17 to 32 years, had a mean weight of 42 kg. Six had recent diagnoses. All patients were undergoing inpatient psychiatric therapy. All had reported gastrointestinal symptoms at some time.

Both the liquid and the solid components of the test meal were

Br. J. Psychiatry 139:550–552, December 1981.

emptied significantly more slowly in patients with anorexia nervosa than in healthy subjects, although the early phase of emptying was comparable in the two groups. There apparently was no impairment of postprandial receptive relaxation of the stomach in the patients.

Whether anorexia nervosa represents a primary hypothalamic disorder or whether hypothalamic dysfunction is secondary to changes induced by inanition or psychologic distress is uncertain. Gastric emptying may improve with weight gain, suggesting that the abnormality is a result of secondary hypothalamic dysfunction. Some symptoms of anorexia nervosa may represent a "normal" perception of abnormal upper gastrointestinal function. Use of a drug that promotes gastric emptying such as metoclopramide may be useful in overall management of patients with anorexia nervosa.

Endocrine Disturbances in Anorexia Nervosa and Depression are discussed by B. Timothy Walsh (Columbia Univ.). The possibility of a link between anorexia nervosa and major depressive illness has aroused much interest. Some patients with anorexia respond to antidepressant therapy; also, an increased rate of major affective illness has been found in the families of anorectic patients. Adrenocortical function is similar in patients with anorexia or major depressive illness. At least half of the patients have elevated plasma cortisol levels, which decline as recovery takes place. In anorectic patients only, cortisol is broken down more slowly than in normal individuals. A slight rise in the plasma thyroxine level is noted occasionally in depressed patients, and about 25% of depressed patients have a subnormal thyrotropin response to thyrotropin-releasing hormone (TRH). Anorectics exhibit a number of clinical features suggesting hypothyroidism; plasma triiodothyronine levels are reduced, but the thyrotropin response to TRH is generally normal.

There are certain endocrinologic similarities between anorexia nervosa and major depressive illness, but available data do not suggest an identical neuroendocrine dysfunction in these states. The depression seen in anorexia nervosa patients might be a result of severe psychologic and biologic illness, or it could have a role in the development of anorexia nervosa. The illness may represent an attempt at restoration of affective equilibrium in persons who are susceptible because of their psychosocial environment, early experiences, or a biologic predisposition. Studies of patients who exhibit only a few specific features of anorexia nervosa might help in determining to what degree the endocrine abnormalities are attributable purely to physiologic factors (e.g., weight loss) and to what degree they are due to psychologic factors, e.g., depression.

▶ [This incisive review article summarizes some important endocrine similarities and the differences between patients with anorexia nervosa and those with depressive psychoses. It cuts many of the facile analogies that have been drawn between the two groups of patients.—H.W.] ◀

Psychosom. Med. 44:85–91, March 1982.

Neurochemical Abnormalities in Anorexia Nervosa: Similarities to Affective Disorders. It has been suggested that anorexia nervosa (AN) is a form of hypothalamic disturbance. Some patients have been reported to escape from dexamethasone suppression, and it has been reported that the urinary 3-methoxy-4-hydroxyphenylglycol (MHPG) level, an indirect measure of CNS norepinephrine, is low in acute AN and increases nearly to normal after refeeding. Harry E. Gwirtsman and Robert H. Gerner (Univ. of California, Los Angeles) examined the relation between the dexamethasone suppression test (DST) and MHPG in 13 female patients with AN, having a mean age of 23.5 years. All were free from medical illness and were in an early weight-gain phase of treatment at the time of study. Escape from suppression was defined as a plasma cortisol level of more than 6 μg/dl the day after oral administration of 1 mg of dexamethasone.

Eleven of the 13 patients had low MHPG levels, and this was significantly associated with failure of dexamethasone suppression. The mean MHPG level in the 11 patients weighing less than 80% of ideal body weight was substantially lower than that in 15 female control subjects of normal weight. Five patients had first-degree relatives with either primary affective disorder or alcoholism. None of the patients was hypothyroid by standard tests.

The finding of a relationship between failure to suppress cortisol and a low urinary MHPG level supports the hypothesis that a hypothalamic disturbance is present in AN. It remains to be determined whether this is responsible for low body weight in anorexia or merely is an epiphenomenon. Patients in this study frequently had relatives with either primary affective disorder or alcoholism. Similar biochemical abnormalities are observed in primary affective disorder, suggesting a link between such disorder and AN.

▶ [This article should be read along with the preceding article. There are analogies between depressive disorders and anorexia nervosa, but the differences are also glaring!—H.W.] ◀

Continuous Infusion of Luteinizing Hormone-Releasing Hormone (LHRH) in Patients with Anorexia Nervosa. Anorexia nervosa is characterized by a disturbance of the hypothalamic-pituitary-gonadal axis. P. J. V. Beumont and Suzanne F. Abraham (Univ. of Sydney) examined gonadotropin and estradiol responses to exogenous LHRH in 1 male and 13 female patients with anorexia nervosa. The average age was 20 years. An average minimum weight of 60% of standard had been reached in the course of the illness. The average duration of secondary amenorrhea in 11 patients was 2 years 5 months. The average time since onset of weight loss was 3 years 5 months. The patients were treated by refeeding and supportive psychotherapy only. Five healthy young women also were evaluated.

Biol. Psychiatry 16:991–995, October 1981.
Psychol. Med. 11:477–484, August 1981.

Twenty-two LHRH tests were done during refeeding. Six patients were restudied after weight gain and 4 after a course of bromocriptine.

The luteinizing hormone (LH) response to LHRH infusion was reduced initially but increased progressively as weight was regained. The response patterns suggested deficient stimulation by endogenous LHRH at low weight and impaired estrogen feedback at intermediate weights. Bromocriptine did not enhance the LH response in patients with normal prolactin levels. The mean follicle-stimulating hormone response did not differ significantly at different weight levels. Plasma estradiol levels were lower at the outset than when weight was regained. One patient resumed menstruating after the last infusion of LHRH, and 7 others resumed menstruating after 3 to 12 months, all when they were at 95% or more of standard weight. Only 2 of 5 patients who were still amenorrheic when last seen had reached a weight of 75% of standard.

The plasma LH value and the LH response to LHRH are depressed in patients with anorexia nervosa at low body weight but increase as weight is regained. The feedback effects of estrogen on LH secretion are impaired in anorexia. The amenorrhea of anorexia is probably not directly related to changes in prolactin secretion.

▶ [Considerable controversy exists as to the LH response to LHRH in anorexia nervosa. Some investigators find normal responses despite marked weight loss, or they may find a delayed LH response to LHRH. This study again shows that this LH response is reduced when LHRH is continually infused into patients. Yet, when it is intermittently infused, the responses are normal despite marked weight loss.

The difference in administration may be the key to the controversy. Intermittent or pulsed stimulation of LH release by LHRH may simulate the natural situation.—H.W.] ◀

Additional Reading

Anderson, H., et al.: Treatment of girls with excessive height prediction: Follow-up of 40 girls treated with intramuscular estradiol and progesterone. *Acta Paediatr. Scand.* 69:293, 1980.

Burrow, G. N.: Truth and fancy in the management of the solitary thyroid nodule. *Yale J. Biol. Med.* 53:325, 1980.

Cahill, G. F., Jr., and McDevitt, H. O.: Insulin-dependent diabetes mellitus: Initial lesion. *N. Engl. J. Med.* 304:1454, 1981.

Cohen, L. F., et al.: Cystic fibrosis and pregnancy: A national survey. *Lancet* 2:842, 1980.

Congden, P. J., et al.: Vitamin status in treated patients with cystic fibrosis. *Arch. Dis. Child.* 56:708, 1981.

Dalterio, S., et al.: Δ^9-Tetrahydrocannabinol increases plasma testosterone concentrations in mice. *Science* 213:581, 1981.

Easton, P. A., and Wall, J. R.: Graves' hyperthyroidism and ophthalmopathy following treatment of spontaneous hypothyroidism with levothyroxine. *Can. Med. Assoc. J.* 125:65, 1981.

Eliaschar, I., et al.: Sleep apneic episodes as indications for adenotonsillectomy. *Arch. Otolaryngol.* 106:492, 1980.

England, W. L., and Roberts, S. D.: Immunization to prevent insulin-dependent diabetes mellitus? The economics of genetic screening and vaccination for diabetes. *Ann. Intern. Med.* 94:395, 1981.

Further analyses of mortality in oral contraceptive users: Royal College of General Practitioners' oral contraception study. *Lancet* 1:541, 1981.

Garrison, R. J., et al.: Obesity and lipoprotein cholesterol in the Framingham offspring study. *Metabolism* 29:1053, 1980.

Glass, D., et al.: Early-onset pauciarticular juvenile rheumatoid arthritis associated with human leukocyte antigen-DRw5, iritis, and antinuclear antibody. *J. Clin. Invest.* 66:426, 1980.

Goerz, G., et al.: Urticaria in association with etiocholanolone fever. *Br. J. Dermatol.* 105:109, 1981.

Haugejorden, O., and Helöe, L. A.: Fluorides for everyone: A review of school-based or community programs. *Community Dent. Oral Epidemiol.* 9:159, 1981.

Hay, I. D., et al.: Familial cytomegalic adrenocortical hypoplasia: X-linked syndrome of pubertal failure. *Arch. Dis. Child.* 56:715, 1981.

Hendricks, S. A., et al.: Hypothalamic atrophy with progressive hypopituitarism in an adolescent girl. *J. Clin. Endocrinol. Metab.* 52:562, 1981.

Hermansson, G., et al.: Beat-to-beat variation in children and adolescents with juvenile diabetes mellitus. *Opuscula Med.* 26:54, 1981.

Kopelman, P. G., et al.: Effect of weight loss on sex steroid secretion and binding in massively obese women. *Clin. Endocrinol.(Oxf.)* 14:113, 1981.

Langdon, D. R., et al.: Comparison of single- and split-dose insulin regimens with 24-hour monitoring. *J. Pediatr.* 99:854, 1981.

Levy, G., et al.: Relationship between saliva salicylate concentration and free or total salicylate concentration in serum of children with juvenile rheumatoid arthritis. *Clin. Pharmacol. Ther.* 27:619, 1980.

Linde, R., et al.: Reversible inhibition of testicular steroidogenesis and spermatogenesis by a potent gonadotropin-releasing hormone agonist in normal men: Approach toward the development of a male contraceptive. *N. Engl. J. Med.* 305:663, 1981.

MacGillivray, M. H., et al.: Acute diabetic ketoacidosis in children: Role of stress hormones. *Pediatr. Res.* 15:99, 1981.

Mirouze, J., et al.: Servo-controlled versus continuous insulin infusion as a factor of remission in juvenile diabetes. *ASAIO J.* 3:133, 1980.

Okita, N., et al.: Suppressor T lymphocyte deficiency in Graves' disease and Hashimoto's thyroiditis. *J. Clin. Endocrinol. Metab.* 52:528, 1981.

Parkin, J. L.: Familial multiple glomus tumors and pheochromocytomas. *Ann.. Otol. Rhinol. Laryngol.* 90:60, 1981.

Petersen, N. T., et al.: Respiratory infections in cystic fibrosis patients caused by virus, *Chlamydia,* and *Mycoplasma:* Possible synergism with *Pseudomonas aeruginosa. Acta Paediatr. Scand.* 70:623, 1981.

Reindollar, R. H., et al.: Delayed sexual development: Study of 252 patients. *Am. J. Obstet. Gynecol.* 140:371, 1980.

Rizza, R. A., et al.: Control of blood sugar in insulin-dependent diabetes: Comparison of an artificial endocrine pancreas, continuous subcutaneous insulin infusion, and intensified conventional insulin therapy. *N. Engl. J. Med.* 303:1313, 1980.

Shangold, M. M., et al.: Acute effects of exercise on plasma concentrations of prolactin and testosterone in recreational women runners. *Fertil. Steril.* 35:699, 1981.

Sherwin, R. S., and Koivisto, V.: Keeping in step: Does exercise benefit the diabetic? *Diabetologia* 20:84, 1981.

Stokes, D. C., et al.: Sleep hypoxia in young adults with cystic fibrosis. *Am. J. Dis. Child.* 134:741, 1980.

Sutton, M. G. St. J., et al.: Prevalence of clinically unsuspected pheochromocytoma: Review of 50-year autopsy series. *Mayo Clin. Proc.* 56:354, 1981.

Tamborlane, W. V., et al.: Insulin infusion pump treatment of diabetes: Influence of improved metabolic control on plasma somatomedin levels. *N. Engl. J. Med.* 305:303, 1981.

Tom, L. W. C., et al.: Hemoptysis in children. *Ann. Otol. Rhinol. Laryngol.* 89:419, 1980.

Trompeter, R. S., et al.: Gonadal function in boys with steroid-responsive nephrotic syndrome treated with cyclophosphamide for short periods. *Lancet* 1:1177, 1981.

Vannasaeng, S., et al.: Endocrine function in thalassemia. *Clin. Endocrinol. (Oxf.)* 14:165, 1981.

West, R., et al.: Prospective study of insulin-dependent diabetes mellitus. *Diabetes* 30:584, 1981.

White, N. H., et al.: Reversal of neuropathic and gastrointestinal complications related to diabetes mellitus in adolescents with improved metabolic control. *J. Pediatr.* 99:41, 1981.

Yovos, J. G., et al.: Thyrotoxicosis and a thyrotropin-secreting pituitary tumor causing unilateral exophthalmos. *J. Clin. Endocrinol. Metab.* 53:338, 1981.

Neurology

"To do is to be."—ARISTOTLE

To "do" requires the nervous system to be functioning to full capacity. It is surprising the number of articles in various journals which deal with neurologic malfunction in adolescents and young adults. Many of the conditions which begin in childhood end in adolescence, and many of the conditions which start in adolescence plague the adult. The health care professional working with this age group must have a healthy understanding of the neurologic abnormalities that present in the adolescent years.

A number of articles in this section deal with seizure disorders and their diagnosis and treatment. Of special interest is the article by Emerson et al. on stopping medication in children with epilepsy. Since this becomes an issue in the adolescent years, it is important that we have various guidelines to follow. As noted in this article a waiting period of four years is arbitrary. Whether two years would be reasonable for low-risk patients is not determined; however, in certain instances it might be indicated. A child with epilepsy who has had no seizures for at least two years while taking anticonvulsants has about a 70% chance of remaining seizure-free when the drug is withdrawn. In the adolescent years, once biological maturity has occurred, a two-year seizure-free period seems reasonable. The key is to follow these patients for a period of time before making a final decision. Sometimes medication may have to be reinstituted.

Also of interest is the article on diagnostic evaluation of pseudoseizures. Pseudoseizures and epileptic seizures in adolescents and young adults can present a dilemma. Prolonged video-EEG recording to document pseudoseizures and to differentiate them from epileptic seizures is an important diagnostic tool. The clinician should be aware of this technique and also be willing to use it to differentiate a pseudoseizure from a true seizure. This fact obviously becomes important with respect to medication and further treatment.

Multiple sclerosis and myasthenia gravis are also discussed here. In particular, the article from Johns Hopkins University discusses the pathogenesis of multiple sclerosis. The authors concluded that acquisition of an exogenous factor, such as infection, and the onset of host factors related to pubescence which allow the pathogenesis to proceed are part of a two-stage process in development of this condition which affects adolescents and young adults.

Stopping Medication in Children With Epilepsy: Predictors of Outcome. Ronald Emerson, Bernard J. D'Souza, Eileen P. Vining, Kenton R. Holden, E. David Mellits, and John M. Freeman (Johns Hopkins Hosp.) undertook a study to evaluate reports that 75% of children with epilepsy remain free from seizures without anticonvulsants if their seizures have been controlled fully for 4 years before discontinuation of medication and to identify factors that can predict safe withdrawal or recurrence of seizures.

Between 1973 and 1979, anticonvulsants were discontinued routinely in all patients followed at Johns Hopkins Hospital who had had two or more afebrile seizures but who had been seizure-free for 4 or more years. Medication was gradually withdrawn during a 2–3 month period. The 68 patients in the study were aged 6–22 years when their medications were discontinued. Patients were followed for 6 months to 6 years after drug withdrawal.

Of the 68 patients, 50 (74%) remained seizure-free after drug withdrawal. Risk of relapse was greatest soon after initiation of drug withdrawal. Patients with an IQ below 70 had a significantly increased risk of relapse, and more patients with a known organic cause of their epilepsy had a relapse than did those with disease of unknown cause. No relation was apparent between risk of relapse and presence of abnormal neurologic examination. A striking relation was observed between early age of seizure onset and increased risk of recurrence upon drug withdrawal and also between number of gener-

Fig 23.—Cumulative probability of continued freedom from seizures in 64 patients (calculated from Kaplan-Meier curves). The four variables of normal EEG, abnormal EEG, history of 30 or fewer seizures, and history of more than 30 seizures are shown in four combinations. (Courtesy of Emerson, R., et al.: N. Engl. J. Med. 304:1125–1129, May 7, 1981.)

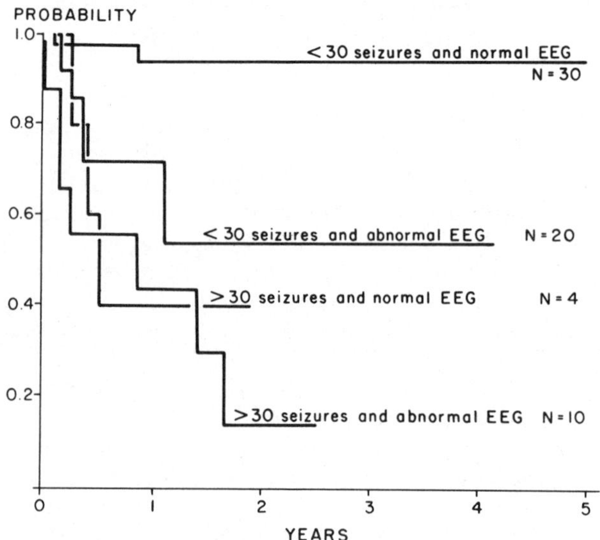

N. Engl. J. Med. 304:1125–1129, May 7, 1981.

alized tonic/clonic seizures before control and risk of recurrence. An EEG obtained just before drug withdrawal was useful as a predictor of outcome. Figure 23 shows risk of relapse with use of Kaplan–Meier curves.

A child with epilepsy who has had no seizures for several years while taking anticonvulsants has about a 70% chance of remaining free from seizures when drugs are withdrawn. From a psychosocial view, termination of medication implies wellness and removes the stigma of epilepsy. A waiting period of 4 years is arbitrary. Whether 2 years would be reasonable for "low-risk" patients has not been determined.

▶ [Trying to see whether a young patient with epilepsy really needs protracted treatment is highly sensible. The criteria suggested by this study for predicting successful withdrawal from anticonvulsant drugs also make sense.—L.E.H.] ◀

Pseudoseizures: Diagnostic Evaluation. Episodes that superficially resemble epileptic seizures but are not epileptic in origin have long been noted. Don W. King, Brian B. Gallagher, Alice J. Murvin, Dennis B. Smith, Donald J. Marcus, Lawrence C. Hartlage, and L. Charles Ward, III (Med. College of Georgia) evaluated prolonged video-EEG recording for the diagnosis of pseudoseizures in 60 patients, 33 with a history of episodes of uncertain status and 27 with uncontrolled seizures presumed to represent epilepsy. Seventeen patients in the first group had had episodes of questionable nature, whereas 16 were thought to have had both epileptic seizures and episodes of uncertain nature. All patients were aged 16 years or older and had had an average of at least two episodes a month in the 3 months prior to video-EEG.

Pseudoseizures were recorded in 16 patients and epileptic seizures in 17. Twenty-three patients, 4 of whom also had pseudoseizures, had consistently epileptiform interictal discharges, but epileptic seizures were not recorded. Of the 17 patients with a questionable history, epileptic seizures were recorded in 2 and pseudoseizures in 8. Epileptic seizures and pseudoseizures each were recorded in 4 of the 16 patients thought to have had both types of episodes. All but 4 of the 27 patients with a history of epilepsy exhibited evidence of epilepsy. Four patients in this group, 2 of whom had interictal evidence of epilepsy, had pseudoseizures recorded. The mean age at onset of pseudoseizures was 24 years, compared with 13 years at the onset of epileptic seizures. Ten patients with pseudoseizures alone were on an anticonvulsant regimen when admitted: all drugs were discontinued in 7 without subsequent evidence of epilepsy.

Pseudoseizures occur frequently in patients evaluated for seizures or episodes of uncertain mechanism. They are often present where they are not suspected. Differentiation of epileptic seizures from pseudoseizures often is inaccurate but is facilitated by prolonged video-EEG recording.

▶ [Pseudoseizures occur frequently in patients being evaluated for epilepsy and sus-

Neurology (NY) 32:18–23, January 1982.

pected epilepsy. The differentiation between true epileptic attacks and pseudoseizures is often difficult to make and is best done by prolonged video-EEG recording.—R.N.D.J.] ◄

Status Epilepticus Caused by Solvent Abuse. Glue sniffing may present in a number of ways and may be fatal. Charles Allister, Michael Lush, John S. Oliver, and Joyce M. Watson (Glasgow) describe an adolescent with severe status epilepticus caused by solvent abuse.

Boy, 15, presented with a grand mal seizure followed by severe uncontrolled status epilepticus. Two febrile seizures had occurred in early childhood. He was comatose when admitted but localized painful stimuli; no focal signs were noted. Skull films and a CT study were normal. A frontal lobe biopsy specimen taken on the third day gave no evidence of encephalitis. An anonymous telephone call suggested that the boy might have sniffed glue, and the biopsy sample was found to contain 14.5 μg of toluene per gm of tissue. Frequent seizures continued despite therapeutic serum concentrations of various anticonvulsant combinations. Intermittent positive-pressure ventilation, muscle relaxants, and sedation also were used, and a tracheostomy was performed. Improvement began at 2 weeks; frequency of seizures decreased without any major change in treatment. A CT study at 10 weeks showed ventricular dilatation and several low-density areas resembling infarcts. The boy was discharged after 5 months. Follow-up 2 years later showed no focal deficit or definite psychometric impairment. He continued to have 1 or 2 seizures a month and also had major behavioral problems.

Hypoxia may have influenced the neurologic disorder in this case, but the illness probably was initiated by solvent intoxication. A latent predisposition to seizures may have been a significant factor. Solvent intoxication should be considered in cases of epilepsy or encephalopathy of unknown etiology that arise for the first time in adolescence.

► [These clinicians suspected herpes simplex encephalopathy, thus the brain biopsy. Solvent abuse is something to keep in mind as a cause of unexplained seizures in a youth.—R.D.C.] ◄

Multiple Sclerosis: A Two-Stage Process? Harvey R. Fischman (Johns Hopkins Univ.) investigated the hypothesis that the pathogenesis of multiple sclerosis (MS) depends on both an environmental factor and host factors associated with puberty. Data for the Faroe Islands "epidemic" was used in the study. Although this epidemic affected only 25 persons, it is unique in that the disease previously had been nonexistent in the Islands until the British military occupation during WW II (1940 to 1945).

An age-associated bimodality was observed in the affected population. The midpoint of the British occupation (1942) was used as the time of onset in the older group; the overall mean incubation period for this group was 5 years. In the younger group, with puberty used as the time of onset, the mean incubation period was 5 years for female subjects and 6.3 years for male subjects (overall mean, 5.7 years). The similar incubation periods for male and female subjects

Br. Med. J. 283:1156, Oct. 31, 1981.
Am. J. Epidemiol. 114:244–251, August 1981.

in both groups provided a check of internal validity. Although 10 of the individuals were below the age of puberty at the time of the occupation, none exhibited MS before reaching puberty. This suggests that the onset of the pathogenesis of MS depends on passing or having passed through puberty. It also explains why MS rarely develops before age 10, is unusual in persons younger than age 15, and why age 15 is considered a critical time in studies of the risk of MS in migrant populations. It also explains why female subjects have an earlier onset than male subjects. The data further show that susceptibility to MS may be acquired across a wide range of ages. Individuals below the age of puberty can acquire susceptibility to MS at a younger age, although pathogenesis does not become evident until puberty occurs. The abrupt rise in incidence that coincides with puberty and the relative rarity of occurrence after age 45 to 50 years suggest that the classic age-incidence curve may not describe an infectious curve, but rather represents the waxing and waning of a host factor related to sexual maturation and aging. This is supported by the fact that many aging curves, such as those for estrogen, testosterone, and 17-hydroxycorticosteroid, are strikingly similar to the MS incidence curves.

Analysis of the data for the Faroe Islands epidemic of MS suggests a two-stage process in the pathogenesis of MS: (1) acquisition of an exogenous factor, and (2) the onset of host factors related to pubescence that allow the pathogenesis to proceed.

▶ [The fact that many aging curves, such as those for estrogen, testosterone, and 17-hydroxycorticosteroid production, are strikingly similar to those showing the incidence of the onset of multiple sclerosis suggest that both environmental factors, such as infection, and host factors associated with puberty may play a part in the pathogenesis of multiple sclerosis.—R.N.D.J.] ◀

Etiology of Multiple Sclerosis: Temporal-Spatial Clustering Indicating Two Environmental Exposures Before Onset. The highest known prevalence rates in the world for multiple sclerosis (MS) occur in the Orkney and Shetland Islands north of Scotland. These rates are at least twice as high as those for the Highland areas of Scotland. The available evidence suggests that an environmental factor figures prominently in the etiology of MS. David C. Poskanzer, Alexander M. Walker, Lewis B. Prenney, and Jean L. Sheridan (Massachusetts Gen. Hosp.) report the results from a subsection of an extensive epidemiologic study of MS in the Orkney and Shetland Islands conducted from 1974 to 1977. Cases in the study were identified by reference to previous surveys and interviews with health professionals.

In Orkney, 42 patients with probable MS were identified, and 29 such patients were identified in Shetland. The patient groups yielded 861 and 406 pairs, respectively, for analysis of temporal and spatial associations. When the data were analyzed by each year of birth, at each chronological age, for each calendar year of onset, there was no

Neurology (NY) 31:708–713, June 1981.

evidence of clustering. However, when the parishes of residence of the Orkney patients were analyzed by years before onset of disease, a striking bimodal pattern of association was observed. The association was seen at 21 to 23 years before onset and just prior to the onset of MS. No clustering was seen in the Shetland patients. Each of the two episodes of clustering in time occurred on three separate islands, two of which showed clustering in both episodes. A control group was matched for age, sex, and parish of birth. Analysis of the control subjects for clustering showed clustering 2 decades before onset in Orkney, although no clustering immediately before onset occurred. Previous attempts to demonstrate clustering may have failed because of a lack of specific data or use of inappropriate methods.

Although the results may suggest that MS is, in fact, two diseases, there was no clinical, epidemiologic, or laboratory evidence to support this hypothesis. It is more likely that there are two points of susceptibility to MS, one that occurs at least 21 years before onset and the other that occurs shortly before or at onset. This suggests that the pathogenesis of MS is a two-stage process that represents environmental exposure (infectious or toxic) to the same agent at two points in time or to two different agents at different times prior to the onset of MS.

▶ [These investigators present strong evidence that environmental exposure (infectious or toxic) is paramount in the etiology of multiple sclerosis. They further express the belief that two exposures, one at least 12 years prior to onset and one just prior to onset of symptoms, may be responsible for the development of the disease.— R.N.D.J.] ◀

Pathogenesis and Treatment of Myasthenia Gravis are discussed by Glenis K. Scadding and C. W. H. Havard (Royal Free Hosp., London). Myasthenia gravis is an uncommon disease of neuromuscular function caused by a reduction in available acetylcholine receptors at the neuromuscular junction. Two thirds of patients are women, with a peak age at onset of 20 to 29 years. Generalized myasthenia may be associated with thymoma when there is no clear HLA association; with thymitis in patients less than age 40 years in whom there is an association with HLA B8 or DRW3, or both; and with thymitis in patients more than age 40 who have a high incidence of HLA A3 and B7 or DRW2, or both.

There is increasing evidence that antibodies to acetylcholine receptors are important in the pathogenesis of myasthenia gravis. Although the antibodies appear to cause muscle weakness, correlation with the severity of disease is poor. Antibodies could act through complement-mediated lysis, modulation, or direct blocking of acetylcholine-binding sites. The thymus is an active site of antibody production in most patients with thymitis.

Myasthenia gravis is treated symptomatically with anticholinesterase drugs, which prolong the action of acetylcholine at the postsynaptic membrane. Azathioprine has led to clinical improvement and

Br. Med. J. 283:1008–1012, Oct. 17, 1981.

reduced antibodies to acetylcholine receptors. The effects occur more slowly than with steroid therapy. Men, patients more than age 35 years, and those with the disorder for less than 10 years are especially likely to respond to azathioprine therapy, as are patients with evidence of a thymoma or thymic hyperplasia and those with a high titer of antireceptor antibody. Plasma exchange may be indicated in severely ill patients while other forms of treatment become effective. Thymectomy has become increasingly important in the management of myasthenic patients, but the mechanism of its beneficial effect is unclear.

Myasthenia may become worse with a change in hormonal state or with some drugs, and myasthenic crisis with respiratory failure and virtual paralysis may result. Other forms of treatment that have been tried in refractory cases include low-dose, total-body irradiation and antithymocyte globulin. Administration of anti-iodiotype antibodies to acetylcholine receptors could prove to be of value and might also restore normal control mechanisms.

▶ [This is a concise current summary.—R.D.C.] ◀

A Case of Sporadic Juvenile Parkinson's Disease. Juvenile Parkinson's disease is rare, and virtually all reported cases have been associated with either a family history of the disease or other neurologic findings. Christopher G. Clough, Marina Mendoza, and Melvin D. Yahr (Mt. Sinai School of Medicine) report a sporadic case of classic Parkinson's disease with no other neurologic abnormalities in a patient who became symptomatic at age 15 years.

Woman, 22 had had, at age 15, a tremor of both hands that failed to respond to simple sedatives. Difficulty walking was noted the following year, when there was a tremor in both arms, as well as "cogwheel" rigidity. In the next 5 years, the patient practically became housebound, with a virtually constant tremor. Levodopa-carbidopa therapy had led to dramatic improvement. There was no family history of Parkinson's disease or other movement disorders. Mild orofacial dyskinesia was observed, as well as hypotonia and nearly imperceptible trunk movements. A parkinsonian tremor appeared in the arms within 3 hours of stopping medication, and after 24 hours the patient lay immobile and had a pill-rolling tremor in both hands and greatly increased muscle tone of the cogwheel type. Mentation was normal. Normal function rapidly returned on the resumption of levodopa-carbidopa therapy. Recurrent symptoms between 4-hourly doses were overcome with the use of deprenyl.

This patient had classic findings of Parkinson's disease with an onset at age 15 years. Sporadic juvenile Parkinson's disease is rare but does occur. The findings in the present patient were similar in all respects to those in patients with disease of later onset.

▶ [This looks like an airtight case of juvenile Parkinson's disease. If, as the twin studies tell us, the hereditary component in Parkinson's disease is small or nonexistent, what causes it here? The patient had experienced no prior events that might damage the brain, and one of the usual precipitating drugs, chlorpromazine hydro-

Arch. Neurol. 38:730–731, November 1981.

chloride, had been used only a week. Perhaps there is a rare (recessive) gene?—R.D.C.] ◄

Encephalopathy of Reye's Syndrome: Review of Pathogenetic Hypotheses is presented by G. Robert DeLong and Thomas H. Glick (Harvard Med. School). The encephalopathy of Reye's syndrome is reversible, noninflammatory, and stereotypic in its early progression and can be characterized as toxic or metabolic in nature. Its basis remains unclear. Initially the pathologic condition of the liver and hyperammonemia suggested a hepatic encephalopathy as the cause, and later the role of fatty acidemia came under consideration. Recently, a generalized disorder of cell energetics caused by mitochondrial dysfunction has been proposed.

The time course of hyperammonemia correlates closely with the course of the disease in most cases, and hyperammonemia correlates better with the severity of disease than do other measures. Experimental hyperammonemia in animals reproduces features of Reye's syndrome. Treatments aimed at the direct removal of ammonia have proved to be ineffective, and measures to increase ammonia disposal have not been adequately evaluated. Increased serum concentrations of free fatty acids are consistently found in Reye's syndrome, but these concentrations have not been determined in relation to cerebral neuropathologic markers in patients. Interactions between fatty acids and ammonia metabolism may provide a basis for treatment to reduce fatty acidemia. It remains unclear how viral illness might lead to mitochondrial dysfunction in the liver, or what mitochondrial functions are disordered and in what pathogenetic sequence. Hyperlactatemia also has been implicated in Reye's syndrome encephalopathy, but the neuropathology of lactic acidosis differs from that of Reye's syndrome.

Strong evidence is available implicating hyperammonemia as a cause of the encephalopathy of Reye's syndrome, but the lack of an efficient means of reducing the toxic burden of ammonia in the brain has made it difficult to prove this. Treatment of the encephalopathy awaits an effective metabolic intervention.

► [The authors purposefully have emphasized the role of ammonia in this review and discuss possible therapeutic metabolic intervention, which so far has not been successful.—R.D.C.] ◄

The Relationship Between Learning Disability, Neurologic Impairment, and Delinquency: Results of a Follow-up Study. Proposed relationships between learning disability and delinquency rest chiefly on retrospective reports. Otfried Spreen (Univ. of Victoria) has reviewed the findings in a prospective follow-up study of 203 children with learning handicaps who had a full neurologic workup at age 8 to 12 years and then were interviewed extensively at a mean age of 18.9 years. Sixty-four of the 203 children initially had definite neurologic indications of brain damage, 82 had neurologic indications

Pediatrics 69:53–63, January 1982.
J. Nerv. Ment. Dis. 169:791–799, December 1981.

of suggested brain dysfunction, and 57 had no neurologic indications of brain dysfunction. Most of the children in the first two groups had been affected since birth.

In all, 55% of the subjects indicated they had come to the attention of the police, with no significant differences among the three groups and a group of control subjects. The total number of first, second, third, and fourth offenders also did not differ significantly among the groups. Subjects with learning disabilities but no neurologic indications of brain damage received somewhat more penalties and more severe penalties than the other groups for first and subsequent offenses. Subjects with lower IQs tended to show a somewhat greater number of more serious offenses, whereas those with higher IQs tended to receive a slightly greater number of more serious penalties.

Learning handicap in itself did not significantly increase the risk of encounters with police or the number of offenses committed in this prospective study. The findings provide little support for an association between learning disability and delinquency on the one hand and neurologic deficit on the other. It seems unlikely that organicity or neurologic impairment has more than an accidental role as a precursor or cause of delinquency. Discrepancies with previous studies may be related to differences in research design and to the use of test vs. clinical indicators of neurologic impairment.

▶ [This is a surprising conclusion based on a prospective study and is at variance with the general assumption that the delinquent is more likely to have a learning disability. No doubt the argument will continue.—R.D.C.] ◀

Additional Reading

Cloyd, J. C., et al.: Status epilepticus: Role of intravenous phenytoin. *J.A.M.A.* 244:1479, 1980.

Davis, A. G., et al.: Once-daily dosing with phenobarbital in children with seizure disorders. *Pediatrics* 68:824, 1981.

Davis, C. H., and Joglekar, V. M.: Cerebellar astrocytomas in children and young adults. *J. Neurol. Neurosurg. Psychiatry* 44:820, 1981.

Honig, P. J., and Charney, E. B.: Children with brain tumor headaches: Distinguishing features. *Am. J. Dis. Child.* 136:121, 1982.

Jennings, M. T., and Bird, T. D.: Genetic influences in the epilepsies: Review of the literature with practical implications. *Am. J. Dis. Child.* 135:450, 1981.

Rogers, M. P., et al.: Giggle incontinence. *J.A.M.A.* 247:1446, 1982.

Mental Health

"I don't think the present psychiatric diagnostic system fits most people who are labeled by it. I have therefore, in response to popular demand, created my own. If for some reason or another a person can't be described as normal, then one of these four categories will most assuredly fit: tight-assed, smart-assed, boring, or mean."—SOL GORDON, in *The New You.*

The present psychiatric diagnostic system certainly has trouble with labelling many of the mental conditions in the adolescent. By the "nature of the beast," mood swings, impulsiveness, and vulnerability confuse the classification. In many circumstances we would like to use one of Dr. Gordon's categories to describe an adolescent and his parents. Hopefully we don't.

Mental health problems certainly constitute one of the major concerns in this age group. Depression and suicide together account for significant morbidity and mortality. Clinical observations and research today are trying to make our jobs easier as we try to work to reduce these statistics. Of the many articles included in this section, those on suicide, its recognition, and its management are of particular interest. In the article entitled "Are young women who attempt suicide hysterical?" it was pointed out that the study group of suicide attempters had more obsessoid personalities but did not necessarily exhibit marked hysterical traits. Therefore the author cautions against diagnosing young women who attempt suicide as hysterical even though they may seem hysterical at the time of the attempt. The relationship between suicide and depression and the diagnosis of depressive states in children and adolescents are also covered. The article by Carlson and Cantwell on masked depression points out that depressive disorders in children and adolescents may present as hyperactivity, aggressive behavior, and some antisocial behavior. The ability to unmask the depression which may be underlying these conditions is extremely important.

Cults are another contemporary problem, and the article by Levine provides some useful insights. Many times we are confronted with an adolescent or young adult who has been part of a cult. Mental health professionals as well as general health care providers should become acquainted with cults and cult practices in their particular area. Neither the automatic acceptance of these groups nor their rejection is indicated, for some cults may prove supportive to adolescents in times of stress. Understanding the cult as it relates to the adolescent and to his or her family can be extremely important in working with young people.

Anorexia nervosa is included in this section because of its psychosocial aspects. Of particular interest is the article by Swift whose review of seven outcome studies provides little support for the view that onset of anorexia nervosa at an early age is associated with a good prognosis. However, the author believes that the apparent increase in prevalance of anorexia may provide for development of greater insight into the relationship between age at onset and outcome of the disorder.

Follow-up of Adolescent Psychiatric Inpatients. Psychiatric hospital services for adolescents have steadily increased in recent years, but there is not much information on the effects of hospital treatment of adolescents. Dave M. Davis, Victor Gonzalez, and James Piat (Peachtree-Parkwood Mental Health Center, Atlanta) report a 1-year follow-up of 74 adolescents, aged 14–19, based on structured follow-up interviews and standardized psychologic testing. The program from which subjects were selected for study is geared toward 3–6 months of intermediate-term care and is designed as a specialized therapeutic community. Social learning theory is used to emphasize responsibility for self, accountability for one's actions, and the importance of feedback from persons in the community. Members participate in group therapy, family and individual therapy, and community meetings and attend a school within the hospital.

Most subjects were white. Over half had antisocial personality disorders, whereas 15% were schizophrenics and 14% were depressive neurotics. At follow-up, 84% of patients were living with their families and 40% were enrolled in school. About one-third were employed full- or part-time, and most described their work adjustment as good. Most subjects described their relationship with their families as good. Nearly one-third are currently in treatment. One-fifth have been rehospitalized at least once, and the same proportion are on psychotropic medication. Current functioning was described as good or very good by 68% of subjects. The more alienated the subject was initially, the less likely he was to be enrolled in school at follow-up. The more external the locus of control, the less likely the subject was to be employed and the poorer the family and peer relations. Treatment after discharge was more likely with greater emotional discomfort at the outset.

Most of the relationships between discharge measures and outcome variables in this study are consistent with clinical expectations. Perhaps the most striking finding was the importance of the locus of control scale as a predictor of outcome. The subjects will continue to be evaluated annually in an attempt to determine patterns of treatment response over time.

▶ [The proliferation of literature about malfunctioning adolescents reflects the significant pressure for more attention and services for them. Particularly in the larger cities, day and inpatient programs for adolescents are unable to keep abreast of the demand for treatment. As shown in the statistics of the Davis, Gonzalez, and Piat

South. Med. J. 73:1215–1217, September 1980.

report, most of the patients in these therapeutic centers are difficult-to-control youngsters with personality disorders that cannot be dealt with in traditional outpatient treatment programs. Although drug problems in this group appear to be declining, they are still found in considerable numbers, whereas alcohol-related difficulties are increasing. At the same time, there has been a greater emphasis on neurotic and depressive symptoms in teenagers who are found to be malfunctioning in the classes now mandated by law for emotionally disturbed and learning disabled students. Adolescent medicine specialists also have increasing sophistication about the needs of malfunctioning youth. In addition, one must credit the greater availability of coverage for these services by third-party payments, including state education and mental health departments. However, it is also becoming apparent that without follow-up treatment programs, the gains from day and inpatient therapeutic approaches only too often disappear.—R.S.L.] ◄

► ↓ The greater awareness of depressive syndromes in adolescents is reflected in the emphasis placed on their accurate diagnosis by Meeks and by Bowden and Sarabia. The recent proliferation of studies of bipolar illness has created increased awareness of depression in teenagers, although its manifestations are more usually masked and easily misdiagnosed. Lithium as a treatment modality in this age group is still not completely worked out, but its trial is not contraindicated.

Meeks provides an important set of criteria for treatment of adolescent depressions, including dealing with unresolved developmental distortions that are resurfacing for better resolution, with depression as the presenting manifestation. The most serious aspect of depression in this age group is the possibility of suicide. Eisenberg makes an eloquent case for greater emphasis on the prevention and treatment of suicidal attempts. The frequent ambivalence of such attempts can be outweighed by their being made on impulse, at a time when rescue is unavailable. Greater awareness of the earlier, but too often disregarded, calls for help is necessary if the alarming rise in the adolescent suicide rate is to decline.—R.S.L. ◄

Diagnosis and Treatment of Common Adolescent Depressive States are discussed by John E. Meeks (Washington, D. C.). It often is stated that adolescent depressions are usually reactive, but there now is growing recognition that manic-depressive illness may develop during the adolescent years. Pure reactive depressions in otherwise healthy adolescents are not an important treatment problem as they are basically self-correcting. Major psychotic depressions are relatively easy to diagnose if a diligent history is taken. Treatment is chiefly biologic and is improving rapidly. Most depressed adolescents who require psychotherapy have a long history of self-doubt, dysphoria, and social isolation, which, however, may not be grossly obvious. Often the precipitating event seems to be a self-generated part of the illness. Lack of hope for the future is frequently apparent.

Classic insight-oriented intervention often fails in these cases. A significant majority of depressed adolescent patients who come for treatment exhibit cognitive deviations such as distorted time perspectives or very poor psychosocial adaptive capacity. Intense depressive themes may resurface during treatment after what is understood as effective conflict resolution. Treatment of depressed adolescents often must include the mobilization of family support systems, and techniques of helping parents should be systematically implemented. The therapist must interpret the difference between not getting what was wished for and losing a loved one, and he must emphasize the newly

South Med. J. 73:920–923, July 1980.

reestablished psychotherapeutic relationship. Later, treatment can become more insight oriented. Extended periods of continuous individual treatment and collaborative family work are necessary. The final phase of therapy is difficult in that, whereas it is the therapist who is idealized, the idealization must occur according to terms constructed by the adolescent. This is especially important for patients with developmental deviations, whose sense of connectedness with real persons must replace the identity and defense of depression.

Diagnosing Manic-Depressive Illness in Adolescents is discussed by Charles L. Bowden and Fermin Sarabia (Univ. of Texas, San Antonio). Manic-depressive illness, manic type, occurs in adolescence but appears to be seriously underdiagnosed, whereas schizophrenia is overdiagnosed. At least 4% of all psychiatric outpatients appear to have manic-depressive illness, and Loranger and Levine (1978) found evidence of illness in adolescence in about one fifth of the adults diagnosed as having manic disorder. In affected adolescents, the diagnosis of adolescent adjustment reaction may be made in order to minimize harm to the patients' reputations. In others, the problems are misdiagnosed as hyperactivity or are incorrectly diagnosed because of the preference of some child psychiatrists to avoid the use of drugs. An accurate diagnosis of manic-depressive illness in adolescents is important, as it influences the attitude of the treating staff and indicates that neuroleptic drugs should be avoided in favor of lithium carbonate, which provides superior symptom control and relapse protection and which does not appear to be associated with long-term toxicity.

Experience with four cases indicates that the Research Diagnostic Criteria for manic-depressive illness can be applied to adolescents. Restlessness and hyperactivity tend to be more episodic in manic-depressive illness than in hyperactive children. A positive family history may be diagnostically helpful. A wide range of developmentally related symptoms may be present, including school refusal, fluctuations in learning ability, irregular aggressive outbursts, and suicide attempts. Episodic delinquent behavior may be a product of manic symptoms. A clear response to lithium is extremely helpful diagnostically. The premorbid personality characteristically is energetic and outgoing; some patients have had mild cyclothymic mood swings or mild hyperactivity. Usually, psychosocial precipitants of illness are not identified.

Reported cases of adolescent manic-depressive illness have responded to lithium treatment. Lithium therapy appears to be safe in adolescents, but must be monitored closely. Thyroid function, glucogenesis, and white blood cell formation shoud be assessed periodically. Lithium therapy should be continued only if the diagnosis is established firmly.

Compr. Psychiatry 21:263–269, July–Aug. 1980.

Use of Lithium Carbonate in Adolescence is discussed by Derek Steinberg (Beckenham, England). Lithium carbonate is effective in the treatment of adult manic-depressive illness, but its efficacy in adolescents with manic-depressive disease is less clear. Kropf and Muller-Oerlinghausen (1979) reported a possible link between the effects of lithium on the brain and an "anti-manic" effect in healthy young male volunteers. Toxic lithium levels may vary considerably among individuals, and single estimates may not give an accurate picture of the level that prevails most of the time. A diuretic effect of lithium and a reduction in thyroid function have been described. Clinical reports on the use of lithium in manic-depressive adolescents have involved fairly few cases, without systematic presentation and follow-up. Apparently, some subjects require a high dose of lithium. Lithium also has been used in children and adolescents with behavior disorders and aggressive behavior.

At least some lithium-responsive disorders of childhood and adolescence may be conceived of as "affective equivalents" in immature personalities, or premorbid behavioral abnormalities of a qualitatively different type. Much remains to be learned about the practical aspects of using lithium. There is little doubt that lithium helps some adolescents with manic-depressive disorder, and it probably helps some with periodic psychotic disorders, especially when they are accompanied by aggressive behavior and excitement; when there is a family history of affective illness; and where endogenous factors are more significant than environmental ones. Other methods of treatment should be tried first unless subjects are classically manic-depressive. The possibility of lithium therapy helping a small minority of disturbed adolescents does not detract from the growing evidence of the external origins of emotional and conduct disorders.

Adolescent Suicide: On Taking Arms Against a Sea of Troubles. Leon Eisenberg (Harvard Med. School) points out that, although the health of American adolescents has improved rapidly in recent decades, mortality for those aged 15 to 24 years has risen in the past 20 years, chiefly because of increasing deaths from violence, including suicides. Suicide is the third leading cause of death in the male population and the fourth in the female population in this age group.

Although suicide rates are quite high from a medical perspective, suicide is infrequent as a statistical event, making assessment of preventive efforts difficult. Even an unusually powerful screening measure would be of dubious value. Restricting access to means of committing suicide can make a difference. Suicides from barbiturates have declined, while those from firearms have increased. Suicide and attempted suicide are more likely in the presence of major psychiatric disorder, alcohol or drug abuse, prior attempts, a turbulent family situation, and recent changes in behavior. Most patients give ample warning of suicide.

J. Child Psychol. Psychiatry 21:263–271, July 1980.
Pediatrics 66:315–320, August 1980.

The first decision facing the physician is whether hospitalization is necessary for behavioral reasons after resolution of the medical sequelae of attempted suicide. Some physicians recommend routine admission to an adolescent inpatient unit at least for a brief time, but it is not clear that this leads to a better outcome than selective hospitalization. Hospitalization is essential in the presence of psychosis. Most suicidal patients are ambivalent, with a hope of being saved accompanying the wish to die. The force of the intent to die can be inferred from the lethality of the means the patient has chosen. Outpatient counseling may be feasible if the parents are understanding and concerned and a wish for rescue predominates. Medication may be indicated for the severely depressed or schizophrenic patient, but is inappropriate most of the time. Drugs can be counterproductive by shifting the focus away from the essential task of modifying family relationships and life stress. A therapeutic context that permits the rebuilding of hope and the reestablishment of healthy ties among family members is essential. Suicide is best regarded as a deficiency of social connections and the ultimate expression of alienation. The goal of treatment is to restore to the patient the sources of emotional sustenance on which all depend for survival.

Are Young Women Who Attempt Suicide Hysterical? The term "hysterical" or some variant frequently has been applied to those who attempt suicide, particularly when the risk to life is low. However, there are few objective data supporting the view that these subjects usually can be described as hysterical and narcissistic and are attempting to manipulate others or win attention. Robert D. Goldney (Univ. of Adelaide) used a questionnaire to assess 110 women, aged 18–30 years, who had attempted suicide by drug overdose and were admitted to a large city general hospital. Twenty-five control women, aged 18–30 years, were attending a community health center. The Hysteroid-Obsessoid Questionnaire (HOQ) was utilized.

The ages of women in the two groups were similar. Age correlated significantly with HOQ scores in the suicidal group. Comparison of age-matched subjects indicated that fewer suicide attempters were married or living in a de facto relationship. Attempters tended to exhibit more obsessoid personalities than the comparison group. High-lethality attempters were the most obsessoid of all. Scores on the Levine-Pilowsky Depression Questionnaire correlated significantly but weakly in a negative way with the HOQ scores, indicating increasing depression associated with an increasingly obsessoid personality dimension. Scores on both questionnaires correlated significantly with age, but the association between the two measures remained when age was controlled for.

Patients in this study who had attempted suicide appeared to be more obsessoid than comparison subjects. The findings fail to support the clinical view that young women who attempt suicide exhibit

Br. J. Psychiatry 138:141–146, February 1981.

marked hysterical traits. Clinicians may have considered these subjects to be hysterical because of the dramatic impact of attempted suicide and because of the pejorative way in which the term has been used. In addition, young women may automatically be labeled as hysterical. Caution is needed before applying a hysterical diagnosis to those who have attempted suicide.

Management of Suicidal Behavior is discussed by H. Gethin Morgan (Univ. of Bristol). A wide range of risk-taking behaviors may be associated with serious damage to self while not being consciously related to a wish for self-destruction; examples include automobile driving and chronic alcoholism. There is much evidence that conscious suicidal behavior is preventable. Most suicidal subjects contact helping agencies within weeks before death and declare their intentions in a variety of ways. They tend to be recognizably ill. Recognition of suicide risk depends on adequate interviewing technique. Empathy and nonjudgmental acceptance are important. When the patient is told that he is obviously upset or in a state of despair, he spontaneously may mention suicidal ideas. Open discussion of suicidal ideas will not implant them in a vulnerable person's mind, although an aggressive challenge is dangerous when suicide risk is present. It can be misleading to rely too much on suicide stereotypes based on averaged data, although it makes sense to take note of individual and social risk factors.

Patients who seem unwilling or unable to give reassurance about their intentions should be admitted for close observation, especially when high risk factors are present and the patient is not well known to the interviewer. With open ward care, failure of communication can lead to inadequate surveillance of high-risk patients, especially when nursing shifts change. Suicidal persons tend to become alienated from help even in the ward situation, often through difficult behavior or a failure to respond to treatment. In outpatient management, regular interviews are important. Scrupulous review of long-term psychotropic medication is essential. Failure to improve is more likely to be related to intractable situational factors than to ineffective pharmacotherapy. The value of audit techniques for helping the ward team to learn from problems encountered in the management of suicidal patients should be explored. An external chairman might review events with senior ward staff.

Fifty-Two Medical Student Suicides. Stress in medical and other professional schools has been of increasing public and institutional concern. The suicide rate for physicians appears to exceed that of nonphysicians, but little is known of suicide rates among younger physicians and medical students. Fran Pepitone-Arreola-Rockwell, Don Rockwell, and Nolan Core (Univ. of California, Davis) surveyed all 116 United States medical schools to determine how often medical

Br. J. Psychiatry 138:259–260, March 1981.
Am. J. Psychiatry 138:198–201, February 1981.

students attempt and complete suicide and seek psychiatric treatment. Responses from 96 schools yielded 52 suicides for the classes of 1974 to 1981. The annual suicide rate for male students was 15.6/ 100,000, comparable to that for the national population. The rate for female students equaled that for male, but it was three to four times that of their general population agemates. The overall annual rate of suicide for medical students was 18.4/100,000 students per year. Three fourths of suicides were committed by sophomore and junior students. Half occurred in November through January.

Further attention by medical school faculty and administration to the mental health needs of students may be necessary. Some medical schools clearly underestimate the need for psychiatric treatment, and schools in general underrecognize suicide attempts. It should be possible to devise a profile of the suicide-prone medical student and to use it in attempts at long-range prevention. The second-year medical school class is at particularly high risk of suicide. The availability of a personal clinical role model earlier in medical school has been suggested as a means of reducing stress on students. It seems to be appropriate to direct preventive and educational programs on depression and suicide at the first and especially the second years of medical school. Such programs should relate not only to cognitive content, but also to attitudinal changes, so as to overcome the help-seeking resistance of students early in medical school.

▶ ↓ Once child psychiatry's eyes were opened to the existence of depression in the prepuberal years, a considerable literature began to appear. It is now an official diagnostic category in DSM-III. Carlson and Cantwell have developed a basis for looking behind the forms of masking that can mislead clinicians about underlying affective disorders.

As an integrated part of the interest in childhood depressions, Pfeffer has reactivated the subject of suicidal preoccupation in the latency years. It had been relatively neglected for nearly 15 years. Her contribution reviews what is known about this symptom complex, including its dynamics, therapeutic approaches, and the areas still to be studied. In addition, with her collaborators she reports her own findings indicating the seriousness of this problem. Even though the actual incidence of suicide in this age group is lower than in adolescence, the children's attempts and their talk or writing about suicide indicate more or less serious underlying conflict. The children so involved have earned themselves at least a diagnostic evaluation. Pfeffer's suicidal potential scale is important in such studies as a basis for intervention.—R.S.L. ◄

Unmasking Masked Depression in Children and Adolescents. Some workers feel that most children do not express depression directly, but that its existence must be inferred from behaviors and symptoms that mask the depressive feelings. Gabrielle A. Carlson and Dennis P. Cantwell (Univ. of California at Los Angeles) examined depressive symptoms and conduct problems in 102 systematically interviewed children aged 7–17 years. One goal of the larger study was to validate the Kovac-Beck Children's Depression Inventory (CDI). Both the child and the parents were interviewed, and school performance was assessed.

Am. J. Psychiatry 137:445–449, April 1980.

Twenty-eight children were diagnosed as having affective disorder according to DSM-III. Depressive neurosis or manic-depressive psychosis was diagnosed in 11 cases. Twelve of these children were thought to have a primary depressive disorder and 16, a secondary one. Children with affective diagnoses had higher CDI scores than the others. Those with behavior disorders or anorexia nervosa alone scored much lower. Global depression ratings showed similar trends. Two thirds of the children with a diagnosis of affective disorder and behavior disorder and only one fifth of those with behavior disorder alone claimed to be unhappy. Impaired school performance did not distinguish the various groups. Depressive behavior was most prominent in the children with anorexia nervosa. Most children with primary affective disorder had behavior problems viewed by the parents as disturbing, but these were not seen as the child's major problem. More serious behavior problems were present in the children with secondary affective disorder or behavior disorder alone. The latter children rated themselves as more irritable than did those with affective disorder alone.

Depressive disorder is present in some children with hyperactivity, aggressive behavior, and some antisocial behavior, but it may be overshadowed by the behavior disturbance. These children can be detected by means of adult research diagnostic criteria. Not all children with behavior disorders or anorexia nervosa are depressed. Further follow-up is needed to determine the continuity, if any, between childhood affective disorder and adult psychopathology.

Suicidal Behavior of Children: Review With Implications for Research and Practice. Cynthia R. Pfeffer (Cornell Univ. Med. College) reviewed the environmental and psychologic factors associated with suicidal behavior in children aged 6 to 12 years. The incidence of completed suicide in this age group may be relatively low, but suicidal behavior appears to be increasing. This may be partly a function of more thorough clinical evaluations. The influence of age, sex, and ethnicity or race on suicidal behavior in latency-age children requires further study. Conflicts with the mother as the key person often form a background for a suicidal act. Empirical studies support the importance of deprivation of love or loss of significant love objects, parental depression and suicidal behavior, and parental rejection of the child.

The relation between depression and suicidal behavior in children is difficult to define because of controversy over whether depression exists in children. Depression is, however, a major correlate of suicidal behavior in children. Few studies have systematically attempted to clarify the suicidal child's concepts of death, and few have attempted to identify and correlate specific types of ego functioning in children with suicidal behavior. There appear to be similarities between the suicidal motivations of children and of adults.

Educating clinicians in the suicidal behavior of children will im-

Am. J. Psychiatry 138:154–159, February 1981.

prove early evaluation and intervention. Work with potentially suicidal children is hampered by the unfounded belief that children are unable to plan and effect a suicide attempt. The supportive role of such community resources as teachers, clergy, and police cannot be minimized. Intrapsychic and social variables that may be associated with the future risk of suicidal behavior in children should be studied prospectively. Further studies of the relation between accidents and childhood suicidal behavior also are needed. Techniques must be developed for evaluating the potential for suicidal behavior in young children seen in pediatric and psychiatric emergency services.

Suicidal Behavior in Latency-Age Children: An Outpatient Population. Previous reports have estimated that 7% to 10% of latency-age children in psychiatric outpatient care are suicidal. Cynthia R. Pfeffer, Hope R. Conte, Robert Plutchik, and Inez Jerrett (New York) evaluated 39 children, aged 6 to 12 years, in a municipal hospital psychiatric outpatient clinic for suicidal behavior. A battery of structured child suicide potential scales was administered as a supplement to the standard clinical evaluation. Suicidal behavior was defined as thoughts or actions that may lead to death or serious injury to the child.

Thirteen children (33%) exhibited suicidal ideas, threats, or attempts. Eleven of 29 boys (38%) and 2 of 10 girls (20%) were suicidal. The suicidal and nonsuicidal children did not differ in race-ethnicity, sex, or diagnoses. Acute environmental stresses were also similar in these groups. The suicidal children had greater psychomotor activity in the 6 months preceding the evaluation than the nonsuicidal group. No difference in parental psychopathology was evident, and there were no differences in marital tension, separations, or child abuse. Parents of the suicidal children had significantly more suicidal ideation than those of nonsuicidal children, but no difference in suicidal threats or attempts was noted. Suicidal children were more preoccupied with death, but there was no difference in the perception of death as permanent or temporary or in affective perceptions of death as pleasant or unpleasant. Parameters of ego function did not differ significantly in the suicidal and nonsuicidal children, and no differences in defense mechanism profiles were observed.

A much higher rate of suicidal behavior was observed among latency-age children in psychiatric outpatient care in this group than previously has been reported. This may reflect a trend paralleling the increase in completed suicides observed in adolescents. Parents of suicidal children appeared incapable of appropriately responding to their children's developmental needs. The suicidal children frequently blamed themselves for family problems and felt they were bad and in need of punishment. Fantasies of escape were prevalent. All children who are evaluated psychiatrically should be assessed for suicidal potential.

J. Am. Acad. Child Psychiatry 19:703–710, Autumn 1980.

Single-Car Road Deaths: Disguised Suicides? If many single-car, single-occupant road deaths are suicides, as is often claimed, the epidemiologic implications would be serious, because most such deaths are recorded as accidents and are excluded from the suicide rate. If they are suicides, their seasonal variation and age distribution should resemble those of suicides, and they should occur independently of road conditions. J. Jenkins and P. Sainsbury (Univ. of Surrey, Guildford England) reviewed data on single-car accidents in 1969 to 1970. There were 528 such road deaths in Great Britain in this 2-year period.

The peak time of road deaths was November, compared with April for suicides, and the seasonal distributions of the two events differed significantly. Road deaths were most common in the younger age groups, whether or not passengers were present, whereas suicides increased with age, and the age distribution of the two events differed significantly. Adverse road conditions affected all types of accidents to a similar degree.

Single-car, single-occupant road deaths differ from suicides in several respects. It appears that no large proportion of these road deaths can be viewed as suicides. Much work that imputes suicidal intent is based on extremely small samples, anecdotal evidence, or speculative argument. The present findings agree with those of Schmidt et al., who investigated 300 single-vehicle fatalities in Baltimore and found only 2.7% to be suicides. They also agree with the finding of Tabachnick et al. that the psychologic state of drivers involved in road accidents is "close to normal."

▶ [Because suicide of a family member often places a heavy burden of guilt on all the surviving family members, this bit of evidence that single-car road accidents usually are not suicides may be helpful in counseling a bereaved family.—P.G.C.] ◀

Cults and Mental Health: Clinical Conclusions. Few issues in recent years have led to as much controversy as the membership of thousands of young persons in intense fringe religious movements, or cults. Saul V. Levine (Univ. of Toronto) reviewed personal and others' experience with 453 young persons in a variety of cults. About 100 parents of cult members were interviewed, and extensive work was done with 83 ex-cult members. Many meetings and rituals were attended, and cult leaders and deprogrammers were interviewed.

It is concluded that cults do not attract more disturbed persons than do other intense, dedicated movements, but they do attract persons who experience specific painful feelings, which make them amenable to groups with simplistic solutions to the complexities and ambiguities of modern life. Cults do significantly reduce symptoms of anxiety, depression, and confusion and at times serve as a haven and even a therapeutic milieu for persons with serious psychiatric or behavior disorders. Cults may contribute to the appearance of emotional problems in ex-cultists. They may contribute to

Br. Med. J. 281:1041, Oct. 18, 1980.
Can. J. Psychiatry 26:534–539, December 1981.

cognitive and behavior patterns that cause considerable concern, though not falling strictly into psychopathologic nosology. Cults fulfill critical and basic needs of believing and belonging. Potential members are captivated through personal susceptibility and potent recruitment techniques. Cults wield great power over their "true-believing" members.

Mental health professionals should become acquainted with cults and their practices. Neither automatic acceptance of all these groups nor their absolute condemnation is indicated. A substantial number of young persons, especially those with low self-esteem, will be vulnerable to cults unless the family or society can instill in youth some degree of purpose and sense of community.

Anorexia Nervosa. Anorexia nervosa is a disorder of unknown cause that primarily affects younger women and is characterized by substantial, self-induced weight loss, psychologic disturbances, and secondary physiologic abnormalities. The incidence of anorexia nervosa in white women around the age of puberty in Western countries may be as high as 1 in 200. Arthur D. Schwabe et al. (Univ. of California, Los Angeles) reviewed the literature on the clinical features, associated menstrual abnormalities, and nutritional and psychologic aspects of anorexia nervosa.

The clinical and physiologic features of anorexia nervosa appear to result from a complex interaction among psychologic disorders, endocrine disturbances, and malnutrition. The psychologic presentation is diverse, suggesting an anorexia nervosa spectrum syndrome, with distortion of body image, weight phobia, disordered perception of hunger and satiety, and a sense of ineffectiveness being the most frequently encountered abnormalities. The diminished secretion of LH-releasing factor, release of gonadotropins, and estrogen production in anorexia nervosa reflects a disturbance in the hypothalamic-anterior pituitary-gonadal axis. However, since improved nutrition reverses most of the endocrine abnormalities, the latter are likely secondary to malnutrition rather than to hypothalamic dysfunction. The presence of hypercarotenemia in 16 of 21 patients recently studied appears to be of value in differentiating anorexia nervosa from other forms of malnutrition and weight loss. An integrated therapeutic approach, including behavior modification, family therapy, and environmental manipulation, has dramatically reduced mortality from anorexia nervosa. However, some fundamental questions remain unanswered. Do the behavioral and psychologic changes precede the clinical presentation of anorexia nervosa, and how do these changes relate to the ensuing clinical and physiologic alterations? Does critical body weight by itself determine the diminished sensitivity of the hypothalamus to gonadal feedback or, more precisely, why do some patients have persistent amenorrhea after normal body weight has been restored? What is the exact nature of the relation between cate-

Ann. Intern. Med. 94:371–381, March 1981.

cholamines and fuel mobilization in fasting? Answers to these and other questions may lead eventually to more successful management of this complex disorder.

▶ [Diagnostic criteria for anorexia nervosa include onset of illness before age 25, at least 25% weight loss with anorexia, denial that the thinness is pathologic, and no other medical or psychiatric illness that would account for the weight loss. In addition, the patient should have at least two of the following: amenorrhea, lanugo, tachycardia, emesis, episodes of overactivity or episodes of bulimia. These patients should have extensive psychiatric and medical treatment.—P.G.C.] ◀

Some Recent Observations on the Pathogenesis of Anorexia Nervosa are reviewed by Paul E. Garfinkel (Univ. of Toronto). Anorexia nervosa remains a puzzling disorder, but it appears to be a discrete entity characterized by the relentless pursuit of a thin body frame despite emaciation. Patients who diet have been distinguished from those who rely heavily on vomiting and laxative use to control their weight.

Bulimic patients are more likely to have been obese previously and to induce vomiting and misuse laxatives to lose weight. They exhibit a variety of impulse-related behaviors such as alcohol and street drug use, stealing, self-mutilation, and attempted suicide. Bulimic patients are more outgoing and sexually active than restricting patients. Their mothers often are obese. Observations suggest that a distinct subgroup of women are predisposed to development of the bulimic type of anorexia nervosa. Bulimia has regularly been found to be a poor prognostic sign in anorexia nervosa.

Social pressures that encourage slimness and dieting may encourage the expression of anorexia nervosa by predisposed persons. About 10% of normal women score in the anorexic range on a test evaluating the range of behaviors and attitudes characteristic of anorexia nervosa. Anorexic subjects have exhibited a tendency to overestimate their body size more frequently than young women of normal weight do. Body image disturbance is related to several measures of psychopathology. The disturbance is quite stable in anorexic subjects and is related to a poor prognosis. Successful psychotherapy may facilitate cognitive change, permitting the patient to adapt to refractory misperceptions of her body. Emphasis should be placed on the patient's acceptance of herself and her body, regardless of how it appears to her. Development of such a cognitive framework may be possible only if the patient trusts in herself, and this may require the formation of a trusting therapeutic relationship.

▶ [This review article by one of the leading authorities on anorexia nervosa focuses on psychologic and sociocultural factors in anorexia nervosa and bulimia nervosa. It correctly points out that the current criteria for their diagnoses are too restrictive, and that too much emphasis (especially by Russell) has been placed on body image disturbances in the pathogenesis of anorexia nervosa. Many psychobiologic disturbances occur in both, yet they remain unexplained. In fact, our understanding of the etiology and pathogenesis of anorexia and bulimia nervosa remains rudimentary. It is still impossible to disentangle which disturbances precede and which follow their

Can. J. Psychiatry 26:218–223, June 1981.

onsets. In addition, neither anorexia nor bulimia nervosa is likely to be a homogeneous disease entity.—H.W.] ◄

Family Issues in the Pathogenesis of Anorexia Nervosa are discussed by Joel Yager (Univ. of California, Los Angeles). There are wide differences of opinion regarding the role of the family in the pathogenesis of anorexia nervosa. A "typical" family is an upper middle class, highly achievement-oriented unit that values physical exercise and slimness. It is superficially healthy but excessively concerned with external appearances and with avoiding social shame. The parents experience a lack of fulfillment as a couple, and chronically depressed, they strive for other fulfillments but rigidly deny anger with anyone else. The mother becomes excessively involved with the children, and a vulnerable daughter may become more concerned with parental approval than with her own internal satisfactions. There are several limitations to this formulation, however, and methodologic shortcomings beset the literature on family studies.

Further work is needed to isolate possible genetic contributions to familial anorexia nervosa. A variety of illnesses commonly related to stress have been noted in parents of patients with anorexia nervosa. Great diversity of personality is observed in both mothers and fathers. Family systems theorists have proposed relations between family structure and anorexia nervosa, but these hypotheses remain to be critically tested. Presumptions that anorexia nervosa is caused primarily by the "anorexogenic mother" are presently losing adherents. As with many psychiatric disorders, the sickest patients usually come from the sickest families.

Biologic vulnerability with a genetic component has not been adequately ruled out. Family pedigree studies of anorexia nervosa would be helpful, as would prospective studies of children at high risk. Family assessment instruments should be applied further to anorexia nervosa. Future family-oriented research should be planned in conjunction with projects that simultaneously consider the specific vulnerabilities of the affected family member.

► [This is by far and away the most sophisticated review of the role of the family in anorexia nervosa. It points out the many fallacies in past work on this complex disorder. Many of the etiologic formulations about the role of the family are suspect because families were studied when the girl was already sick; only a heartless mother would not be involved ("enmeshed") with a daughter who was starving herself (to death). This article is also constructive, in that it points out the way for future studies.—H.W.] ◄

Depression in Anorexia Nervosa. Mood changes, especially depression, are frequent in patients with anorexia nervosa, and it has been claimed that the condition is essentially a form of depressive illness. Elke D. Eckert, Solomon C. Goldberg, Katherine A. Halmi, Regina C. Casper, and John M. Davis evaluated 105 hospitalized females with anorexia nervosa for depressive symptoms with the use of a variety of rating instruments. All met the rigid research diagnostic

Psychosom. Med. 44:43–60, March 1982.
Psychol. Med. 12:115–122, February 1982.

criteria of Feighner et al. The patients were randomized to receive cyproheptadine or placebo, as well as behavior modification; the latter was essentially an operant conditioning program with negative reinforcement of isolation and positive reinforcement of activities contingent on weight gain. All patients received individual psychotherapy and ward milieu therapy as well.

The patients as a group were somewhat more depressed than anxious neurotic patients and less depressed than depressed neurotic patients on the Hopkins Symptom Checklist. Minnesota Multiphasic Personality Inventory ratings indicated mild to moderate depression. The more depressed patients had more bizarre food habits and were more bothered by the approach of mealtimes and by eating food. They also had more of a thin ideal than the other patients and were more bothered by their self-images. The more depressed patients exhibited more denial of illness by self-report. Initial depression could not be related to the percentage of weight gain, but patients who gained more weight experienced a greater decrease in depression.

These patients were mildly to moderately depressed as a group. The more depressed patients were more likely to exhibit disturbed eating attitudes and patterns. The degree of depression is reduced, but not eliminated, over time. Patients with the most improvement in depression gain more weight. It remains unclear whether the depression is a result of emaciation, or whether weight loss is produced by depression. A study of the effects of antidepressant therapy might help to resolve this question.

▶ [A number of claims have been made that there are strong links between affective disorders and anorexia nervosa (AN). The families of AN patients are said to have an increase in affective disorders. Analogies have been drawn between some of the pathophysiologic changes in AN and depressive psychoses. But these arguments are based on analogical thinking; the differences are also striking. The depression in AN patients has not been fully described and characterized; this report begins to do so. The results indicate that the depression in this group of patients is mild. But is it really a depressive affect? Starving persons without AN are often lethargic, apathetic, and disinterested in their environments. These feelings disappear on weight recovery, as did the "depression" in the patients described in this series.—H.W.] ◄

Long-Term Outcome of Early-Onset Anorexia Nervosa: Critical Review is presented by William J. Swift (Univ. of Wisconsin). Some clinicians believe that early onset of anorexia nervosa predicts a good prognosis. Evidence from later-onset studies to support this belief is limited; most such studies have indicated that age at onset is not predictive of the long-term outcome. Review was made of 7 outcome studies focusing on an early-onset population, patients aged 11 to 15 years. Of 186 patients in these studies, 3.2% were dead at follow-up, typically of suicide and inanition. Nutritional outcomes were variable. Few of the studies reported the menstrual outcome. No mention was made of vomiting or laxative abuse at follow-up. Psychiatric symptoms were fairly common at follow-up. Psychosis was not rare in 3 of 5 studies.

J. Am. Acad. Child Psychiatry 21:38–46, January 1982.

There is insufficient evidence from long-term outcome studies to support the view that early age at onset of anorexia nervosa is associated with a good outcome. The long-term results of the present studies of early-onset cases were closely similar to those of later-onset studies. The reported psychosocial outcome was variable. More insight into this question may soon be gained because of the apparent increase in prevalence of the disorder. It is no longer necessary to wait for years to collect enough patients for a statistically sound follow-up study. It may be that more and better outcome research will show that early onset does predict a good outcome of anorexia nervosa.

▶ [Swift's review of outcome in early onset of anorexia nervosa reflects greater awareness of the existence of this challenging syndrome so that there is less reluctance to make the diagnosis early. The variable outcome indicates from one viewpoint that, as in many other clinical syndromes, the underlying psychopathology can be quite variable and at different levels of seriousness in each teenager involved. Therefore, there is no single therapeutic approach which is effective in most of these patients.—R.S.L.] ◀

Pseudoseizures: Diagnostic Evaluation. Don W. King, Brian B. Gallagher, Alice J. Murvin, Dennis B. Smith, Donald J. Marcus, Lawrence C. Hartlage, and L. Charles Ward III (Med. College of Georgia) examined the efficacy of prolonged video-EEG recording for the diagnosis of pseudoseizures. Study was made of 17 patients with episodes of questionable nature only, 16 believed to have had both epileptic seizures and episodes of uncertain nature, and 27 with a history of uncontrolled epileptic seizures. All were aged 16 and older and had had at least 2 episodes a month in the past 3 months. Video-EEG recordings were obtained for 6–8 hours on at least 3 occasions.

At least 1 episode was recorded in 33 patients; 16 had pseudoseizures, and 17 had epileptic seizures. No patient had both epileptic seizures and pseudoseizures recorded. A definitive diagnosis of questionable episodes was made in 10 patients, 2 of whom had recorded epileptic seizures and 8 of whom had recorded pseudoseizures. A definitive diagnosis of questionable episodes was made in half of the patients who were thought to have had both types of episodes. Four of them had epileptic seizures recorded, and 4 had pseudoseizures. All but 3 of the 27 patients with a history of epilepsy only had evidence of epilepsy. Four patients, 2 of whom had interictal evidence of epilepsy, had pseudoseizures recorded. Pseudoseizures tended to begin at a later age than epileptic seizures. A correct prediction by the admitting neurologist was related to the presence or absence of motor activity for pseudoseizures, but not for epileptic seizures.

Pseudoseizures occur frequently in patients evaluated for seizures or episodes of uncertain mechanism. They often are present in patients in whom they are not suspected, and the differentiation of pseudoseizures and epileptic seizures often is inaccurate. The differentiation is aided by prolonged video-EEG recording, particularly in patients with frequent episodes.

Neurology (NY) 32:18–23, January 1982.

▶ [Pseudoseizures, or hysterical seizures, have been described for centuries. They are poorly understood and a source of consternation to patients, physicians, and other observers. Their frequency is well documented in this study, but their diagnosis remains a negative one—predominantly, the absence of focal or generalized EEG changes, during or after a seizure episode, or interictal EEG abnormalities. However, subcortical abnormal EEG activity may not reveal itself by scalp recordings. The matter of pseudoseizures remains a moot one.—H.W.] ◀

▶ ↓ It is encouraging that developmental studies of adolescence continue. The investigation by Mattsson's group of the level of plasma testosterone in male delinquents puts to rest a well-worn theory that it is a major determinant in aggressive behavior. The report of the Wellesley College investigators, Koff, Rierdan, and Jacobson, adds important dimensions to the preparation of girls for menarche. Despite the adolescent girl's better intellectual understanding of menarche, unresolved earlier stages, such as her fear of body damage and giving up dependency, still need greater emphasis at this developmental point. An important crisis could be missed in the resolution of these earlier stages, as it is when menarche appears that the underlying conflicts are closer to the surface.—R.S.L. ◀

Plasma Testosterone, Aggressive Behavior, and Personality Dimensions in Young Male Delinquents. Previous reports on a relation between plasma testosterone and male aggressive behavior have often noted labile testosterone production. Åke Mattsson, Daisy Schalling, Dan Olweus, Hans Löw, and Jan Svensson attempted to relate the plasma testosterone levels of young male delinquents to several parameters of aggressive behavior, including delinquency records, self-assessments of physical and verbal aggression and other personality variables, and clinical ratings of aggression and other behavioral dimensions.

Forty male delinquents aged 14–19 years, with a mean age of 16, were studied at an institution in Sweden for serious recidivist youth offenders. They were in good general health and of at least normal intelligence. The average time of confinement was 10 months. Nineteen subjects had committed only property offenses, whereas 14 had committed assault and battery as well, and 7 had repeated assault charges and had committed armed robbery at least once.

The mean testosterone level was 587 ng/100 ml in the delinquent group, compared with 544 ng/dl in a group of boys from a normal Swedish high school, not a significant difference. The mean coefficients of variation were 23% and 15%, respectively. Individual plasma testosterone levels did not correlate with age or weight in either group. Puberal development correlated with testosterone in the nondelinquent group only. Plasma testosterone did not correlate with age at the first known offense or with the number of escapes from institutions. Subjects with more serious records tended to have higher testosterone levels than the others. Testosterone levels were related to verbal aggression and aggressive attitude scores on testing. Staff ratings of aggressiveness did not correlate significantly with mean testosterone values.

The relationships found in this study between plasma testosterone levels and behavioral and personality variables in male delinquents

J. Am. Acad. Child Psychiatry 19:476–490, Summer 1980.

were small in degree. The findings suggest that increased testosterone production in puberty is only one factor that may contribute to antisocial behavior in certain vulnerable boys with previous psychosocial and organic trauma. Longitudinal studies are needed to confirm suggestive evidence of a relation between rising testosterone production at puberty and adolescent aggressive behavior.

Personal and Interpersonal Significance of Menarche. There have been few systematic studies of the psychologic correlates of menarche. It has been suggested that menarche leads to a greater articulation of body image and an acceptance of womanhood. Elissa Koff, Jill Rierdan, and Stacy Jacobson (Wellesley College) examined the psychosocial impact of menarche in 43 girls aged 12.2 to 14.8 years, in the seventh and eighth grades of a private girls' school. Of the girls with known menarchal status, 18 identified themselves as postmenarchal and 16 as premenarchal. Their respective mean ages were 13.6 and 13.0 years. A sentence completion task structured around themes suggested by both clinical observations and theoretical considerations was used.

Postmenarchal girls described primarily negative thoughts as responses to menarche. Most reported having felt "sick," "strange," and "scared." Premenarchal girls anticipated the dismay of postmenarchal girls, but to a lesser degree. A fantasy of instant change from child to adult with the onset of menstruation was implicit in the responses of most girls in both groups. Menarche was perceived rather universally as imposing limitations such as a certain loss of freedom and an inability to be as "carefree" as before. The mother was portrayed as responding positively to being told of the event. A mutual lack of communication with the father concerning menstruation was reported and anticipated. Agonizing self-consciousness characterized many girls as they considered whether to tell their best friends about the event.

There is increasing evidence that young adolescent girls perceive and experience menarche as a primarily negative event. Menstruation, however, can be an important focus for positive developmental progress. Our culture may paint an unrealistic, ultimately counterproductive picture of menarche for adolescent girls. For menarche to function as a focus for reorganization and integration of a more mature, well-defined, positive female identity, ways must be found to ameliorate its perceived negative consequences.

Hyperventilation Syndrome in Children and Adolescents: Long-Term Follow-up. Stephen P. Herman et al. (Mayo Clinic) reviewed the records of 34 children seen during 1950–1975 in whom hyperventilation syndrome was diagnosed. Age at outset was 6–18 years, with 53% aged 13–15 years. Sex distribution was equal. Thirteen patients had chronic and acute signs and symptoms of anxiety; in 6, no associated factors were noted; in 5, the history suggested

J. Am. Acad. Child Psychiatry 20:148–158, Winter, 1981.
Pediatrics 67:183–187, February 1981.

SYMPTOMS AT TIME OF FOLLOW-UP IN 30 PATIENTS

Symptom	Patients	
	No.	%
Anxiety	16	53
Hyperventilation	12	40
Depression	11	37
Cold sweats	10	33
Headaches	10	33
Nail biting	10	33
Gastrointestinal disorders	8	27
Light-headedness	8	27
Ochlophobia	5	17
Chest pain (functional)	6	20
Necrophobia	5	17
Dry mouth	7	23
Choking sensations	5	17
Breathlessness	5	17
Palpitations	4	13
Paresthesias	4	13
Sexual difficulties	3	10
"Nervous" cough	1	3
Lip biting	1	3

marked psychopathology or a severely disturbed family situation, or both; 5 had only isolated hyperventilation related to an obvious life event; and 5 had postexertional hyperventilation. About half of the patients had a prior medical problem that often had resulted in long hospitalization. Eight had a psychiatric history preceding onset of hyperventilation.

Most children simply were reassured that they had a benign disorder. A few were advised to rebreathe into a paper bag when an epi-

Fig 24.—Pathophysiologic mechanisms of hyperventilation. (Courtesy of Herman, S. P., et al.: Pediatrics 67:183–187, February 1981. Copyright American Academy of Pediatrics 1981.)

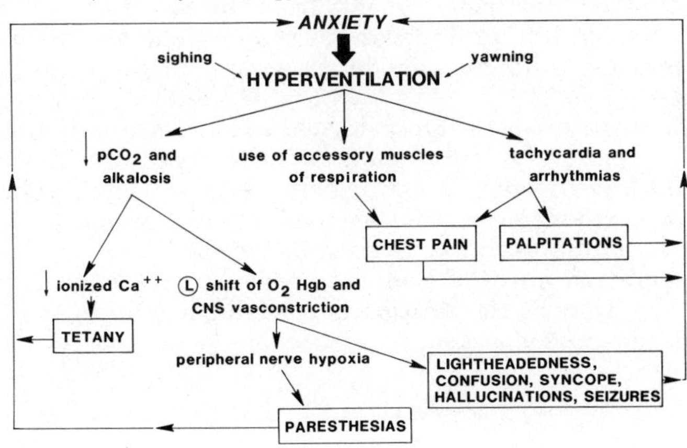

sode was felt to be coming on. Twelve of the 30 patients with follow-up had episodes of hyperventilation well into adulthood (table). The proposed pathophysiologic mechanisms of hyperventilation help explain the signs and symptoms (Fig 24). The syndrome is a signal suggesting that the child's adjustment at the personal, social, and school levels and the family situation should be investigated.

Pharmacologic therapy is not indicated without some consideration of the child's fears and anxieties. Several types of hyperventilation apparently exist. Treatment has been varied and empirical. Some children require psychiatric consultation. Where conflicts are identified in the child and family, they must be dealt with therapeutically.

▶ [When the hyperventilation syndrome is recognized, laboratory tests should be kept to a minimum, for they may augment the anxiety and increase the hyperventiia-tion.—P.G.C.] ◀

Bimanual Coordination in Adolescent Boys With Reading Retardation. Considerable disagreement continues regarding the functional relationship between motor development and specific learning disabilities. Only some young children with learning disabilities exhibit significant motor impairment; many others perform at age-appropriate levels on conventional neuromotor measures. Christian Klicpera, Peter H. Wolff, and Charles Drake examined the motor performance of 30 boys, aged 11½ to 14½ years, who were at least 1½ years delayed in reading proficiency but had psychometric intelligence values in the normal range. Fifteen boys in a nearby school for normal students served as controls. Studies were done by having the boys tap on brass touchplates in time to a metronome beat with the index fingers of either or both hands.

Retarded readers had substantially more difficulty than the control children in maintaining a steady tapping rhythm, but the deficit was limited to tasks requiring asymmetric timing commands to the two hands. Retarded readers intermittently moved both hands simultaneously for three or four taps in a sequence, as if they could not suppress unintended mirror movements from the leading to the nonleading hand. No group differences were apparent in the bimanual simultaneous or unimanual mode on testing in the symmetric tapping mode.

These findings indicate that retarded readers are impaired significantly on a relatively "pure" manual motor task and that complex motor skills reveal such motor deficits, even at adolescence, when they are not evident on testing by conventional measures. Other coordinated bimanual skills and nonmotoric measures of interhemispheric cooperation must be examined before it can be concluded that impaired hemispheric cooperation is related causally to specific reading retardation.

Dev. Med. Child. Neurol. 23:617–625, October 1981.

Boyhood Behavior Problems as Precursors of Criminality: A 15-Year Follow-up Study. Many attempts have been made to relate childhood experiences and behavior to subsequent involvement in criminal activities, but most such studies have been retrospective. Sheila Mitchell and Peter Rosa (Univ. of Stirling) reviewed data obtained in 1961 in a large-scale survey of schoolchildren in Buckinghamshire, England, and examined the subsequent convictions of those regarded by their parents and teachers as particularly troublesome. Convictions of these subjects during 15 years for indictable offenses were compared with those of a matched control group originally exhibiting "normal" behavior. The "deviator" group consisted of the 10% of boys, totaling 3,258, who had the highest deviation scores on parent and teacher questionnaires concerning behavior and health.

Deviators were significantly more likely than the comparison subjects to become offenders and to become recidivists. Parental reports of antisocial behavior such as stealing, lying, destructiveness, and wandering from home carried the worst prognosis for subsequent conviction, especially when teacher reports accorded with the parental reports. Deviators were more likely to have been convicted of theft, damage to property, violence toward persons, and fraud. They also were more likely than control subjects to appear in court on several occasions. Two of 3 boys described by their parents as having stolen on several occasions had appeared in court, and over half were recidivists. Lying, wandering, and destructive behavior also were associated strongly with subsequent conviction for theft.

Like most other studies, the present one does not provide accurate information on what the child actually does, but only on how parents and teachers see his behavior. Further research based on random samples of "normal" children is needed to identify at risk groups. Subjects seen by parents or teachers as being thieves, liars, destroyers, wanderers, or antisocial in other ways could be evaluated in more detail in a longitudinal manner.

Additional Reading

Anthony, E. J.: The paranoid adolescent as viewed through psychoanalysis. *J. Am. Psychoanal. Assoc.* 29:745, 1981.

Ballot, N. S., et al.: Anorexia nervosa: A prevalence study. *S. Afr. Med. J.* 59:992, 1981.

Bishop, D. V. M.: Comprehension of spoken, written, and signed sentences in childhood language disorders. *J. Child Psychol. Psychiatry* 23:1, 1982.

Chess, S.: Selectivity of treatment modalities. *Can. J. Psychiatry* 26:309, 1981.

Farberow, N. L.: Suicide prevention in the hospital. *Hosp. Community Psychiatry* 32:99, 1981.

J. Child. Psychol. Psychiatry 22:19–33, January 1981.

Gruber, A. R., et al.: Children who set fires: Some background and behavioral characteristics. *Am. J. Orthopsychiatry* 51:484, 1981.

Hoeffer, B.: Children's acquisition of sex role behavior in lesbian mother families. *Am. J. Orthopsychiatry* 51:536, 1981.

Johnson, D. A. W.: Studies of depressive symptoms in schizophrenia: I. The prevalence of depression and its possible causes. *Br. J. Psychiatry* 139:89, 1981.

Kellerman, J., et al.: Psychologic effects of illness in adolescence: I. Anxiety, self-esteem, and perception of control. *J. Pediatr.* 97:126, 1980.

Liberman, R. P., and Eckman, T.: Behavior therapy vs. insight-oriented therapy for repeated suicide attempters. *Arch. Gen. Psychiatry* 38:1126, 1981.

Lloyd, K. G., et al.: Biochemical evidence of dysfunction of brain neurotransmitters in the Lesch-Nyhan syndrome. *N. Engl. J. Med.* 305:1106, 1981.

Macaskill, N. D.: Therapeutic factors in group therapy with borderline patients. *Int. J. Group Psychother.* 32:61, 1982.

Manuck, S. B., et al.: Behaviorally induced cardiovascular reactivity among sons of reported hypertensive and normotensive parents. *J. Psychosom. Res.* 25:261, 1981.

McDermott, J. F., Jr.: Indications for family therapy: Question or nonquestion? *J. Am. Acad. Child Psychiatry* 20:409, 1981.

Meares, R., et al.: A sex difference in the seasonal variation of suicide rate: A single cycle for men, two cycles for women. *Br. J. Psychiatry* 138:321, 1981.

Mitchell, J. E., et al.: Frequency and duration of binge-eating episodes in patients with bulimia. *Am. J. Psychiatry* 138:835, 1981.

Mogul, K. M.: Overview: The sex of the therapist. *Am. J. Psychiatry* 139:1, 1982.

Moss, G. R., and Rick, G. R.: Overview: Applications of operant technology to behavioral disorders of adolescents. *Am. J. Psychiatry* 138:1161, 1981.

Nuttall, E. A., et al.: Patients of a public state mental health system who commit suicide. *J. Nerv. Ment. Dis.* 168:424, 1980.

Pfeffer, C. R.: The family system of suicidal children. *Am. J. Psychother.* 35:330, 1981.

Phipps-Yonas, S.: Teenage pregnancy and motherhood: Review of literature. *Am. J. Orthopsychiatry* 50:403, 1980.

Rapoport, J., et al.: Childhood obsessive-compulsive disorder. *Am. J. Psychiatry* 138:1545, 1981.

Sakinofsky, I.: Suicide in doctors and wives of doctors. *Can. Fam. Physician* 26:837, 1980.

Schachar, R., et al.: The characteristics of situationally and pervasively hyperactive children: Implications for syndrome definition. *J. Child Psychol. Psychiatry* 22:375, 1981.

Shaffer, D., and Fisher, P.: The epidemiology of suicide in children and young adolescents. *J. Am. Acad. Child Psychiatry* 20:545, 1981.

Silver, L. B.: The relationship between learning disabilities, hyperactivity, distractibility, and behavioral problems: A clinical analysis. *J. Am. Acad. Child Psychiatry* 20:385, 1981.

Singer, M. T., and Larson, D. G.: Borderline personality and the Rorschach test. *Arch. Gen. Psychiatry* 38:693, 1981.

Smith, B., and Phillips, C. J.: Age-related progress among children with severe learning difficulties. *Dev. Med. Child Neurol.* 23:465, 1981.

Stallone, F., et al: Statistical predictions of suicide in depressives. *Compr. Psychiatry* 21:381, 1980.

Stewart, M. A., and Culver, K. W.: Children who set fires: The clinical picture and a follow-up. *Br. J. Psychiatry* 140:357, 1982.
Swanson, L.: Vigilance deficit in learning-disabled children: A signal detection analysis. *J. Child Psychol. Psychiatry* 22:393, 1981.
Werkman, S., et al.: The psychologic effects of moving and living overseas. *J. Am. Acad. Child Psychiatry* 20:645, 1981.

Substance Use and Abuse

"To use or abuse: that is the question."—To paraphrase HAMLET

Substance use in many forms is part of our lives today. Unfortunately many adolescents use substances to alleviate the "pain of living." The health care professional dealing with adolescents and young adults in all walks of life must constantly have a high index of suspicion for substance use and abuse. Recurrent somatic complaints, poor school performance, peer rejection, family difficulties, and difficulty in accomplishing the psychosocial tasks of adolescence should call attention to possible substance use and/or abuse. Many articles are offered in this section dealing with use of marihuana, cigarette smoking, and alcohol as well as other types of chemicals. The article by Roush is of particular interest because it points out that nonmedicinal drug use was associated with a number of factors including a low level of religious activity and parental use of alcohol, cigarettes, and psychoactive drugs. There was also an association between nonmedicinal drug use and the recommendation of psychoactive drugs by a physician, and heavy nonmedicinal use was strongly correlated with the frequency of a physician's recommendation. The commenter cautions, however, that this report should not be interpreted that physicians have caused nonmedicinal drug use.

In the Finnish study of the role of drugs in traffic accidents, it is noted that alcohol was the chief risk factor in the largest number of traffic accidents. Women and young drivers in general were more frequently involved in accidents than other age groups. The major thrust of this report was that illness and alcohol are more important potential causes of injury from traffic accidents than are prescription drugs in general.

Depression, Demographic Dimensions, and Drug Abuse. Recent reports indicate that a significant proportion of drug abusers have depressive symptoms. Walter Dorus and Edward C. Senay (Chicago) used a multivariate approach to relate depressive symptoms to patterns of drug use and various demographic features in 432 applicants for treatment in a drug abuse program. Interviews were repeated about 4 and 8 months after intake. Depression was measured with the Beck Depression Inventory, the Hamilton Rating Scale for Depression, and the Current and Past Psychopathology Scales.

A history of opioid addiction for 2 years or longer was present in 266 cases, whereas 100 patients had used opioids for less than 2

Am. J. Psychiatry 137:699, June 1980.

years, and 66 were not opioid dependent. At intake, 46% of subjects reported moderate or high levels of depression on the Beck scale, and 29% scored in the high or moderate range of depression on the Hamilton scale. Female patients were significantly more depressed than male patients. Educational level was related inversely to Beck Scale depression levels. Less than 10% of the total variance on these scores were attributable to the substance abuse subgroup and to demographic variables. After 8 months, depression scores were significantly lower in all drug abuse subgroups. The changes were not related to the type or length of treatment received. The most important determinant of elevated depression scores at 8 months appeared to be a history of episodes of depression or anxiety.

These findings are in accord with those of other studies in which heroin addicts exhibited high levels of depressive symptoms, particularly when entering treatment. This is true of both recently addicted subjects and long-term opioid addicts. A decrease in depression scores was noted at follow-up in all substance-abusing subgroups in the present study. Tricyclic drugs should be used cautiously in this setting, in light of the substantial improvement observed in patients in and out of treatment, the potential for abuse of these drugs, and the risk of drug abusers' attempting suicide or accidentally over-dosing.

▶ [Although depression is common in substance abusers when they initially are examined, the depressive symptoms frequently improve without specific antidepressant medications while the patients are involved in drug rehabilitation programs. Clearly, such depressants should be used sparingly and only when depressive symptoms do not respond to the drug management program itself.—J.C.N.] ◀

▶ ↓ Although there have been no recent significant advances in the management of substance abuse, articles published on the subject indicate that it continues to be a serious and widespread problem in modern American society. This is documented strikingly by Pope and his colleagues in their survey of drug use by a college senior class. Of particular interest is the recent significant rise in the abuse of cocaine. Surprisingly, the drug behavior of these young men and women appeared to have little deleterious effect on their overall performance. Roush and his co-authors similarly point to the potential seriousness of drug abuse in the high school population.— J.C.N. ◀

Drug Use and Life-style Among College Undergraduates: Nine Years Later. Walters et al. observed drug use in two thirds of a senior class at a New England university but no relation between drug use and grades, athletic participation, or other "official" college activities. Harrison G. Pope, Jr., Martin Ionescu-Pioggia, and Jonathan O. Cole compared drug use in 1978 with that observed by Walters et al. in 1969 at the same institution. The questionnaire was completed by 710 of 740 seniors who received it, 507 men and 203 women. It was identical with that used in the previous study.

Many of the drug categories showed little change over the decade of review. There was no change in the proportion of students who had tried alcohol or marihuana at least once, but there was a modest rise in regular users of alcohol and a striking rise in regular users of mar-

Arch. Gen. Psychiatry 38:588–591, May 1981.

ihuana from 16% to 26%. Use of cocaine more than 10 times was reported by 8.5% of respondents, and nearly one third of subjects reported having used it at least once. Virtually no significant differences were found between drug users and nonusers with respect to grades in the first 3 years, and there was no significant relation between any category of drug use and participation in college activities. Career plans did not differ between users and nonusers. There was no evidence that drug users had more psychiatric problems. No strong relation was evident between drug use and subjective alienation. Increased heterosexual activity was characteristic of all drug users. Homosexual activity was not significantly more common in any category of users compared with nonusers.

A moderate increase in marihuana use and a dramatic rise in use of cocaine were apparent in this follow-up study of college students. Differences between drug users and nonusers, modest 9 years ago, have narrowed further. Differences in psychiatric visits and sexual activity probably are related to differences in self-concept, attitudes, and values, rather than to drug use itself.

Psychoactive Medicinal and Nonmedicinal Drug Use Among High School Students. It has been suggested that the use of medicinal and nonmedicinal psychoactive drugs might be interrelated. George C. Roush, W. Douglas Thompson, and Rosalie M. Berberian (Yale Univ.) examined correlates of nonmedicinal drug use by high school students in an urban area and attempted to determine whether such drug use is associated with physician recommendations of psychoactive drugs. A cross-sectional study was made of 1,094 high school students in the New Haven area in 1972–1973; a self-administered questionnaire was used. Only students in grades 10 through 12 were included in the survey.

Use of nonmedicinal drugs was 2 to 11 times greater among students who had had three or more recommendations of a psychoactive drug by a physician than among those with no such recommendation. The relationship was significant for cigarettes, marihuana, amphetamines, barbiturates, and heroin. The relation of cigarette, marihuana, amphetamine, and heroin use to physician recommendations appeared to be as strong as that of previously identified correlates of nonmedicinal drug use, and the findings were not attributable to artifacts of reporting. Fifteen percent of students reported physician recommendations of psychoactive drugs. Over half of those for whom amphetamines or sleeping pills were recommended were also told to take a tranquilizer. Socioeconomic status was not a potentially confounding variable in this study. Gender, race, religious activity, and parental drug-taking habits did not explain the findings. The type of physician recommendation bore little relation to the type of nonmedicinal drug use reported.

Although causal mechanisms cannot be inferred from these data,

Pediatrics 66:709–715, November 1980.

the findings may have implications for preventive programs aimed at reducing nonmedicinal drug use. If the physician is a causal factor, there might be a need for more careful patient evaluation, rigorous prescribing criteria, and nonpharmacologic approaches to neuroses.

▶ [Although there appears to be a relation between drug abuse and the prescription of medication by physicians in this group of subjects, the authors rightly refrain from making a directly causal connection, because the same underlying factors may have been responsible among the drug abusers for their initially seeking medical help and their propensity for the abuse of drugs. At the same time, these findings should make physicians cautious in prescribing medications, particularly psychoactive drugs, to adolescents without making a careful assessment of their psychologic state for possible addictive tendencies.—J.C.N.] ◀

Plasma Δ^9-Tetrahydrocannabinol Concentrations and Clinical Effects After Oral and Intravenous Administration and Smoking. A. Ohlsson, J.-E. Lindgren, A. Wahlen, S. Agurell, L. E. Hollister, and H. K. Gillespie obtained kinetic data and data on systemic availability of Δ^9-tetrahydrocannabinol (THC) after administration by three routes and evaluated clinical drug effects in 11 men aged 18 to 35 years, all of whom had had previous experience with marihuana. All were in good physical and mental health. A cigarette containing about 19 mg of THC was smoked in a way designed to obtain the maximum desired "high." Tetrahydrocannabinol was given orally in cookie form in a dose of 20 mg and intravenously in a dose of 5 mg over 2 minutes with a normal saline infusion. The studies were done at intervals of at least a week.

Plasma concentrations of THC fell rapidly after intravenous injection; the 4-hour values were 1.7 to 4.6 ng/ml. Peak plasma THC concentrations after smoking ranged from 33 to 118 ng/ml. The plasma curve after smoking paralleled the intravenous curve at about half the concentration. Peak plasma concentrations after oral ingestion of THC were 4.4 to 11 ng/ml. The range of systemic availability after oral administration was 4% to 12%. Conjunctival injection occurred later after oral ingestion than after injection or smoking. Pulse rate changes were least marked after ingestion of THC. Correlation of the plasma concentration with subjective rating of intensity of intoxication was more positive after smoking than after intravenous injection. A moderate correlation was found with oral ingestion; the "high" was delayed until the plasma concentration began to fall.

A delay in the "high" behind the rise in plasma concentration after administration of THC suggests that the brain concentration is increasing as the plasma concentration declines. Clinical effects began more slowly and lasted longer after oral ingestion of THC, but the effects occurred at much lower plasma concentrations than after smoking or intravenous injection.

▶ [Smoking marihuana is obviously an effective way of getting active drug into the body, and a lot better than the oral route.—L.C.L.] ◀

Clin. Pharmacol. Ther. 28:409–416, September 1980.

Ingestion of Hashish Oil-Filled Condoms is discussed by Michael Vowels and Patricia M. Harvey (Sydney). Ingestion of drug-filled condoms, or balloons, for purposes of concealment is a new medical problem in Australia. Short flight times from Asia permit safe delivery of drug per rectum at a convenient time after transit through customs, unless complicated by intestinal obstruction or rupture of the casing, which results in intoxication or, with more potent substances such as cocaine, possible death.

Three cases of ingestion of condoms containing hashish oil are reported. The subjects, after being apprehended, reported having ingested a large number of the condoms 36 hours before a flight from Bombay to Sydney. The subjects appeared to be normal, except for drowsiness attributed to LSD. Abdominal x-rays showed positive results in only 1 subject. Minor abdominal cramps developed, but the subjects otherwise remained well. A total of 66 intact condom packages, each containing 20–30 gm of hashish oil, was recovered from the subjects' stools.

Conservative management of these subjects was successful. No deaths from toxicity after cannabis ingestion have been described. Drug-filled condoms usually traverse the normal gastrointestinal tract uneventfully. Nonintervention is advisable, however, only when the ingested drug is known to be cannabis. The presence of more potent substances such as cocaine calls for operative management, as does intestinal obstruction. Ingestion of cocaine-containing condoms or balloons may be fatal if rupture occurs. Endoscopy is considered a risky procedure. Radiologic examination may be helpful, but characteristic appearances may not be observed.

▶ [Airport clientele sometimes present baffling diagnostic or therapeutic challenges to physicians. The rupture of drug-filled condoms that have been swallowed for smuggling purposes can lead to either marked sedation or to excitement and convulsions, depending on the drug ingested.—L.C.L.] ◀

Long-Term Toluene Abuse. Jonathan D. Lewis, Dennis Moritz, and Linda P. Mellis (Univ. of Illinois) report 2 cases of long-term toluene abuse.

Case 1.—Man, 28, had CNS difficulty as evidenced by coarse tremors, staggering gait, and scanning speech. He had been inhaling toluene since age 14 years. He had also tried other substances including heroin, LSD, alcohol, and pills. At age 20, after 6 years of toluene abuse, his condition began to deteriorate. A tremor of the upper extremities that interfered with ability to hold objects began 8 years after the beginning of toluene abuse.

Neurologic evaluation revealed marked horizontal nystagmus, no visual field defect or optic atrophy, coarse tremors of all extremities, and a wide-based and titubant gait. Sensory examination was normal except for mildly decreased vibratory sense in lower extremities. Abdominal and left cremasteric reflexes were absent, and the finger-to-nose test showed poor coordination. The EEG revealed a moderate degree of slow wave abnormality in the temporal areas. A computerized tomography scan showed symmetrically en-

Med. J. Aust. 2:509–510, Nov. 1, 1980.
Am. J. Psychiatry 138:368–370, March 1981.

larged lateral ventricles and prominent cortical sulci. Psychologic testing revealed that the patient was mentally defective, with an IQ in the range of mental retardation.

In summary, the current degenerative brain condition of the patient superseded previous development and colored his entire personality.

CASE 2.—Man, 30, was hospitalized because of an acute psychotic episode, including religious hallucinations. He had begun sniffing glue at age 12 years. At 18, after glue sniffing, he had jumped out of a second-floor window and sustained minor injuries. At 23, he first showed signs of religious grandiosity and left home to join a religious group. At 26, he increased the frequency of glue sniffing. At 28, he was admitted to a psychiatric institution. When admitted for the most recent episode he was agitated, abusive, and suspicious. He was oriented, but his judgment and insight were impaired. Neurologic examination revealed symmetrically decreased deep tendon reflexes, slight horizontal nystagmus, moderate dysdiadochokinesia, and mildly impaired finger-to-nose testing. He was treated with antipsychotic medications and later discharged. However, he continued his glue sniffing. No follow-up could be carried out.

Most cases of toluene abuse are short-term and rarely extensive enough to cause neurologic damage. In each of the cases of long-term abuse, the patient was completely aware of increasing physical problems, which he attributed to toluene.

▶ [It is always hard to tell what is chicken and what is egg in weird folks like these patients, but toluene obviously can be bad news when it is sniffed for long periods of time.—L.C.L.] ◀

Reliability of the Toxic Screen in Drug Overdose. Joseph A. Ingelfinger, Gordon Isakson, Daniel Shine, Catherine E. Costello, and Peter Goldman evaluated laboratory reliability in detecting drugs taken by overdosed patients. Twenty consecutive patients with signs and symptoms of drug overdose were studied. Blood and urine samples were obtained soon after patients entered the emergency room. Three times the usual volume of blood was collected through a single venipuncture. The staff notified three commercial laboratories that STAT toxic screen samples were ready. Preliminary results were telephoned to the hospital within 3 to 12 hours. Written reports were mailed to the hospital within 24 hours. Samples also were analyzed by an academic research laboratory with extensive experience in identifying drugs in body fluids by gas chromatography-mass spectrometry. The directors of each laboratory were aware of the nature of the study.

Of the 20 patients, 11 were hospitalized because of overdose. Of these, 5 were admitted to the intensive care unit. Laboratory A detected no drug (except ethanol or salicylates) in 4 patients; laboratory C and the research laboratory detected no drug in 3 patients; and laboratory B detected no drug in 1 patient. Twenty-three drugs were reported as being present in the 11 patients, but all laboratories agreed on only 6 of the drugs (26%). Three laboratories agreed on 8 drugs (35%), two laboratories on 3 drugs (13%), and only one labora-

Clin. Pharmacol. Ther. 29:570–575, May 1981.

tory reported a drug as present 6 times (26%). Clinical evaluation implicated a single drug as the major cause of the overdose in 10 of the 11 patients. False positive results were obtained in 7 instances when a laboratory reported concentrations of drugs that credible patients specifically denied taking. Laboratories sometimes reported substantially different concentrations for the same specimen. The inconsistencies in laboratory results for the 9 patients discharged from the emergency room were similar to, though less striking than, those for the admitted patients.

Laboratories using advanced and sophisticated techniques of gas chromatography-mass spectrometry identify drugs contributing to overdose in only 50% to 70% of cases. Emergency qualitative and quantitative analyses of drugs in serum of overdosed patients frequently yield misleading results, and toxic screen testing, although potentially valuable, may not deserve the role it presently is given.

▶ [People who run clinical chemistry laboratories take umbrage when it is suggested that their data are imprecise or downright wrong. Although these authors did not "spike" blood with known amounts of drug, the results are nevertheless disquieting. As they put it: "If two laboratories disagree, at least one is incorrect, and when a drug is detected by three laboratories and implicated by clinical history, it seems reasonable to conclude that the one laboratory that "disagrees" is in error. By this criterion, even the research laboratory appears to have missed an occasional drug."—L.C.L.] ◀

Role of Drugs in Traffic Accidents. Therapeutic doses of several drugs impair psychomotor skills related to driving, and some drugs may potentiate the deleterious effects of others or of alcohol. Drug consumption has increased substantially in Western countries in the past 2 decades, and harmful drug effects may increasingly endanger road traffic. Risto Honkanen, Liisa Ertama, Markku Linnoila, Antti Alha, Irmeli Lukkari, Marianne Karlsson, Olli Kiviluoto, and Markku Puro (Univ. of Helsinki) examined the drug use associated with driving in Finland and the role of drugs as a risk factor in accidents. Serum specimens were obtained from 201 drivers seen at emergency departments within 6 hours after injury in a road accident and from 325 control drivers. Specimens were screened for drugs by combined thin-layer and gas chromatography. Blood alcohol concentrations were also estimated. The injured driver was considered to be responsible in about half the accidents.

Women and young drivers were more frequent in the study group than in the control group, but ages were similar. More study subjects had had a driving license for less than 2 years; 6 of these and 1 control had no license. Only the reported use of spasmolytic drugs was significantly more frequent in the study group. Only 1 patient, who had had local anesthesia for dental surgery, indicated that drug use may have played a causative role in the accident. Serum analyses showed psychotropic drugs more frequently in study subjects than in controls. The difference for diazepam was nearly significant. Fewer

Br. Med. J. 281:1309–1312, Nov. 15, 1980.

than half the patients in whom benzodiazepines were detected reported having taken these drugs. Most reported health disorders were unlikely to have affected driving. Health disorders were the likely causes of 4 accidents, anginal pain in 2 cases and epilepsy and poor vision in 1 case each. Thirty patients were intoxicated by alcohol, and 27 of them were considered to be responsible for the accident.

Illness appeared from this study to be a more important traffic hazard than drugs in general. Taking diazepam may increase the risk of being involved in a traffic accident, but alcohol was the chief risk factor in this study. Interviewing is not a reliable means of determining whether drivers have taken psychotropic drugs. Serum concentrations of many drugs decline rapidly below measurable values, thus complicating the interpretation of such determinations.

▶ [The controls in this study were not ideal. Instead of stopping vehicles at the site of accidents, the authors got their control subjects from nearby gas stations. It is disturbing that the controls differed from the patients in significant ways that may or may not account for the other differences observed. I tend to agree, nevertheless, with the conclusion that illness and alcohol are more important potential causes of injury from traffic accidents than are prescription drugs.—L.C.L.] ◀

Additional Reading

Berger, O. G.: Varicocele in adolescence. *Clin. Pediatr. (Phila.)* 19:810, 1980.

Hillbom, M., and Kaste, M.: Ethanol intoxication: A risk factor for ischemic brain infarction in adolescents and young adults. *Stroke* 12:422, 1981.

Modéer, T., et al.: Relation between tobacco consumption and oral health in Swedish schoolchildren. *Acta Odontol. Scand.* 38:223, 1980.

Rinella, V. J., and Goldstein, M. R.: Family therapy with substance abusers: Legal considerations regarding confidentiality. *J. Marital Fam. Ther.* 6:319, 1980.

Saracino, M., et al.: Epidemiology of poisoning from drug products. *Am. J. Dis. Child.* 134:763, 1980.

Sexuality and Gynecology

"The young are in character prone to desire and ready to carry any desire they may have found into action. Of bodily desires, it is the sexual to which they are most disposed to give way, and in regard to sexual desire they exercise no self-restraint."—ARISTOTLE

The issues surrounding sexuality, especially adolescent sexuality, have been present for centuries. The sexual revolution only compounded these issues in recent years. Sexually transmitted diseases, pregnancy, contraception, rape, incest, and abortion are only signs and symptoms of the basic issues of adolescent sexuality. The clinician working with this age group must be knowledgeable in these areas. This section focuses on the specific areas of adolescent sexuality and basic gynecology. Other articles on related subjects are included in the sections on Infectious Diseases and Mental Health. The articles on contraceptive agents cover the major areas of congenital anomalies and thromboembolic diseases. It is important to note here that in the adolescent population these risk factors seem to be minimal.

One article in this section is of particular interest. Accompanying Singleton's discussion of vaginal discharge in children and adolescents is a flow diagram to evaluate vaginal discharge. This is extremely important to the clinician who is trying to deal with a gynecologic problem which also may have psychosexual tones.

The article entitled "Amenorrhea: The modern office evaluation" nicely demonstrates the normal and abnormal physiologic features of menstruation. It separates the causes of amenorrhea into four anatomic compartments, and the disorders that may be associated with each compartment are noted. This should be a useful reference for the primary care physician evaluating an adolescent with amenorrhea.

Oral Contraception and Congenital Abnormalities. Pravin N. Kasan and Joan Andrews (St. David's Hosp., Cardiff) retrospectively investigated the relationship between oral contraceptives and congenital abnormalities in offspring of all women living in the city of Cardiff and the towns of Barry and Penarth in Wales who were delivered of a single child between January 1974 and June 1976. Comparison was made between those who used oral contraception in the 3 months before their last menstrual period or in early pregnancy, either by accident or by design (users, 27.3%), and those who had not taken oral contraceptives during this period (nonusers, 72.7%). It is not

Br. J. Obstet. Gynaecol. 87:545–551, July 1980.

known how long the effects last after oral contraception has been discontinued. The significance of differences in findings between users and nonusers was tested by chi-square analysis. The 20- to 29-year age group accounted for 80% of all pill users and 62% of nonusers. There were greater numbers of nonusers among women aged 16–19 years and women older than 30 years of age. In the user group there was a preponderance of women in social class III. Users also smoked more than nonusers.

There were 81 (2.83%) infants with abnormalities among users and 225 (2.95%) among nonusers. There was no significant difference in the number of infants with one or more abnormalities born to users compared with those born to nonusers. There was no significant difference in the incidence of abnormality of the gastrointestinal tract, cardiovascular system, urogenital system, bones, muscle and connective tissue, or endocrine and hematologic system, or of microcephaly or cleft palate and harelip. There was no increase in the incidence of chromosomal abnormality among users. There were 18 (0.63%) infants with neural tube defects born to users, compared with 19 (0.25%) among nonusers. This difference is statistically significant.

There was no definite evidence found that the difference in incidence of neural tube defects was due to a third factor such as maternal age, parity, social class, or smoking habit. There is a known association between lower social class and increased incidence of neural tube defect, and this study shows a preponderance of pill users in social class III. Either oral contraception has an effect, or some unidentified factor associated with social class exists. Results suggest that the use of mechanical contraception be recommended for 2 to 3 months after elective cessation of oral contraception. There is an urgent need for coordinated prospective studies of the effect of oral contraception on subsequent offspring.

▶ [These results are generally reassuring. The "user" group included both patients with recent oral contraceptive use and those with inadvertent exposure in early pregnancy. Although neural tube defects were more common in users, the overall malformation rate was not. Users differed from nonusers in several respects, including smoking habits. It is too bad that the user group was not characterized by time of exposure to oral contraceptives, i.e., that prepregnancy use was not considered separately from that during pregnancy. Most recent studies have not found an association between recent oral contraceptive use and congenital malformations. For further consideration of the issue, read on.—R.M.P.] ◀

Oral Contraceptives and the Decline in Mortality From Circulatory Disease. Richard A. Wiseman (Burgess Hill, England) and Kenneth D. MacRae (London) report that many publications have claimed that oral contraceptives (OCs) are associated with an increased risk of circulatory disease, in particular, thromboembolism, subarachnoid hemorrhage, and myocardial infarction; yet between 1962 and 1976, when OCs became widely used in the United Kingdom, death rates from circulatory disease in women of reproductive

Fertil. Steril. 35:277–283, March 1981.

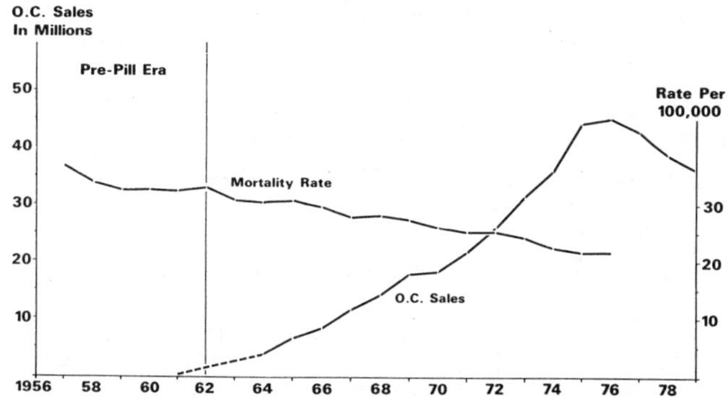

Fig 25.—All circulatory disease. Mortality in women per 100,000 population in England and Wales, aged 15–44 years inclusive. (Courtesy of Wiseman, R. A., and MacRae, K. D.: Fertil. Steril. 35:277–283, March 1981.)

age fell steadily, by 34% (Figs 25 and 26). This decreased mortality was greater in young women than in men of comparable age and did not occur in older women. The mortality attributable to nonrheumatic circulatory disease for the 4 or 5 years before the introduction of the pill was fairly static.

These data tend strongly to refute the belief that OCs are causative of circulatory disease. A plausible mechanism explaining a direct protective effect of OCs is that increased high-density lipoprotein cholesterol levels are protective against coronary heart disease; estrogens have been reported to increase such levels, whereas progestogens tend to decrease them. All the early combined OCs were estrogen-dominated; only in 1973 was a low-estrogen OC introduced. If this hypothesis is correct, a gradual removal of the protective effect might be seen in the future.

It was concluded that OCs could not be completely responsible for

Fig 26.—Cerebrovascular *(CVD)* and ischemic heart disease *(IHD)*. Mortality in women per 100,000 population in England and Wales, aged 15–44 years inclusive. (Courtesy of Wiseman, R. A., and MacRae, K. D.: Fertil. Steril. 35:277–283, March 1981.)

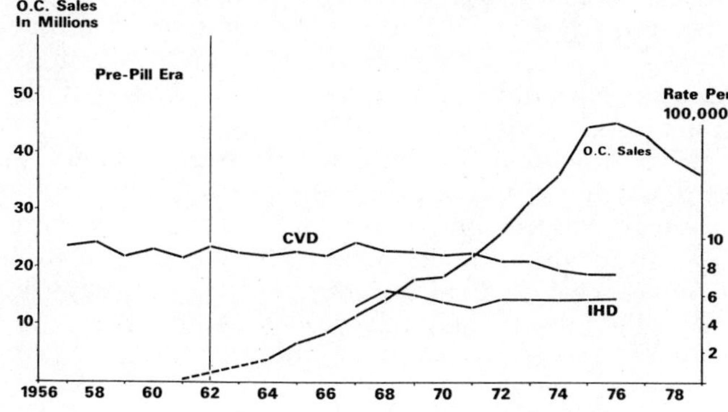

the decreased mortality, although a partial protective effect could not be ruled out. The findings on circulatory mortality are not confined to the United Kingdom. It is suggested that when mortality trends are opposed to results of case-control or cohort studies, doubts are cast on the conclusions about causal relationships.

▶ [Because of several case-control epidemiologic studies, there is a general view that oral contraceptives predispose a patient to thromboembolism, ischemic heart disease, and perhaps to stroke as well (the latter issue is confused by an association in some, but not all, studies with subarachnoid hemorrhage rather than with thrombosis). If that general view reflects reality, one might predict an increase in cardiovascular mortality in a population of women in association with the introduction of oral contraceptives on a large scale. Not so, according to this report. The declining incidence of rheumatic heart disease largely explains the falling mortality rate, but deaths from those conditions allegedly associated with an increased risk in oral contraceptive users have not increased despite the use of oral contraceptives by one third of British women of reproductive age. Other factors are probably operative here, and this death certificate study should not be regarded as the final word; however, these results may make oral contraceptive users and their gynecologists a little more comfortable.—R.M.P.] ◀

DES Story: Review and Report. Diethylstilbestrol (DES) was used for many years to reduce abortions, prematurity, postmaturity, and toxemia, although controlled studies failed to show its effectiveness. The first report of clear cell adenocarcinoma of the vagina in a daughter of a DES-exposed mother appeared in 1966, and more than 400 such cancers have now been registered. Mahmood Yoonessi, Daniel A. Mariniello, Wanda S. Wieckowska, Marieta G. Angtuaco, and Patrick Diesfeld (SUNY at Buffalo) reviewed the findings in 217 patients believed to have been exposed to DES in utero. Most were aged 20 to 29 years. The gross changes included cervicovaginal hood in 20%, adenosis in 8.2%, hood and cockscomb in 12%, hood and adenosis in 3.6%, and cockscomb with or without adenosis in 13%, and 1 case of adenosis and pseudopolyp. There was no gross abnormality in 12.4%. Three patients had Papanicolaou class III smears. Vaginal adenosis was confirmed histologically in 14% of cases. Reviewers confirmed only 25 cases of true dysplasia; 8 were severe. Three of 7 hysterosalpingograms showed hypoplastic uterus; 1 of these had a bicornuate appearance.

Gross and microscopic vaginocervical changes have been observed with variable frequency in DES-exposed daughters. Vaginal and cervical adenocarcinomas have been observed in an approximate ratio of 7:3. Examinations should begin at age 14, or earlier if the patient has symptoms or is menstruating. The estimated risk of clear cell vaginal or cervical adenocarcinoma in DES-exposed daughters is 0.4 to 1.4/1,000. Peak incidence is at age 19 years. Meticulous examination of the entire vagina and cervix is necessary. Elevated serum cathepsin B activity offers hope for earlier detection of these lesions and their recurrences. Radical surgery and radiotherapy have been about equally effective in the early stages. Some recurrent or meta-

N.Y. State J. Med. 81:195–198, February 1981.

static cases have responded partially to chemotherapy, especially when it has been combined with radiotherapy. An increased rate of upper genital tract anomalies has been reported in DES-exposed daughters, but an increased rate of cervicovaginal intraepithelial neoplasia has not been proved.

▶ [The DES story should make all of us humble about our ability to predict the long-term effects of drugs. Prolonged follow-up of everyone exposed to a new drug is manifestly impossible. Animal studies might also have a poor yield or be misleading. How can these risks be reduced when they are so long in becoming evident?—L.E.H.] ◀

Evolution of Diethylstilbestrol-Associated Genital Tract Lesions. Colposcopy is valuable in defining the type, location, and extent of mucosal changes in the cervicovaginal hood (CVH) and vagina in women exposed to diethylstilbestrol (DES). However, there is little information in the literature regarding the stability of these mucosal abnormalities over time. To determine the evolution of the colposcopic manifestations of adenosis involving the CVH and the vagina, Louis Burke et al. (Boston) conducted a long-term follow-up study of 173 women who had been exposed to DES. Changes in colposcopic appearances were correlated with the histopathologic findings.

At initial examination, colposcopic abnormalities of the CVH and vagina were seen in 95.1% and 87.9% of the women, respectively. The most common abnormality was white epithelium, followed by mosaic and columnar patterns. Multiple patterns were seen in 44.4% of abnormal CVHs and in 29.0% of abnormal vaginas. The extent of the lesions was greater in the CVH than in the vagina. Histopathologic analysis revealed either adenosis with variable amounts of squamous metaplasia or squamous nodules consistent with complete metaplasia of adenosis in 98.4% of the CVH biopsy specimens and 92.6% of the vaginal biopsy specimens. Among women followed up 1 year or less, colposcopic examination revealed a changed appearance in 25% of those with CVH columnar epithelium and in none of those with vaginal columnar epithelium. However, among those followed up more than 3 years, 81.8% with CVH columnar epithelium and 100% with vaginal columnar epithelium showed a changed pattern. Most of the changes were to grade I white epithelium (Fig 27). Progression to a different pattern was observed in 3.3% of the women with a CVH mosaic pattern and in 30.4% of those with vaginal mosaic lesions. All of the changes were either to grade I white epithelium or normal-appearing mucosa. As with the pattern of columnar epithelial changes, the frequency of change was related to the duration of observation. In 31.2% of women with CVH white epithelium and 44.4% of those with vaginal white epithelium followed up for more than 3 years, progression to completely normal mucosa was usually observed.

The results show that adenosis is a dynamic lesion that progressively evolves into squamous metaplasia over time. Conversion to

Obstet. Gynecol. 57:79–84, January 1981.

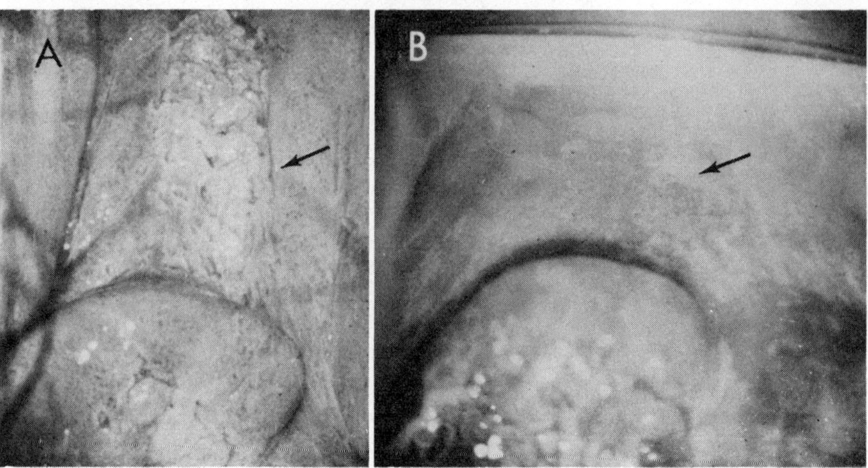

Fig 27.—A, large triangular-shaped area of columnar epithelium in anterior part of vagina is present at initial examination. **B,** follow-up examination at 24 months. The columnar epithelium has been replaced by grade I white epithelium. (Courtesy of Burke, L., et al.: Obstet. Gynecol. 57:79–84, January 1981.)

white epithelium reflects a maturation of the squamous metaplasia, whereas conversion to a normal appearance indicates development of normally glycogenated mucosa. In this study, only 1 patient exhibited squamous cell dysplasia. There were no instances of glandular dysplasia or of carcinoma.

▶ [Diethylstilbestrol (DES) exposure during pregnancy has been studied quite intensively in the past 5 to 6 years. There is now some evidence that DES exposure may not carry as serious a prognosis as was once thought. Clear cell adenocarcinoma of the cervix or vagina is not an invariable consequence of the DES-exposed environment. This article shows that with observation over time, the DES-associated lesions are labile and tend to decrease in extent; in fact, they even may disappear eventually. The final result of remodeling of the cervix is a smooth, contoured cervix with a metaplastic transformation zone and minimal, if any, evidence of previous extensive ectopy. Because the lesion is prone to self-eradication over time, DES-exposed patients should have continued, close follow-up with colposcopic evaluation rather than surgical intervention. Women exposed to DES probably have no greater incidence of squamous dysplasia than non-DES-exposed populations.

In September 1981, a communique from the National Cancer Program appeared offering updated information for physicians about DES exposure. In 1981, DES-exposed daughters and sons ranged in age from the preteens to the late 30s. The mothers of these children were in their late 20s to 60s. It will take more years, perhaps the next decade, to obtain complete and satisfactory answers to all questions regarding the extent of cancer rates and risks and problems of reproduction in DES-exposed offspring. The National Cancer Institute has published booklets, which are free of charge, entitled, "Prenatal Diethylstilbestrol (DES) Exposure: Recommendations of the Diethylstilbestrol Adenosis Project for Identification and Management of Exposed Individuals," and "Questions and Answers about DES Exposure." Also available is a patient education public-alert brochure entitled, "Were You or Your Daughter or Son Born After 1940?" The publications may be obtained from the Office of Cancer Communications, Building 31, Room 10 A-21, Department SC, 9000 Rockville Pike, Bethesda, Maryland 20205.—C.E.D.] ◀

Vaginal Discharge in Children and Adolescents: Evolution and Management; Review. Alice Faye Singleton (Univ. of California, Los Angeles) categorizes patients with vaginal discharge as prepuberal or postpuberal and in the prepuberal group distinguishes physiologic causes, gonococcal infections, and nongonococcal infections, some of which may be associated with foreign body or pinworm infestations.

At birth, because of placental hormone stimulation, the infant vagina is hypertrophied. Desquamation of squamous epithelial cells and mucus from the stimulated cervix accounts for a neonatal physiologic discharge. As hormone effects diminish, endometrial shedding and possibly vaginal bleeding may occur within the first 2 weeks.

Prepuberal girls show vaginal discharge in association with vulvovaginitis, exocervicitis, or both. Their anatomy, neutral to alkaline vaginal pH, and hygienic habits make them particularly susceptible to vulvovaginitis. In prepuberal gonococcal infections, sexual abuse must always be ruled out. Diagnosis and treatment are outlined in Figure 28. With the onset of cyclic ovarian activity preceding menarche, physiologic discharge results from desquamated vaginal cells and cervical secretions. Treatment consists of reassurance, use of frequently changed, loose, cotton panties, and use of talcum powder. The condition improves in several years.

In the postpuberal group, there are three established causes of vaginitis (*Trichomonas vaginalis, Candida albicans,* and *Hemophilus vaginalis*) and three established causes of cervicitis (*Neisseria gonorrhoeae, Chlamydia trachomatis,* and herpes simplex virus). Infections tend to be venereal in origin, but poor hygiene and foreign body, e.g., retained tampon, may be involved. Involvement of the endocervix, beginning after puberty, is characteristic of *C. trachomatis* infection and gonorrhea. Herpes simplex virus tends to involve the endocervix and exocervix with ulcers and inflammation. All three agents may cause asymptomatic infection. Pregnant women with herpes simplex virus infection who are near term should be evaluated for nonvaginal delivery; all infected women should have an annual Papanicolaou smear (risk of cervical dysplasia).

Sexually active postpuberal females should be counseled about methods of preventing infection, e.g., use of condoms, and avoiding pregnancy. Complete physical examination and pregnancy testing are essential.

▶ [The first obvious dictum in dealing with vaginal discharge in children and adolescents is that gynecologic examination will be necessary. Ordering treatment based on the list of symptoms without gynecologic examination is unlikely to be effective. The physician will have to modify his or her approach in the gynecologic examination to ensure comfort both physically and emotionally for the young gynecologic patient. Emans and Goldstein (*Pediatrics* 65:758, 1980) have suggested that the knee-chest position with the child assisting by pulling apart the buttocks may create a situation for an easier examination than the standard lithotomy position. Examination with the parent present may not always be advisable when sexual activity or sexual abuse is

Clin. Pediatr. 19:799–804, December 1980.

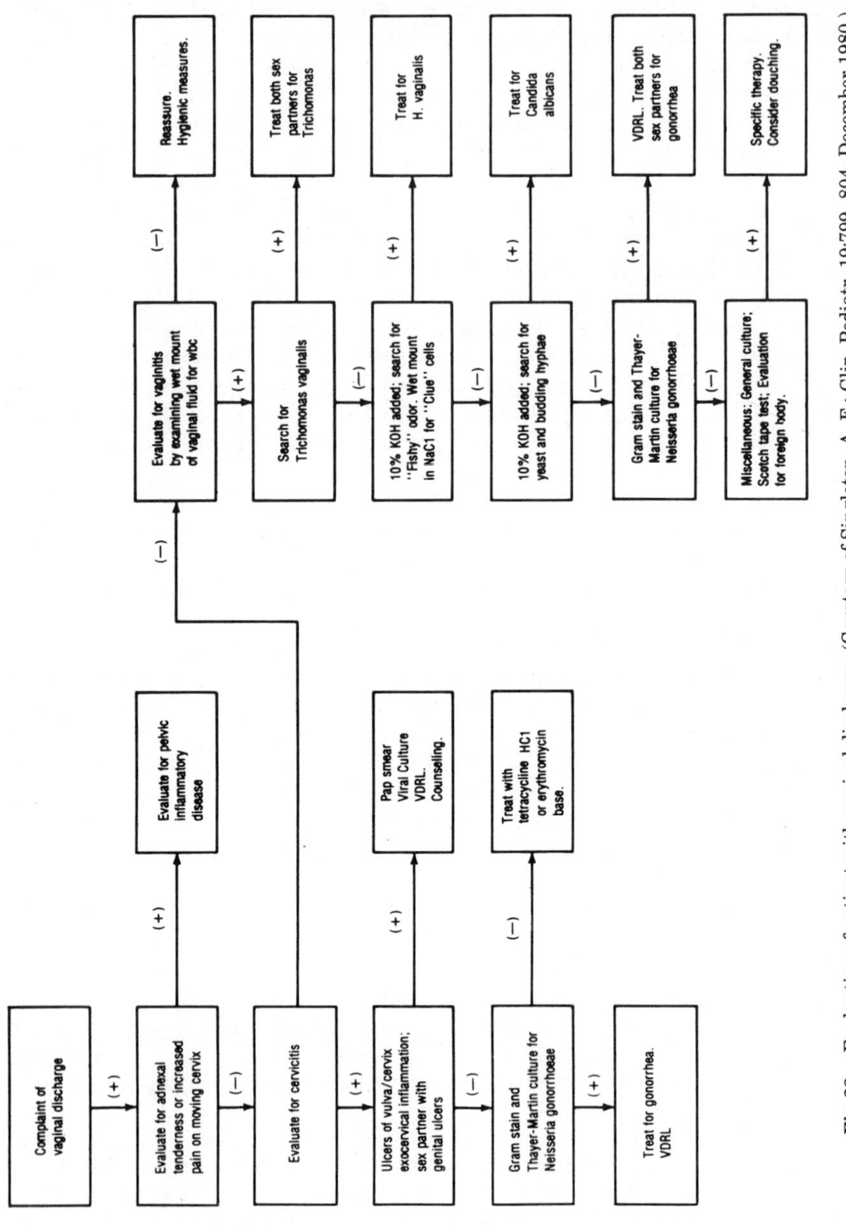

Fig 28.—Evaluation of patient with vaginal discharge. (Courtesy of Singleton, A. F.: Clin. Pediatr. 19:799–804, December 1980.)

suspected. Talking with the child alone may aid the discussion of sexual concerns or questions of the young female patient. In a very young child, some modification of equipment may have to be done. Perhaps the easiest way to investigate vaginal discharge is to adapt the handheld otoscope into a vaginoscope by using veterinary-length otic specula (Billmire et al.: *Pediatrics* 65:823, 1980). The specula, when well lubricated, are long enough and thin enough to enter the vaginal opening without trauma and enable a search for discharge for laboratory examination and to rule out the presence of a foreign body or other lesion. These instruments will serve quite nicely in lieu of the conventional and more costly pediatric vaginoscope.—C.E.D.] ◀

Amenorrhea: The Modern Office Evaluation. The normal menstrual cycle requires an exact synchronization of the endocrine glands and their target organs, as well as the hypothalamus and other CNS centers (Fig 29). Disturbed function of the hypothalamic-pituitary-gonadal axis, with or without an associated lesion, may result in amenorrhea. Marco A. Pelosi (Hahnemann Med. College of Philadelphia) discusses the nature of amenorrhea and its causes and presents an evaluative protocol for the diagnosis of primary and secondary amenorrhea (Fig 30).

To simplify the diagnostic evaluation, the causes of amenorrhea are separated into four compartments: disorders of the outflow genital tract or uterus (compartment I), disorders of the ovary (compartment II), disorders of the anterior pituitary (compartment III), and disorders of the hypothalamus and CNS (compartment IV). Physiologic,

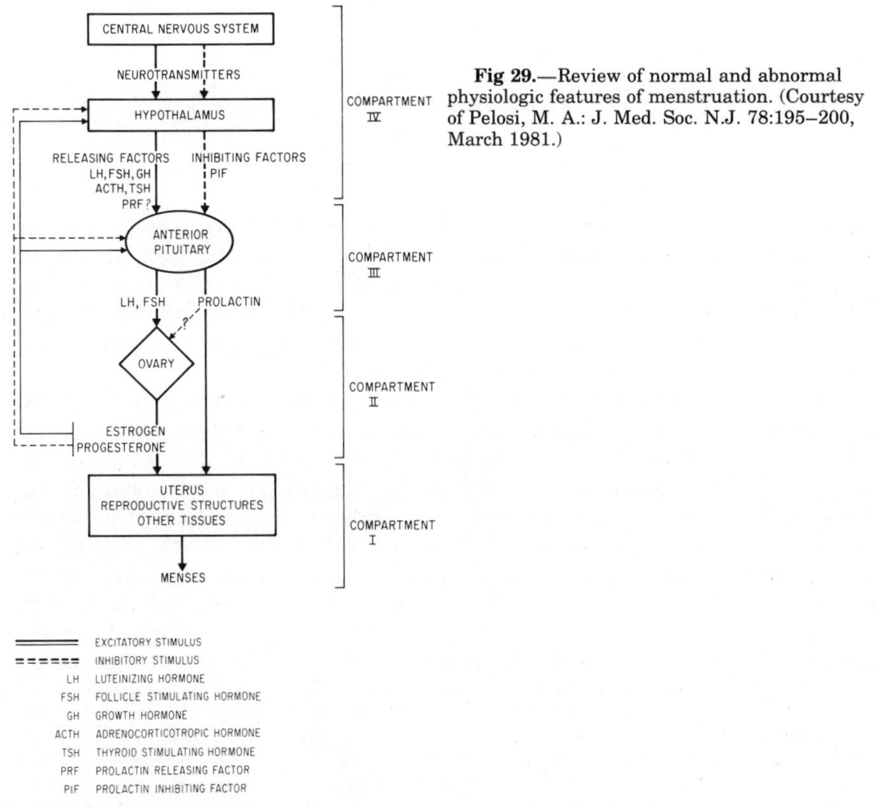

Fig 29.—Review of normal and abnormal physiologic features of menstruation. (Courtesy of Pelosi, M. A.: J. Med. Soc. N.J. 78:195–200, March 1981.)

J. Med. Soc. N.J. 78:195–200, March 1981.

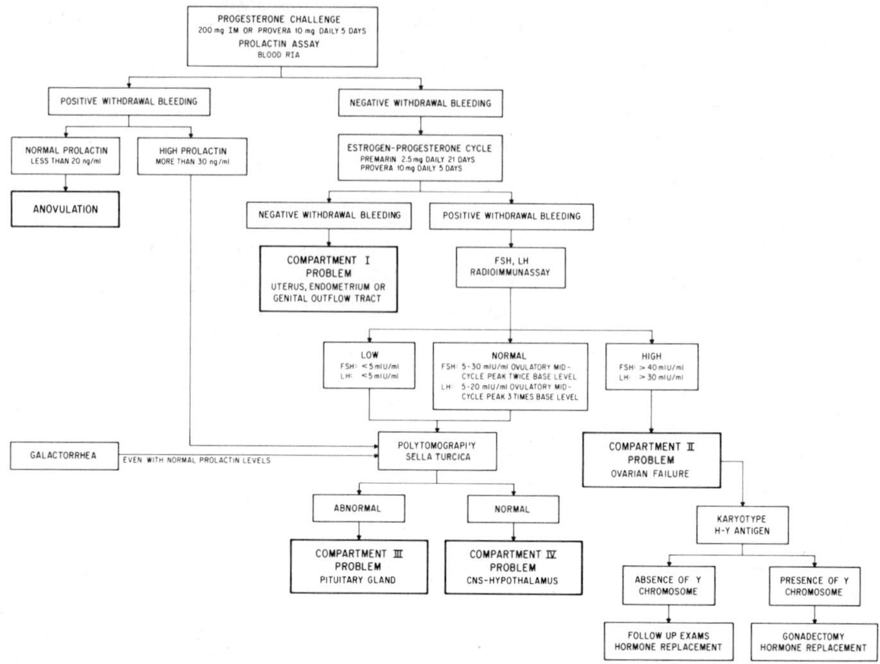

Fig 30.—Modern office workup for amenorrhea. (Courtesy of Pelosi, M. A.: J. Med. Soc. N.J. 78:195–200, March 1981.)

pharmacologic, and pathologic conditions associated with elevated prolactin levels are listed. Approximately 20% of the patients with amenorrhea have elevated prolactin levels, and prolactin-secreting adenomas occur in 65%–79% of those patients with hyperprolactinemic amenorrhea. The diagnostic protocol involves three phases: (1) progesterone challenge and prolactin assay; (2) evaluation of the estrogen-progesterone cycle; and (3) gonadotropins assay. The implications of the findings in these three phases are discussed.

Although it may not be necessary to treat every amenorrheic patient, a specific diagnosis should be attempted in each case. Automatic referral of patients to specialists and initiation of uterine bleeding without investigation of the causes of amenorrhea are considered unjustifiable. Adherence to the diagnostic protocol set forth will readily allow a diagnosis to be made by the primary care physician in most patients.

▶ [Hidden in this article is a nice discussion of the role of prolactin in menstrual disorders. Only in the past decade has this hormone been identified and researched to uncover its physiologic activity. Prolactin is under constant inhibitory control from the hypothalamus (prolactin inhibitory factor, or PIF). Removal of this control factor will lead to increased prolactin secretion. The mean basal prolactin level of normal nonpregnant, nonlactating women has been placed at 9 ± 0.5 ng. per ml. No fluctuation during the menstrual cycle seems to occur, yet a linear rise in prolactin is evident in normal pregnancy. The hormone plays a major role in mammary function and in the establishment of lactation. Excess prolactin may cause amenorrhea or galactorrhea unrelated to pregnancy or lactation. Hyperprolactinemia occurs in approximately 30% of patients with galactorrhea alone and 50% or more of those with amenorrhea and galactorrhea combined. A serum prolactin level above normal (greater than 20 ng/ml) should prompt further evaluation for the presence of a pituitary tumor, and prolactin levels greater than 260 ng in patients with amenorrhea give very strong evidence for a pituitary tumor.—C.E.D.] ◄

► ↓ For the past few years, I have expressed the concern that pelvic inflammatory disease (PID) caused by gonococci and other microorganisms was not getting the attention it warranted. In contrasting the relatively inconsequential acute gonorrhea of male patients with the serious complications in female patients, Rendtorff et al. (*J. Am. Vener. Dis. Assoc.* 1:40, 1974) have pointed out that for every 3 reported cases of gonorrhea in males, 2 females were in the hospital with complications of gonorrhea, primarily PID. Similarly, for every 18 cases of gonorrhea in males, one surgical procedure was being performed on a female because of complications of gonorrhea. The following article documents the growing problem with PID, the factors that favor its occurrence and the variety of sequelae that threaten women who have had it.—D.E.R. ◄

Incidence, Prevalence, and Trends of Acute Pelvic Inflammatory Disease and Its Consequences in Industrialized Countries. Nontuberculous infections of the pelvic organs are common in young women. In some cases, the woman's future reproductive ability will be impaired. L. Weström (Lund, Sweden) discusses the prevalence and trends of pelvic infections and their sequelae.

A lack of simple and specific diagnostic methods is the main obstacle for a true knowledge of the prevalence and trends of salpingitis, a term used here synonymously with pelvic inflammatory disease (PID). Routine use of laparoscopy on liberal clinical grounds has revealed that the commonly used clinical criteria for the diagnosis of tubal infections have a low level of accuracy (Table 1). Many patients with salpingitis have atypical symptoms and signs of disease; some patients with tubal infection have no symptoms at all.

TABLE 1.—CORRELATION BETWEEN CLINICAL CRITERIA FOR PID AND THE FINAL LAPAROSCOPIC DIAGNOSIS

Criteria for suspicion of a tubal infection	Laparoscopic diagnosis per 100 cases		Percent of all salpingitis cases
	Tubal infection	Normal tubes	
Minimum: All three of:			
Signs of genital infection			
Low abdominal pain			
Pelvic tenderness	61	39	16.1
In addition: one or			
more of: ESR > 15 mm/h			
Rectal temp > 38.0°C			
Palpable adnexal mass			
Minimum + 1	68	32	28.3
+ 2	90	10	38.7
+ 3	96	4	16.9

Am. J. Obstet. Gynecol. 138:880–892, Dec. 1, 1980.

TABLE 2.—PERCENT OF INFERTILITY AS RELATED TO NUMBER OF EPISODES OF SALPINGITIS IN WOMEN EXPOSED TO A CHANCE OF PREGNANCY

No. of infections	% Infertility postsalpingitis in age group		
	15-24 yr	25-34 yr	Total
1	9.4	19.2	11.4
2	20.9	31.0	23.1
3+	51.6	60.0	54.3

In modern industrialized countries, the annual incidence of PID in female subjects aged 15–39 years seems to be 10–13 per 1,000 females, with a peak incidence of about 20 per 1,000 women in the age group 20–24 years. Since 1960, an increase in incidence by a factor of 1.6–1.9 has been observed in the age group 20–29 years. The incidence of PID is correlated strongly with the prevalence of sexually transmitted diseases, although a fraction of the infections might be of endogenous origin.

Use of intrauterine contraceptive devices and operations for legal abortions contribute to the increase in incidence of PID. Women who have had PID have a tenfold increased risk for ectopic pregnancy, and 25% of the increase in ectopic pregnancy can be accounted for by the increase in post-PID women. Infertility after PID ranges between 5.8% and 60%, depending on severity of infection, number of infections, and age of the woman. Table 2 shows the rate of infertility in relation to the number of episodes of salpingitis in women exposed to a chance of pregnancy. In women who had had only one infection, the infertility rate increased with the severity of the inflammatory changes (Table 3). The fraction of women rendered infertile because of PID has increased by a factor of about 1.6 since 1960.

▶ [It is important to note that even if PID is treated successfully, there is a continuing

TABLE 3.—PERCENT INFERTILITY BECAUSE OF TUBAL OCCLUSION AFTER DIFFERENT DEGREES OF INFECTION IN WOMEN WITH ONE EPISODE OF SALPINGITIS AND EXPOSURE TO A CHANCE OF PREGNANCY

Inflammatory changes	% Infertility postsalpingitis in age group		
	15-24 yr	25-34 yr	Total
Mild	5.8	7.8	6.1
Moderately severe	10.8	22.0	13.4
Severe	27.3	40.0	30.0

predilection to ectopic pregnancy, infertility, chronic menstrual abnormalities, and recurrent PID (often with gram-negative anaerobes and "normal flora"). This article points out that repeated bouts of PID markedly increase the incidence of infertility (from 9.4% after one episode of PID to 51.6% after three or more episodes). The same is true for ectopic pregnancy (from 3.6% after one episode of PID to 8.7% after two or more episodes). The first problem is sad; the second is life-threatening. These data reinforce the importance of three measures to help prevent recurrence of gonococcal PID and probably PID caused by other agents that are sexually transmitted: (1) finding and treating all the patient's sexual contacts, many of whom will be asymptomatic; (2) educating the patient regarding the risks of another episode of PID; and (3) emphasizing to the patient her right to insist that her sexual partners use condoms.— D.E.R.] ◄

Follow-Up Counseling of Adolescent Rape Victims is outlined by Marianne Felice (Univ. of California at San Diego). Up to half of all rape victims are adolescents, and the adolescent, with a unique set of psychosexual developmental tasks, may be particularly vulnerable to untoward consequences. All adolescent rape victims should be given an opportunity for counseling immediately or in the future. Physicians who are not comfortable in this role should become familiar with rape victim counseling services available in the community. Unnecessary repeated descriptions of the details surrounding the event should be avoided. It is not appropriate to question the subject closely in an attempt to determine whether or not she is telling the truth.

Some adolescent rape victims may attempt suicide, though this is rare, it is important to identify these subjects early so that preventive measures can be taken. Generally the attempt is made within 1 or 2 months after the rape, in subjects who have limited support systems.

A trauma syndrome is discernible in some victims, in which a phobic phase is followed by a phase of denial about 2 or 3 months after the rape, when the subject denies that the rape bothers her anymore, and then, 6–8 months after the event, by a psychosomatic phase. This phase may present as headaches, abdominal pain, or dizzy spells, and the subject may not mention the rape episode to the examining physician.

Teenage girls who have been raped often are made to feel guilty about the assault. Girls who are raped by a family friend, neighbor, or acquaintance are particularly vulnerable to blame. The family members may try to protect the rapist rather than the victim, and boys and men in the neighborhood may treat the subject with leers and lewd comments. The physician may be able to help by aiding the adolescent in planning an appropriate response.

Additional Reading

Antonioli, D. A., et al.: Natural history of diethylstilbestrol-associated genital tract lesions: Cervical ectopy and cervicovaginal hood. *Am. J. Obstet. Gynecol.* 137:847, 1980.

Med. Aspects Hum. Sexual. 14:67–68, March 1980.

Back, D. J., et al.: Interaction of phenobarbital and other anticonvulsants with oral contraceptive steroid therapy. *Contraception* 22:495, 1980.

Bartlett, J. G.: Metronidazole. *Johns Hopkins Med. J.* 149:89, 1981.

Burkman, R. T.: Association between intrauterine device and pelvic inflammatory disease. *Obstet. Gynecol.* 57:269, 1981.

Chowdhury, V., et al.: "Escape" ovulation in women due to missing of low-dose combination oral contraceptive pills. *Contraception* 22:241, 1980.

Chvapil, M., et al.: Preliminary testing of contraceptive collagen sponge. *Obstet. Gynecol.* 56:503, 1980.

Claessens, E. A., and Cowell, C. A.: Acute adolescent menorrhagia. *Am. J. Obstet. Gynecol.* 139:227, 1981.

Crabbé, P., et al.: Injectable contraceptive synthesis: Example of international cooperation. *Science* 209:992, 1980.

Davis, J. P., et al.: Toxic shock syndrome: Epidemiologic features, recurrence, risk factors, and prevention. *N. Engl. J. Med.* 303:1429, 1980.

Dietz, C. A., and Craft, J. L.: Family dynamics of incest: A new perspective. *Soc. Casework* 61:602, 1980.

Duguid, H. L. D., et al.: *Actinomyces*-like organisms in cervical smears from women using intrauterine contraceptive devices. *Br. Med. J.* 281:534, 1980.

Felman, Y. M.: Repeal of mandated premarital tests for syphilis: Survey of state health officers. *Am. J. Public Health* 71:155, 1981.

Furgyik, S., and Åstedt, B.: Gonorrheal infection followed by an increased frequency of cervical carcinoma. *Acta Obstet. Gynecol. Scand.* 59:521, 1980.

Goette, D. K., and Odom, R. B.: Vaginal medications as a cause for varied widespread dermatitides. *Cutis* 26:406, 1980.

Goldstein, D. P., and Miler, U.: Breast masses in adolescent females. *Clin. Pediatr. (Phila.)* 21:17, 1982.

Graham, C. A., and McGrew, W. C.: Menstrual synchrony in female undergraduates living on a coeducational campus. *Psychoneuroendocrinology* 5:245, 1980.

Jick, H., et al.: Vaginal spermicides and congenital disorders. *J.A.M.A.* 245:1329, 1981.

Kaufman, D. W., et al.: Decreased risk of endometrial cancer among oral contraceptive users. *N. Engl. J. Med.* 303:1045, 1980.

Klein, J. R., and Litt, I. F.: Epidemiology of adolescent dysmenorrhea. *Pediatrics* 68:661, 1981.

Lähteenmäki, P., et al.: Return of ovulation after abortion and after discontinuation of oral contraceptives. *Fertil. Steril.* 34:246, 1980.

Mann, E. H.: Self-reported stresses of adolescent rape victims. *J. Adolesc. Health Care* 2:29, 1981.

Minkowski, W. L., et al.: Single oral dose metronidazole therapy for *Trichomonas* vaginitis in adolescents. *J. Adolesc. Health Care* 2:41, 1981.

Mukherjea, M., et al.: Long-term contraception with Depo-Provera: Clinical evaluation. *Int. J. Fertil.* 25:122, 1980.

Nilsson, G., et al.: Intrauterine contraception with levonorgestrel: A comparative randomized clinical performance study. *Lancet* 1:577, 1981.

Noble, A. D., and Letchworth, A. T.: Treatment of endometriosis: A study of medical management. *Br. J. Obstet. Gynaecol.* 87:726, 1980.

Pizzo, S. V., et al.: Fibrinolytic response and oral contraceptive-associated thromboembolism. *Contraception* 23:181, 1981.

Plymate, S. R., et al.: Obesity and its role in polycystic ovary syndrome. *J. Clin. Endocrinol. Metab.* 52:1246, 1981.

Pomeroy, J. C., et al.: Abnormal sexual behavior in prepubescent children. *Br. J. Psychiatry* 138:119, 1981.

Rice, P. A., and Goldenberg, D. L.: Clinical manifestations of disseminated infection caused by *Neisseria gonorrhoeae* are linked to differences in bactericidal reactivity of infecting strains. *Ann. Intern. Med.* 95:175, 1981.

Royal College of General Practitioners' Oral Contraception Study: Further analyses of mortality in oral contraceptive users. *Lancet* 1:541, 1981.

Sadeghi-Nejad, A., et al.: Hyperprolactinemia causing primary amenorrhea. *J. Pediatr.* 99:802, 1981.

Saltz, G. R., et al.: *Chlamydia trachomatis* cervical infections in female adolescents. *J. Pediatr.* 98:981, 1981.

Schydlower, M., et al.: Adolescents with abnormal cervical cytology. *Clin. Pediatr. (Phila.)* 20:723, 1981.

Sparks, R. A., et al.: Bacteriologic colonization of the uterine cavity: Role of tailed intrauterine contraceptive device. *Br. Med. J.* 282:1189, 1981.

Wald, A., et al.: Gastrointestinal transit: The effect of the menstrual cycle. *Gastroenterology* 80:1497, 1981.

Pregnancy

"It is said that teenage girls have babies because of unresolved Oedipal complexes. I say a teenager gets pregnant because she has sexual intercourse."—SOL GORDON, in *The New You.*

Oh, if it were only that simple! The social, medical, and obstetric aspects of this topic are mindboggling. Adolescents continue to get pregnant in large numbers despite the availability of contraceptives and sex education programs. Of special interest in this section is the article "Alternatives to adolescent pregnancy: A discussion of the contraceptive literature from 1960 to 1980." Greydanus offers the clinician a thoughtful, detailed approach to this particular problem and includes a number of interesting concepts. He notes that the mortality from pregnancy and childbirth far exceeds that for any contraceptive method that is offered. Any method selected can be replaced later if complications occur or if circumstances change. Carey's discussion of adolescent age and obstetric risk is also extremely valuable. Because preterm delivery in both whites and nonwhites is most frequent in the group aged 15 and younger, that adolescent who becomes pregnant at an earlier chronologic age is indeed at great risk. Current data indicate that for pregnant girls younger than age 15 years, risk of maternal death is 60% greater than for women out of the teen years. The articles on children of diabetic mothers and on pregnancy and cystic fibrosis are included because these conditions may be present in the adolescent who becomes pregnant.

Alternatives to Adolescent Pregnancy: A Discussion of the Contraceptive Literature From 1960 to 1980 is presented by Donald E. Greydanus (Univ. of Rochester). Coital activity among teenagers is increasing, and many would welcome whatever safe measures effectively can reduce the problem of teenage pregnancy. The mortality from pregnancy and childbirth far exceeds that for any contraceptive method. Careful matching of the individual patient with an appropriate contraceptive method will reduce associated morbidity. Any method selected may be replaced later by other contraceptive methods as the patient matures.

Oral contraception remains one of the most effective methods; it prevents pregnancy in many ways. Many laboratory tests are altered by use of the combined oral contraceptive (Table 1). Contraindications to oral contraceptive use are listed in Table 2. There is a slight risk of thromboembolic disorders in teenagers using oral contraception, and screening for risk factors is important. Use of the oral contracep-

Semin. Perinatol. 5:53–90, January 1981.

TABLE 1.—LABORATORY TESTS AFFTECTED BY ORAL CONTRACEPTIVES

A. Values which are increased (serum values, unless otherwise stated)
1. Erythrocyte sedimentation rate (sometimes the hematocrit, white blood count and platelets)
2. Serum iron and iron-binding capacity
3. Sulfobromophthalein and sometimes bilirubin
4. Serum glutamic oxaloacetic transaminase, serum glutamic pyruvic transaminase and serum gamma-glutamyl transpeptidase
5. Alkaline phosphatase
6. Clotting factors I, II, VII, VIII, IX, X and XII; also: increased antiplasmins and antiactivators of fibrinolysis
7. Triglycerides, phospholipids and high-density lipoproteins (sometimes serum cholesterol)
8. Serum Copper and ceruloplasmin
9. Increase in various binding proteins (transferrin, transcortin, thyroxine-binding Globulin)
10. Renin, angiotensin, angiotensinogin and aldosterone
11. Insulin, growth hormone and blood glucose
12. C-reactive protein
13. Globulins (alpha-1 and alpha-2)
14. Alpha-1-anti trypsin
15. Total estrogens (urine)
16. Coproporphyrin (Feces and urine) and porphobilinogen (urine)
17. Vitamin A
18. Xanthuric acid (urine)
19. Positive antinuclear antibody test and LE preparation
20. Others

B. Values which are decreased
1. Antithrombin II
2. LH and FSH
3. Pregnanediol and 17 ketosteroids
4. Folate and vitamin B_{12}
5. Glucose tolerance
6. Ascorbic acid
7. Zinc and magnesium
8. T-3 resin uptake
9. Fibrinolytic activity
10. Haptoglobulin
11. Cholinesterase
12. Others

TABLE 2.—CONTRAINDICATIONS TO ORAL CONTRACEPTIVES

A. Absolute Contraindications
1. History of thromboembolism or thrombotic disease
2. Active acute or chronic liver disease
3. Pregnancy
4. Undiagnosed uterine bleeding
5. Breast cancer
6. Estrogen-depended neoplasia

B. Relative Contraindications
1. Pituitary dysfunction
2. Lactation
3. Fibrocystic breast disease
4. Potential drug interactions
5. Heavy cigarette smoking (over 20/day)
6. Hypertension
7. Hyperlipidemia
8. Diabetes mellitus
9. Epilepsy
10. Sickle cell anemia (other hemoglobinopathies)
11. Uterine leiomyomata
12. Cholelithiasis or cholecystitis
13. History of jaundice of pregnancy
14. Migraine headaches
15. Raynaud's disease
16. Collagen vascular disorder (as rheumatoid arthritis or SLE)
17. Oligomenorrhea
18. Pseudotumor cerebri
19. Chorea
20. Porphyria
21. Bleeding diatheses
22. Major organ disease (heart, lungs, renal)
23. Retinal disorders
24. Depression
25. Severe, chronic monilial vaginitis
26. Various, dermatological problems (as erythema nodosum, melasma, others)
27. Otosclerosis
28. Hemolytic-uremic syndrome
29. Inflammatory bowel disease
30. Others

tive should be avoided or discontinued if the teenage patient has severe migraines or other risk factors for vascular phenomena. Oligomenorrhea need not absolutely contraindicate use of the pill, but a careful search for underlying causes is indicated. There is no evidence that oral contraception causes cancer. Often, oral contraception can be used for a brief time until the patient is psychologically mature enough to accept an alternative. Use of a "low-dose" pill or a "micropill" appears to reduce the risk of thromboembolic phenomena. The risks of hypertension and metabolic changes are less with use of the minipill.

The intrauterine device has a definite role in a limited number of adolescents who have limited risk for sexually transmitted diseases and who will cooperate with careful follow-up. Barrier methods should be the first choice for teenage patients. The condom, with or without vaginal contraceptives, and the diaphragm with vaginal contraceptives can be very effective, safe methods. Unfortunately, most teenagers lack the preparation, skill, emotional development, and self-intimacy needed for successful use of barrier methods. Injectable contraceptives may be considered when the combined oral contraceptive is contraindicated and for some intellectually impaired or mentally ill teenagers.

▶ [Through the help of the knowledgeable and sympathetic clinician, teenagers can choose to avoid pregnancy by selecting a contraceptive method that best fits their needs. Although the oral contraceptive remains the most popular method among teenagers, and it is certainly a very effective method, the physician should stress the safety and efficacy of the barrier methods for the mature and motivated teenager. Also, the use of the condom for contraception will provide the additional benefit of protection against sexually transmitted diseases.

Selecting a contraceptive for a teenager is discussed by Lopez (*Drug Therapy*, p. 92, August 1981). The statistics quoted in this article document the rising incidence of adolescent pregnancy in the United States: 55% of teenage girls younger than age 19 have had sexual intercourse; 1 in every 10 American teenagers will become pregnant before age 18; and about one million 15- to 19-year-olds will become pregnant each year, of whom 600,000 will decide to give birth. One useful feature of this article is patient education instructions for teenagers on how to use various contraceptive regimens.

Contraceptive counseling for teenagers is described in a stepwise fashion by Goldstein and Marean (*Med. Aspect. Human Sexual.* 14:23, 1980). It is suggested that teenagers pass through three behavioral phases in their sexual development: Phase 1 is that of sexual interest and is the first and earliest stage of awareness of sexual attributes of the opposite sex. Phase 2, labeled "sexual activity," is that of being together—dating, touching, kissing, petting, and other activity short of sexual intercourse. Phase 3, sexual intercourse, may occur with or without preparation or precaution and represents the most advanced stage of sexual exploration. Although a teenager usually will work through these stages over a span of years, it can all take place within a matter of months. Physicians should attempt to categorize which stage their teenage patients are in and tailor their counseling approach to the patient's developmental phase. Teenagers are afraid of going to the doctor, afraid of asking for contraceptives at the drug store, and afraid and embarassed to ask questions about sexuality. When the moment for intervention arises, the physician should proceed through interview, examination, and counseling. End with assurance that the staff will be available at any time to discuss problems as they arise and schedule a follow-up visit within 1 to 3 months to handle any concerns that have arisen since the contraceptive method of choice was prescribed. Confidentiality of the patient-physician relationship should be preserved regardless of patient age. It is still advisable to suggest to the teenager that he or she may be confronted by a parent who accidentally discovers the sexual activity or that some medical complication could arise from contraception or sexual activity that would later require parental assistance. The physician can reassure the patient of strict confidentiality while urging the teenager to deal with the parental knowledge issue.—C.E.D.] ◄

Adolescent Age and Obstetric Risk are discussed by William Baldwin Carey et al. Early childbearing has serious demographic and socioeconomic implications for both young parents and society as a whole. Current data indicate that, for pregnant girls younger than age 15 years, the risk of maternal death is 60% greater than for women in their early 20s. Adolescent pregnancy places the mother and infant at social and educational disadvantages that no doubt contribute to higher infant mortality and repeated pregnancies. Prematurity is a major area of concern. Preterm delivery in both white and nonwhite girls is most frequent in the group aged 15 and younger. Pregnancy-induced hypertension is noted in 15%–40% of teenage pregnancies. Iron, vitamin A, and calcium are the nutrients most often deficient in the diets of normal adolescents, and dietary adjustment or supplementation is necessary (table).

The young adolescent needs to accept her appearance, and the appearances of pregnancy may lead to extreme feelings of low esteem. Failure to participate in or comply with proper antenatal care and parenting may result. The decision-making that follows pregnancy may affect the adolescent's mental health. A poor fetal outcome can

ESTIMATES OF DIETARY NEEDS FOR PREGNANT TEENAGERS

Nutrients	Units	Adolescents	During Pregnancy
Calories	KCAL	2400	2700
Protein	g	44	76–100
Vitamin A	IU	4000	5000
Vitamin D	IU	400	400
Ascorbic acid	mg	45	60
Vitamin E	IU	12	15
Folacin	mg	0.4	0.8
Niacin	mg	16	20
Riboflavin	mg	1.3	1.5
Thiamine	mg	1.2	1.3
Vitamin B_6	mg	1.6	2.5
Vitamin B_{12}	mg	3.0	4.0
Calcium	mg	1200	1500
Phosphorus	mg	1200	1200
Iodine	mg	115	125
Iron	mg	18	30–60
Magnesium	mg	300	450
Zinc	mg	15	20

Semin. Perinatol. 5:9–17, January 1981.

be associated with the use of both tobacco and alcohol, as well as drug addiction. The teratogenic potential of marihuana in human beings is unclear. Phencyclidine also is being assessed in this context. Adolescents have a high rate of gonorrhea, and genital herpes is an increasingly common infection in the young.

Pregnant adolescents require a wide range of quality prenatal health care services. Better medical antepartum and intrapartum surveillance would provide an earlier assessment of developing obstetric problems and more effective management. Prenatal classes in parenting also are important.

▶ [Increasing sexual encounters by today's teenagers have led to a substantial increase in adolescent pregnancy. It is reported that 1 in 5 girls has intercourse by age 16 and that 1 in 10 becomes pregnant before age 17. The primary complications of teenage pregnancy are preeclampsia and delivery of low birth weight infants, according to the Committee on Adolescence of the American Academy of Pediatrics (*Pediatrics* 63:795, 1979). Naeye (ibid. 67:146, 1981) studied the consequences of fetal-maternal competition for nutrients in teenage and preteenage pregnancies. In this series, 5% of the urines of mothers aged 10–14 years had 2^+ or greater acetone, versus only 2% of the urines of mothers aged 17–32 years (P <.001). Acetonuria has been shown to be a marker for high perinatal mortality in undernourished gestations, and it correlates with a high perinatal mortality in this study. If growth-retarded newborns of very young mothers survived, they overcame the growth retardation during later childhood.

The entire issue of *Seminars in Perinatology,* vol. 5, no. 1, is devoted to adolescent pregnancy, and it is a good one-night reading assignment for family physicians who deliver adolescent health care.—C.E.D.] ◀

Incidence, Trends, and Risks of Ectopic Pregnancy in a Population of Women were analyzed by L. Weström, L. Ph. Bengtsson, and P.-A. Mårdh (Univ. of Lund). In women in Lund, Sweden, aged 15–39 years, the rate of tubal ectopic pregnancy per 1,000 diagnosed conceptions increased from 5.8 during 1960–1964 to 11.1 during 1975–1979. The mean annual incidence of ectopic pregnancy per 1,000 women increased from 0.6 to 1.2 during the same period. The increase was most pronounced in women aged 20–29. The numbers of ectopic pregnancies per 1,000 diagnosed conceptions increased with increasing age of the women (4.1 in teenagers, 6.9 in those aged 20–29, 12.9 in those aged 30–39). From 1970 on, the mean annual incidence of ectopic pregnancy per 1,000 women in those aged 20–29 became higher than in those aged 30–39.

Intrauterine contraceptive devices (IUCDs) were not used in Sweden before 1965. Among 20- to 29-year-old sexually active women at risk of pregnancy who had never had acute salpingitis, the rates of ectopic pregnancy per 100 woman-years were the same (0.3) in those who did not use contraceptives as in those using nonmedicated or copper-medicated IUCDs. The risk of an ectopic pregnancy increased sixfold to sevenfold after acute salpingitis. It was calculated that if the 20- to 29-year-olds who used IUCDs had used oral contraceptives instead, the increase from 4.6 to 9.7 in ectopic pregnancy rate per 1,000 conceptions from 1960 to 1979 would have stopped at 5.0.

Br. Med. J. 282:15–18, Jan. 3, 1981.

The findings confirm the increased risk of ectopic pregnancy after salpingitis. The use of IUCDs—at least among women aged 20–29 years—seems to account for a substantial proportion of the increased rate of ectopic pregnancy in Lund during the past 2 decades.

▶ [A number of reports have called attention to an apparent increase in the frequency of tubal pregnancy during the past 20 or 25 years. This one from Sweden is particularly important because of the well-defined nature of the population. Except for patients with early spontaneous abortions who do not seek medical attention, all pregnancies in the city of Lund are under the care of the authors' clinics. Thus, the virtual doubling of the total ectopic pregnancy rate (5.8 to 11.1 per 1,000 conceptions) from 1960–1964 to 1975–1979 is undoubtedly real. The data show a close correlation with both salpingitis and the use of intrauterine contraceptive devices, leading the authors to conclude that the intrauterine contraceptive device is at least partially responsible for the increase in tubal gestations.—R.M.P.] ◀

β-Human Chorionic Gonadotropin as a Diagnostic Aid for Suspected Ectopic Pregnancy. Early diagnosis of ectopic pregnancy is complicated by the fact that no single laboratory test is sufficient for differential diagnosis. Radioimmunoassay (RIA) of the serum β-subunit of human chorionic gonadotropin (β-hCG) is recognized as a rapid and unequivocal test for assessing trophoblastic viability. Ronald O. Schwartz and David L. Di Pietro (Vanderbilt Univ. Med. Center, Nashville, Tenn.) evaluated the results of RIA determination of β-hCG in a retrospective study of the hospital records of 234 patients who were tested because of signs and symptoms suggestive of ectopic pregnancy.

One hundred eighty-eight patients (80%) had negative serum β-hCG tests (less than 1 ng/ml); no patient was subsequently found to have an intrauterine or ectopic pregnancy. The most common symptoms were abdominal pain (91%), amenorrhea (76%), irregular bleeding (68%), and adnexal mass (55%). A final diagnosis of ectopic pregnancy was made in 22 patients. All had positive serum β-hCG assays, although 10 did not show the classic triad of symptoms (pain, uterine bleeding, and adnexal mass). There were no false negative β-hCG

SERUM β-hCG AND URINE PREGNANCY TESTS FOR PATIENTS
WITH SUSPECTED ECTOPIC PREGNANCY

No. of patients (N = 86)	Urine pregnancy test*	Serum β-hCG (positive > 1 ng/ml)	Urine test false positive or negative (%)
39	Negative	Negative	
14	Positive	Positive	
14	Negative	Positive	15
19	Positive	Negative	22

*Tests were performed in the hospital clinical laboratories (2-hour tube tests) or in the emergency room (2-minute slide tests).

Obstet. Gynecol. 56:197–203, August 1980.

RIA results, whereas there were 15 false negative and 22 false positive urine pregnancy test results (table). A protocol for diagnosis of ectopic pregnancy is outlined.

The use of β-hCG RIA is recommended in cases of suspected ectopic pregnancy.

▶ [This report concerns the role of a sensitive pregnancy test (radioimmunoassay of β-hCG) in the diagnosis of ectopic pregnancy. Although standard urine pregnancy tests are not helpful in this situation, the serum β-hCG test can be. No patients with ectopic pregnancies had "negative" tests, and all patients with "positive" tests had pregnancies somewhere. Only half of the patients with ectopic pregnancies during the study period had the test performed. Presumably, the others were sick enough or symptoms were clear-cut enough that surgical intervention was indicated immediately and the several hours delay in waiting for the test result was inappropriate. We wonder how many of the positive test results in this series actually were reported "after the fact" to the clinicians involved. A sensitive serum pregnancy test can be helpful in diagnosing ectopic pregnancies, especially in those patients who one is "quite sure" are not pregnant. A positive test result, of course, does not discriminate between an intrauterine and extrauterine location of the pregnancy.—R.M.P.] ◀

Alcohol, Smoking, and Incidence of Spontaneous Abortions in First and Second Trimester. S. Harlap and P. H. Shiono examined the incidence of spontaneous fetal loss at different stages of pregnancy in 32,019 women who completed a questionnaire on alcohol use at their first antenatal visit. Outcomes of pregnancy were ascertained by surveillance of hospital admissions. Of the women participating, 51.7% reported drinking no alcohol in early pregnancy; 44.7% had less than 1 drink daily; and 2.4%, 0.4%, and 0.1% had averages of 1–2, 3–5, or more than 6 drinks daily, respectively. Because drinkers began antenatal care later than did nondrinkers, results were analyzed with life-table methods. The number of women under observation (at risk) each day was calculated from the number who had started antenatal care prior to that day minus those whose pregnancies had already terminated.

Life-table analysis showed that the age-adjusted relative risks of second-trimester losses (15–27 weeks) were 1.03 (not significant: ns), 1.98 (P <.01), and 3.53 (P <.01), respectively, for women having less than 1, 1–2, and more than 3 drinks daily, compared with nondrinkers. The corresponding relative risks for first trimester losses (5–14 weeks) were 1.12 (ns), 1.15 (ns), and 1.15, respectively. Smokers had relative risks of 1.01 (ns) and 1.21 (ns) in the first and second trimesters, respectively, compared with nonsmokers. The increased risk of second-trimester miscarriage in drinkers was not explained by age, parity, race, marital status, smoking, or number of previous spontaneous or induced abortions.

Alcohol use tends to be correlated with smoking. An examination of the combined effects of smoking and drinking on second-trimester losses showed that regular drinkers had a higher incidence of miscarriages in all smoking groups. Within categories of drinkers the effect of smoking per se was weak and inconsistent. The independent effects

Lancet 2:173–176, July 26, 1980.

of both drinking and smoking were confirmed in a linear multiple-regression analysis. Based on regression results, about 69 (10%) of 690 second-trimester abortions were attributed to the effects of drinking or smoking.

These results suggest that alcohol may harm human fetuses not only when it is abused, but also when it is taken in moderation. The findings should not be taken to imply with certainty that alcohol has no effect in the first trimester. The women who initiated antenatal care early in pregnancy (and therefore entered the study early) would have been a selected group and perhaps at higher risk for miscarriage. Therefore, findings for early pregnancy may contain biases which could invalidate the conclusions drawn about first-trimester alcohol effects.

Study on the Effects of Induced Abortion on Subsequent Pregnancy Outcome. Induced abortion is prevalent today, and serious questions have arisen concerning its long-term effects on subsequent pregnancies. Carol Madore, Warren E. Hawes, Frank Many, and Alfred C. Hexter (Univ. of California, Berkeley) have reported evidence that a prior induced abortion is associated with a small but statistically significant increase in the risk of subsequent pregnancy failure. Pregnancy outcome was assessed in 2,081 women who had had one or more previous induced abortions and in 4,098 control subjects matched for race, age, and hospital of delivery. Data were obtained from women delivering spontaneously at nine California hospitals in a 16-month period in 1976–1978. The study and control groups had similar educational levels and first-trimester prenatal care. About 8% of each group had had a previous spontaneous abortion. There were no significant differences in prenatal medical risk factors.

Most pregnancy complications were similar in the study and control groups, with no difference in rates of spontaneous abortion, ectopic pregnancy, congenital anomalies, or low birth weight infants individually. A small but significant increase in incidence of pregnancy failure (i.e., all outcomes taken together) was observed in the study group, but the increased risk was substantially smaller than that associated with several social, economic, and behavioral indicators. Previous elective abortion increased the risk of pregnancy failure by about 45%, with other factors held constant. Mothers who had never practiced contraception had more than double the risk of mothers who had used some method of contraception. Prior therapeutic abortion was not predictive of low birth weight.

Induced abortion appears to have a small adverse effect on subsequent pregnancy outcome. The finding that contraception was the chief variable in this study may indicate that it is a surrogate for self-care. Any effect of prior abortion may reflect unmeasured variables

Am. J. Obstet. Gynecol. 139:516–521, Mar. 1, 1981.

for which prior abortion acts as a surrogate, rather than being a result of the physiologic action of abortion.

▶ [Few questions are as important as that of whether or not induced abortion affects the outcome of subsequent pregnancies. Previous studies have come down on both sides of the issue. The problem is that of separating confounding and intervening variables from the variable of induced abortion. In other words, is an unfavorable outcome a reflection of prior abortion or something(s) about patients who have elected abortion? This study attempted to sort some of the problems out by statistical methods taking into account other factors influencing pregnancy outcome (socioeconomic status, prenatal care, smoking, etc.). The results suggest a modest effect; risk of pregnancy failure (ectopic, spontaneous abortion, and perinatal death) was increased 45% in cases over controls, whereas six other variables carried higher risk. The question can only be answered definitively by a prospective randomized study, but that, of course, is impossible.—R.M.P.] ◀

Prophylactic Antibiotics in First-Trimester Abortions: Clinical Controlled Trial. Stig Sonne-Holm, Lars Heisterberg, Søren Hebjørn, Knud Dyring-Andersen, Jens Thorup Andersen, and Bo Løye Hejl (Univ. of Copenhagen) conducted a double-blind study to determine whether prophylactic administration of penicillin-ampicillin could lower the incidence of infection in 564 women undergoing legalized abortion at up to and including 12 weeks' gestation. They were randomized to receive 2 million IU of penicillin G intramuscularly 30 minutes before and 3 hours after the procedure, followed by 350 mg of pivampicillin three times daily for 4 days or placebo. Median age was 26 years (range, 14 to 45). Abortions were performed by dilation with Hegar dilators and vacuum aspiration after washing with fluid soap and intravaginal rinsing with phenosalyl 1%. After aspiration, blunt curettage was performed. Patients were seen in the outpatient clinic 4 weeks after the procedure.

Forty (7.1%) patients did not attend the follow-up appointment. Of those seen at follow-up, 31 (5.9%) were eliminated from the trial for failure to follow the regimen. The results, based on 493 patients, showed an incidence of infection in the actively treated group of 5.5% (14 of 254), significantly lower than 10.9% incidence in the placebo group. Of the women with a history of pelvic inflammatory disease, (PID), 22.4% developed postabortion infection, in contrast with only 7.2% in the group with no history of PID. Patient age, number of births, number of induced abortions, and insertion of an intrauterine device did not significantly influence the rate of infection, but gestational age did.

Before antibiotic prophylaxis is introduced for any operation, the surgical procedure should have a well-documented high risk of infection; the chosen antibiotic should have a low incidence of adverse effects; and the gains of avoiding infection should be proportional to the risks involved with antibiotic prophylaxis. The total incidence of pelvic infection in induced abortions can be halved by prophylaxis in women who have had PID.

▶ [Infection is the most common complication of induced abortion, but its frequency

---

Am. J. Obstet. Gynecol. 139:693–696, Mar. 15, 1981.

has varied widely in reported series. The 10.9% rate in this reported control group is among the highest, and the protection conferred by the penicillin-ampicillin regimen is similar to an earlier report on the benefits of tetracycline.

I find the authors' retrospective stratification on the basis of previous pelvic inflammatory disease interesting but only partly convincing, because I see no reasons why the infection rate should be 2.1% in antibiotic-treated patients with a prior history of pelvic inflammatory disease and triple that in antibiotic-treated patients *without* such a history. I will stick with the original protocol and the overall analysis, which involved no post hoc statistical second thoughts.—L.C.L.] ◄

Obesity in Pregnancy: Risks and Outcome. Obesity has been associated in the literature with other pregnancy risks such as hypertension and diabetes mellitus, but disagreement persists about the expected course and complications of labor. Moreover, the effects of obesity on intrauterine growth and gestational duration have not been well defined. Thomas Gross, Robert J. Sokol, and Katherine C. King (Cleveland Metropolitan Genl. Hosp.) studied 2,746 consecutive deliveries using a computer-based uniform perinatal record to compare 300 pregnancy risk and outcome factors for obese and nonobese patients. The 279 obese women (i.e., those weighing over 90 kg at some time during pregnancy) were older and of higher parity than the 2,467 nonobese women. The obese patients were at increased an-

---

TABLE 1.—COMPARISONS OF OBESE AND NONOBESE PATIENTS FOR
LABOR ABNORMALITY AND INTRAPARTUM MANAGEMENT
(FREQUENCIES IN %)*

	Obese ($N = 249$)	Nonobese ($N = 2371$)
Labor abnormality		
Nulliparas	35.8	37.2
Multiparas	31.2	29.9
Dysfunctional labor patterns		
Prolonged latent phase	1.2	2.8
Protracted active phase dilatation	26.9	26.5
Secondary arrest of dilatation	4.4	5.3
Prolonged deceleration phase	0.8	1.3
Protracted descent	4.4	5.0
Arrest of descent	3.6	3.4
Labor durations		
Labor > 20 hours	4.4	5.9
Precipitous labor (< 3 hours)	7.2	8.1
Second stage > 2.5 hours	1.6	1.5
Labor and delivery management		
Oxytocin augmentation	20.3	20.8
Low forceps	8.0	10.0
Midforceps	1.7	1.5
Primary cesarean section	12.0	9.6

*There were no significant differences for any of these factors.

Obstet. Gynecol. 56:446–450, October 1980.

TABLE 2.—MATERNAL AND FETAL-INFANT COMPLICATIONS AND OUTCOME FOR THE OBESE AND NONOBESE GROUPS (FREQUENCIES IN %*)

	Obese (N = 279 mothers and 284 infants)	Nonobese (N = 2467 mothers and 2481 infants)	P
Maternal complications			
Vaginal laceration, fourth degree	1.1	4.2	< .025
Postpartum hemorrhage	13.6	10.9	NS
Fetal–infant problems			
Meconium staining	21.8	17.8	NS
Breech presentation	3.0	3.3	NS
Intrapartum trauma	0.3	0.1	NS
Shoulder dystocia	1.1	1.0	NS
Low Apgar score (< 7)			
1 minute	19.6	16.5	NS
5 minutes	2.1	2.3	NS
Perinatal mortality	7.0	16.5	NS

NS = not significant.
*Except perinatal mortality, given as rate per 1,000 births.

tepartum risk and had increased frequencies of chronic hypertension, inadequate pregnancy weight gain, twin gestation, and diabetes mellitus.

Upon admission for delivery, obese patients were more likely to require medical induction of labor and to have been delivered previously by cesarean section. Comparisons of labor abnormalities among women who were not delivered by repeat cesarean section (Table 1) showed that dysfunctional labor patterns occurred with similar frequency in the two study groups; the need for oxytocin augmentation and incidence of primary cesarean section did not differ in the two groups. Maternal and fetal-infant complications in obese and nonobese groups are shown in Table 2. Trauma to the infant, Apgar scores, and perinatal mortality were similar in the two groups, but there were fewer infants of low birth weight (under 2,500 gm) and more macrosomic babies (over 4,000 gm) born to the obese patients. The increase in birth weight was accounted for not only by an increase in the birth weight percentile, but also by a significant lengthening of the period of gestation.

The increased incidences of oxytocin induction of labor and repeat cesarean section may be related to the increased number of antepartum medical problems found in obese women on entering labor. A lack of increase in perinatal mortality in the obese group may be related to a lower incidence of preterm delivery and intrauterine growth retardation. The obese patient was half as likely to be delivered preterm, and 3.5 times more likely to be delivered post term, than the nonobese mother. The obese mother was half as likely to be delivered of an infant small for gestational age and 2.5 times more likely to be delivered of an infant large for gestational age. It appears that the obese patient is at less risk for labor complications than previously was believed. With careful antepartum and intrapartum management, these patients can be delivered vaginally of larger infants, who are less likely to be preterm or small for gestational age.

▶ [Obese patients fared as well in labor as did control patients in this study. Although dysfunctional labor patterns occurred with similar frequency in both groups, nulliparity was less common in obese patients. It would have been interesting to characterize the individual labor progress abnormalities by parity in comparing the two groups. We're not surprised that neonatal macrosomia was more common in the obese group, but we would have expected this to be reflected in more frequent shoulder dystocia. This was not the case.—R.M.P.] ◀

Effect of Pregnancy on Idiopathic Scoliosis. Walter P. Blount and David D. Mellencamp (Med. College of Wisconsin, Milwaukee) followed 10 patients with idiopathic scoliosis through 19 pregnancies. There were 1 lumbar, 7 thoracic, and 2 double thoracic curves. All patients were treated with a Milwaukee brace. At the start of treatment the curves measured 33 to 74 degrees. A full standing anteroposterior roentgenogram of the spine was obtained prior to conception, soon after delivery, and 1 year later.

Three patients lost 2, 6, and 18 degrees of correction during their initial pregnancies, but the curves remained the same or improved with later pregnancies. The curves of the other 7 women, which had stabilized before conception, did not progress. Scoliosis stability was not related to patient age. Stable scoliotic curves did not progress with pregnancy in teenagers, whereas unstable scolioses progressed in patients older than age 20 years. The amount that the curve increased was not related to the initial size of the curve.

▶ [This study indicates that scoliosis does not progress during pregnancy if it has stabilized prior to conception, information that will be of value in counseling patients with the condition. Two additional aspects of scoliosis that may be of importance obstetrically are (1) the possibility of abnormalities of the pelvis, and (2) cardiac disease secondary to impaired pulmonary function with prolonged and severe kyphoscoliosis.—R.M.P.] ◀

Cystic Fibrosis and Pregnancy: National Survey of 119 cystic fibrosis (CF) centers in the United States and Canada was made by Lawrence F. Cohen, Paul A. di Sant'Agnese, and Jacquelyn Friedlander (Natl. Inst. of Health). The survey identified 129 pregnancies in 100 women with CF. Mean age at pregnancy was 20.7 years (range, 17–32), which is similar to that of normal women. Mean age at diagnosis of CF was 11 years, compared with a mean age of 3½ years for all CF patients.

J. Bone Joint Surg. [Am.] 62-A:1083–1087, October 1980.
Lancet 2:842–844, Oct. 18, 1980.

Of the 129 pregnancies, 97 (75%) were completed, 6 (5%) ended in spontaneous abortion, and 25 (19%) ended in therapeutic abortion. Death within 24 months of delivery occurred in 18% of the women, a mortality rate not exceeding that for all CF women of the same age. The women who died soon after delivery had moderate to severe pulmonary disease before pregnancy, with exacerbation of it during pregnancy. Perinatal death and shortened gestation were also significantly associated with maternal death within 2 years of delivery.

Congestive heart failure complicated 13% of the pregnancies. Maternal weight gain was less than 4.5 kg in 41% of the women; this greatly exceeds the expected rate of 7%. Antibiotics were required to manage pulmonary disease in 65% of the women, and aminoglycosides were given to half of these. Of the 97 completed pregnancies, 86 (89%) resulted in viable infants, a rate that differs significantly from the expected rate of 97.8%. Of the 86 viable infants, only 1 (0.8%) had CF, which confirms the recessive nature of the transmission of CF. None had congenital anomalies. The pregnancies lasted less than 37 weeks in 26.8% of the women, compared with an expected rate of about 6.5%. The 11.3% perinatal death rate was significantly greater than the 3% rate reported in unselected pregnancies. Of the 11 perinatal deaths, 10 were in pregnancies that lasted less than 37 weeks. Cyanosis and dyspnea were each associated with increased maternal and perinatal mortality. There were no significant correlations between age at diagnosis of CF or interval between diagnosis and pregnancy, and maternal or perinatal outcome.

Pregnancy normally causes increased respiratory and cardiac work and hypervolemia, and these may be a serious threat to women with CF if they already have significant pulmonary disease. Thus, pregnancy should be avoided if the Schwachman or Taussig clinical score is below 80, indicating serious pulmonary disease. If this advice is not followed, antibiotics may be necessary; if so, penicillin or its derivatives are less toxic than aminoglycosides. The mother should consider the impact of her shortened life span on her child, the fact that reduced exercise tolerance with progressive disease may prevent her from caring for her child, and the fact that her risk of having a child with CF is 1 in 40, compared with 1 in 1,500–2,000 in the general population.

▶ [This review highlights the adverse effects of cystic fibrosis on pregnancy and of pregnancy on cystic fibrosis. Mortality rates, both perinatal and maternal, were high. Forty-one percent of patients gained less than 10 lb during gestation. Serious pulmonary disease prior to conception predicted poor outcome. We recently cared for a gravida with cystic fibrosis; pregnancy was completed and a living infant resulted, but the mother died 3 months post partum.

This problem is becoming more frequent as more cystic fibrosis patients survive into adulthood. At present, it seems that pregnancy is relatively contraindicated.—R.M.P.] ◀

Infants of Adolescent Mothers: Perinatal, Neonatal, and Infancy Outcome. It remains unclear whether biologic or social inad-

Semin. Perinatol. 5:19–32, January 1981.

equacies best explain the apparent reproductive disadvantage of the American teenager and the well-being of her infant. Ruth A. Lawrence and T. Allen Merritt (Univ. of Rochester) previously reviewed neonatal data from 5,711 pregnancies collected by the Collaborative Perinatal Project of the National Institute of Neurological and Communicative Disorders and Stroke, and from 4,000 pregnancies at the University of Kansas Medical Center, including 770 in teenage mothers. Preliminary review was made of data from 6,087 pregnancies at the Regional Perinatal Center of the University of Rochester, New York. An additional 9,000 patients giving birth in Monroe County in 1979 also were reviewed.

Prematurity is especially prevalent in infants of young black mothers. Adolescent women exhibit a disproportionate number of complicating factors in both the medical and behavioral areas. Low birth weight infants are not in excess in adolescent births when these factors are controlled for. Analyses of perinatal mortality fail to support the traditional view that biologic immaturity is the chief factor in the poor outcome of infants of adolescent mothers. In the Rochester series, infants of black adolescent mothers had more neonatal complications than the control subjects, and neonatal mortality was increased in this group. The relationship of biologic maturity to outcome remains unclear, but the data suggest that gynecologic age may correlate better.

Infants of adolescent mothers are said to do less well in school and to be more subject to child abuse and neglect. The health status of children is related not only to maternal age at the time of birth, but to the mother's marital status and basically to family structure. Parenting by the young mother has not been investigated in depth. It appears that age is not the critical factor in adolescent pregnancy unless the mother is aged 14 or younger. Although the intellectual, developmental, and educational expectations of children of adolescents have been lower than those for children of older mothers; these children are disproportionately poor, black, and living in extended, often disrupted families with multiple care-givers. Parenting skills and maternal readiness may well be the critical determinants in the long-term outcome of infants born to adolescent mothers.

▶ [This article represents another attempt to confront the "epidemic" of adolescent pregnancies. This study, utilizing collective data and representing a very large series of patients, concludes with the statement that the ideal time to give birth from a medical viewpoint would appear to be between the ages of 16 and 19, provided the mother is given adequate prenatal care and rears the child in a stable environment. From a psychosocial viewpoint, however, the adolescent parent has no advantage and may suffer from a lack of intellectual and affective skills needed to cope with child rearing. The medical health of the infant at birth would be of secondary importance to the long-range outcome of these infants being reared by young and usually single parents.—C.E.D.] ◀

Follow-up of Children of Diabetic Mothers. Mary Cummins and

Arch. Dis. Child. 55:259–264, April 1980.

Mary Norrish present results of a follow-up study of infants of 51 diabetic mothers who attended the combined antenatal and diabetic clinic at Hammersmith Hospital, London, and delivered 73 infants (one set of twins) of more than 24 weeks' gestation between 1964 and 1972. There were no intrauterine deaths. In 58 pregnancies the mothers required insulin; 1 mother required chlorpropamide. In the other 13 pregnancies, mothers controlled their diabetes with diet alone. Complications of pregnancy included retinopathy (8 patients), renal involvement (1), and severe neuropathy (1). There were 5 deaths from hyaline membrane disease and 2 deaths caused by lethal congenital abnormalities. Sixty-six children survived the neonatal period; there were 3 later deaths. Of the 63 surviving children, 51 were traced in 1977. A medical and developmental history was obtained from the parents. Psychologic assessment (Wechsler Intelligence Scale for children for those aged 6 years or older and the Wechsler Preschool and Primary School Scale of Intelligence for those younger than age 6) was carried out, together with general and neurologic examination, urinalysis, and growth measurements.

Full-scale IQ scores were distributed normally. All but 2 children attend schools for normal children. One child with an IQ below 70 at age 4½ years had delayed speech, poor concentration, and hyperactivity. There was no significant difference between the IQ of children hypoglycemic at birth and those who were not hypoglycemic. The major abnormalities noted at follow-up were severe deafness in 1 child, myopia (1 child), low IQ and hyperactivity (1 child), and epilepsy and urinary infection (1 child). These 4 children had normal neonatal periods without hypoglycemia or other complications. The distribution of height and head circumference centiles was near normal, but one fifth of the children had skinfolds greater than the 90th centile, with very few less than the 10th centile. Obesity correlated well with maternal obesity but not with birth weight.

Lethal congenital malformations remain a serious problem for the infant of the diabetic mother. Congenital malformations were responsible for 20% of the neonatal deaths in this series and 1 of 3 post-neonatal deaths. Although there is a greater tendency toward the development of diabetes in children of diabetic mothers, no children in this series have become overtly diabetic, nor have any siblings. The handicaps found at follow-up apparently did not relate to maternal diabetes.

▶ [This report provides long-term follow-up data on children aged 5–13 years born to diabetic women. Generally, the outcome of surviving children does not seem to have been affected by maternal diabetes. Of particular interest is neuropsychological development; mean IQ was 97.5 and school performance appears similar to that of the general population. Previous studies have related intellectual impairment to maternal acetonuria and neonatal hypoglycemia, neither of which was particularly common in this series. There was a suggestion of an increased tendency to childhood obesity in this series, which could be due to influences during diabetic pregnancy but more likely reflects growing up in a household with an overweight mother.— R.M.P.] ◀

Additional Reading

Garn, S., et al.: Effect of maternal cigarette smoking on Apgar scores. *Am. J. Dis. Child.* 135:503, 1981.

Grimes, D. A., et al.: Fatal septic abortion in the United States, 1975 to 1977. *Obstet. Gynecol.* 57:739, 1981.

Johnson, S., et al.: Immune deficiency in fetal alcohol syndrome. *Pediatr. Res.* 15:908, 1981.

Key, T. C., et al.: Automated erythrocytopheresis for sickle cell anemia during pregnancy. *Am. J. Obstet. Gynecol.* 138:731, 1980.

Khuroo, M. S., et al.: Incidence and severity of viral hepatitis in pregnancy. *Am. J. Med.* 70:252, 1981.

Kline, J., et al.: Drinking during pregnancy and spontaneous abortion. *Lancet* 2:176, 1980.

Miller, J. F., et al.: Fetal loss after implantation: Prospective study. *Lancet* 2:554, 1980.

Wong, V. C. W., et al.: Transmission of hepatitis B antigens from symptom-free carrier mothers to the fetus and the infant. *Br. J. Obstet. Gynaecol.* 87:958, 1980.

Dentistry

"A smile costs nothing but gives much."—AUTHOR UNKNOWN

If that smile belongs to an adolescent, parents know it can cost plenty for it to be beautiful. Health care professionals are forced to consider the mouth, especially the teeth, while delivering total health care to this age group. Medical school taught us little about dentistry, but it is so important in a clinical setting. Therefore this section covers a variety of dental and related conditions.

In the discussion of sports dentistry, Smith notes that mouthguards and splints must protect not only the teeth but also the temporomandibular joint, the carotid blood supply, and the brain. Clinicians therefore must urge their patients who participate in contact sports to use properly fitted mouthguards.

All the articles on the temporomandibular joint (TMJ) are useful in evaluating the adolescent who presents with a headache. It is important that the clinician understand the pathology of the TMJ and be aware that TMJ dysfunction can cause recurrent headaches.

Adolescents who are very sexually active may acquire condyloma accuminatum with involvement of the oral mucosa. The pictures accompanying this article and the discussion of treatment are essential information.

Experience in Providing Orthodontic Treatment in England was reviewed by J. P. Moss, D. W. Williams, and A. M. Cohen (Univ. College, London). In England, orthodontic treatment is available through the National Health Service to all who require it, in general dental services, hospital clinics, and school dental clinics. The demand for treatment has increased in the past decade, but there still is an 18% wastage rate of patients who fail to complete treatment. Review was made of a total of 152,239 cases approved for orthodontic treatment in 1979 in general practices. Initially, 13.5% of subjects did not begin treatment, and 16%–18% had dropped out before treatment was completed. In the past 3 years, dental health education has been provided for orthodontic patients. Patients with a buccal-lingual plaque score of more than 10% have been referred to their general dental practitioners for instruction in oral hygiene. A plaque score chart (Fig 31) is provided to aid in assessing the patient.

In a group of 146 patients considered likely to benefit from orthodontic treatment, who received three appointments to see a hygienist for instruction in dental health, 18% achieved a plaque score below

Eur. J. Orthod. 3:135–139, 1981.

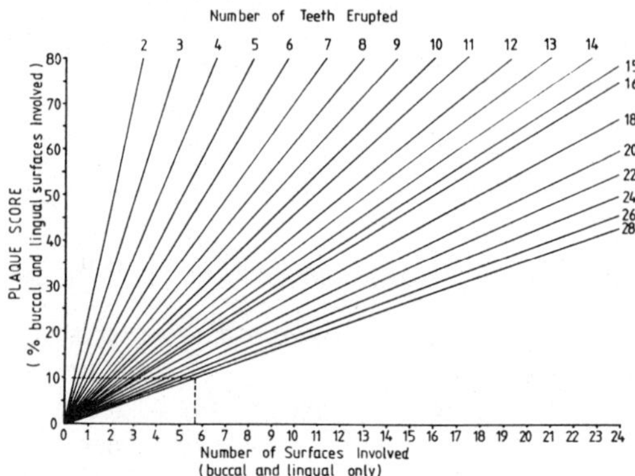

Fig 31.—Form used to indicate the plaque score. The number of surfaces, buccal and lingual, which have plaque on them, are counted and are assessed against the line representing the number of teeth erupted in the mouth. The plaque score can then be read as a percentage on the left-hand side. (Courtesy of Moss, J. P., et al.: Eur. J. Orthod. 3:135–139, 1981.)

10% initially. The mean score was 49%. The mean plaque score was reduced to 29% at the second visit. Of 58 patients seen at the third visit, 34 were not accepted for treatment because of persistently high plaque scores. An overall 14.6% improvement in plaque scores occurred between the second and third visits, but 6 patients showed a mean worsening of 14%.

Patients motivated to practice good oral hygiene appear to become good orthodontic patients. Oral hygiene assessment before orthodontic therapy is a good means of assessing patient motivation and may help reduce wastage resulting from failure to complete treatment. Orthodontic treatment should be provided only if backed up by general dental health education, with the patient becoming fully aware of his responsibility to maintain his own dental health.

Unilateral Face-Bows: A Theoretical and Laboratory Analysis. Orthodontic treatment often requires an extraoral face-bow that predictably will deliver a greater distal force to one side of the dental arch than to the other. The proper use of these devices remains unclear. H. Garland Hershey (Univ. of North Carolina), C. W. Houghton (Roanoke, Va.), and Charles J. Burstone (Univ. of Connecticut) compared the effectiveness of 5 face-bow types in delivering unilateral distal forces to their inner-bow terminals. The bilaterally symmetrical face-bow was compared with four unilateral designs, the power-arm face-bow, the soldered-offset device, the swivel-offset device, and the spring-attachment face-bow. A theoretical analysis was carried out, and the results were compared with those of a laboratory analysis using a strain-gauge transducer system. The theoretical method proved to be a reliable means of approximating the distribution of distal forces to the inner-bow terminals. The net lateral forces also were determined reliably.

Am. J. Orthod. 79:229–249, March 1981.

The power-arm unilateral face-bow and the swivel-offset design were found to be effective in delivering a clinically significant unilateral distal force. The bilaterally symmetrical face-bow and the unilateral soldered-offset and spring-attachment designs were not effective in this regard. All designs that deliver effective unilateral distal forces will also deliver a net lateral force to the inner-bow terminals. The magnitude of the net lateral force increases with the unilateral effectiveness of the face-bow. There is concern about moving teeth on the favored side into lingual cross-bite with their mandibular antagonists, and there also should be concern about moving the maxillary teeth on the nonfavored side facially into buccal cross-bite with their mandibular antagonists. The effects of lateral forces can be manipulated by expansion or constriction of the inner bows. The same clinical results can be achieved by fabricating a power-arm unilateral face-bow in the office as by purchasing a swivel-offset unilateral face-bow. The swivel acts only to allow the outer-bow tips to seek a geometric configuration where they are asymmetrical with one another about the midsagittal plane.

A Survey of Adults' Attitudes Toward Orthodontic Therapy. Orthodontic treatment of adults for malocclusion problems no longer is unusual. Barton H. Tayer and Mitchell J. Burek (Boston Univ.) attempted to determine adult attitudes toward orthodontics in a survey of 20 patients who were questioned at informal meetings. Subsequently, 33 patients were questioned regarding attitudes toward therapy, and the reaction of close personal contacts during and after treatment was assessed. Most of these subjects were women. The age range was 18–58 years. The great majority had attended college.

Some subjects had contemplated orthodontic treatment for 1–3 years, and others had considered it for 6–13 years. In the vast majority of cases, the family dentist had mentioned a need for orthodontic therapy. Most subjects reported having had initial doubts about treatment, but most found their relatives and friends to be highly supportive of their decision to enter treatment. Both relief and satisfaction were expressed near the completion of treatment. The most difficult time was weeks 1 through 4. One third of patients occasionally felt discouraged during treatment because of the length of treatment, the inconveniences involved with the use of appliances, and discomfort. However, most felt that improvement was evident almost immediately and that progress outweighed the feelings of discouragement. Extraoral headgear was viewed most negatively. Removable appliances and elastics also were viewed negatively. No patient reported feeling that treatment would not be acceptable were the decision to be made again.

Orthodontics should not be restricted to children. The present findings indicate that properly motivated and educated adults are excellent candidates for orthodontic treatment. Dentists must be convinced

Am. J. Orthod. 79:305–315, March 1981.

of the importance of orthodontics in overall oral health in order to direct patients properly toward orthodontic treatment.

▶ [I have taught adult orthodontics to graduate students in periodontics and crown and bridge restorative dentistry for about 10 years, and I have a good percentage of adult patients in my private practice. My own experience is much like that of Tayer and Burek. It is very interesting to realize how long a time adults may yearn for orthodontic therapy, contemplating it but never undertaking it until someone pushes them toward treatment. Frequently, that supportive person is a friend, member of the family, or a dentist. One cannot help but wonder how many other adults still want orthodontic treatment and need it, but haven't yet been urged to do so.—R.E.M.] ◀

Sports Dentistry: Protection and Performance From Mouthguards and Bite Splints are discussed by Stephen D. Smith (Philadelphia College of Osteopathic Medicine). The basic use of mouthguards in sports has been for protection and safety during physical contact, but recently, improved athletic performance has been related directly to bite therapy and the use of physiologically designed mouthguards. Mouthguards provide protection to the teeth and the temporomandibular joint (TMJ), the carotid blood supply, and the brain. Protection of the jaw and the TMJ in football is important.

Various commercially available stock mouthguards are available in sports stores. Custom vinyl mouthguards can be constructed. The back teeth must contact the mouthguard evenly to provide proper neuromuscular perception. The vinyl mouthguards do not prevent the jaw from moving side to side or backward on jaw closure. The customized white rubber mouthguard is useful in any sport that involves trauma or contact, such as boxing, ice hockey, football, and skiing. Its only disadvantage is that it makes talking difficult. The orthopedic acrylic repositioning bite splint allows maximum freedom of jaw movement and provides a bite table mainly on the back teeth. Either a maxillary or a mandibular appliance can be made. This splint is ideal for some of the sports with less contact, such as tennis, basketball, cycling, ice skating, running, wrestling, track and field, and baseball. Muscle testing in football players has shown that properly balanced mouthguards improve muscle strength.

In both the athlete and the TMJ patient, the same therapeutic approach to orthopedic appliance construction and mouthguard design applies. This approach offers much potential for reducing pain, improving stress resistance, and improving overall performance.

▶ [Use of properly designed and constructed mouthguards has long been known to reduce dental injury significantly during contact sports. Recent studies showing reduced musculoskeletal stress through use of mouthguards should be of great interest to anyone involved in sports medicine.—D.F.R.] ◀

Changes in Recurrent Headaches and Mandibular Dysfunction After Various Types of Dental Treatment. It has been suggested that more than half of chronic headache suffers can obtain relief by dental treatment. Tomas Magnusson and Gunnar E. Carlsson (Univ. of Göteborg) attempted to determine whether stomatog-

Athletic Training 16:100–106, Summer 1981.
Acta Odontol. Scand. 38:311–320, 1980.

nathic treatment has a demonstrable effect on dysfunction and on recurrent headaches. Review was made of data on 58 patients referred for the treatment of mandibular dysfunction and 70 seen for conventional dental treatment. In only a few of the dental cases did treatment influence the occlusion.

Headaches were less frequent at follow-up in 70% of patients with mandibular dysfunction who had had them. Only 1 patient reported having headaches more often than before. The dental patients improved and became worse with about equal frequency. The clinical dysfunction index decreased in the group with mandibular dysfunction, but did not change in the dental patients. The prevalence of dysfunction remained higher in the former group. These patients still had more frequent and more severe headaches than the dental patients a year after the start of treatment. Headaches lasted longer in this group, and analgesic consumption was greater than in the dental group. Clenching and grinding of teeth both were reported significantly more often by the patients with mandibular dysfunction.

Headache is a frequent symptom with many causes. In many cases, mandibular dysfunction is unrelated to headaches, but many patients with such dysfunction have a reduction in the frequency and severity of headaches after they have received stomatognathic treatment. Functional evaluation of the masticatory system is indicated in patients with recurrent headaches unless tension headache can be ruled out definitely. Patients with clinical signs of mandibular dysfunction should receive stomatognathic treatment.

▶ [Those of us who treat a significant number of patients with temporomandibular dysfunction have long heard from happy patients that headache symptoms often diminish after temporomandibular therapy. This article documents well that additional effect of therapy.—R.E.M.] ◀

Effects of Occlusal Treatment and Intra-articular Injections on Temporomandibular Joint Pain and Dysfunction. Sigvard Kopp and Bengt Wenneberg (Univ. of Göteborg) compared the effects of 2 years of occlusal therapy and intra-articular injections of a steroid-local anesthetic mixture in patients with local pain and tenderness on palpation of the temporomandibular joint (TMJ). Fifteen patients in whom conservative treatment had failed received injections of 3 mg of betamethasone with 5 mg of lidocaine-chloride-anhydrate weekly for 3 weeks. Eighteen patients received occlusal adjustment by splinting for molar support or, in 2 cases, occlusal correction with acrylic resin. The latter patients had complete dentures, and the dentures were relined.

The mean subjective dysfunction score decreased by about half in the patients given intra-articular injections, and 14 of 15 patients improved. The mean clinical dysfunction score was reduced to about one third of baseline. With occlusal treatment, subjective dysfunction was reduced in 78% of patients, but the mean clinical dysfunction score did not change markedly. Maximal mouth opening increased signifi-

Acta Odontol. Scand. 39:87–96, 1981.

cantly after both types of treatment, and with both treatments the number of painful mandibular movements decreased significantly. Temporomandibular joint tenderness also decreased with both treatments.

In this study, marked clinical improvement was apparent 2 years after intra-articular injection of a steroid-local anesthetic, but not consistently after occlusal treatment. Both treatments were associated with long-term relief of subjective symptoms in patients with tenderness to palpation of the TMJ. The prognosis after intra-articular injections is most favorable in patients without radiographic evidence of TMJ remodeling or general joint symptoms.

Description of Population and Progress of Symptoms in a Longitudinal Study of Temporomandibular Arthropathy. Temporomandibular arthropathy (TMA) is considered a monarticular disease of the temporomandibular joint (TMJ) with a marked tendency to heal spontaneously. Ole Collin Rasmussen (Rigshospitalet, Copenhagen) reviewed the course of 119 consecutive patients seen in 1971–1977 with TMJ pain and/or constriction and erosion of the mandibular condyle on transpharyngeal radiography. No general connective tissue, muscle, or joint disease was present. Female patients constituted 85% of the series. The age distribution is shown in Figure 32. Eliciting factors were noted at onset of the intermediate stage of TMA in 20% of cases. Nine patients had bilateral TMA.

An initial stage of functional disturbance of the TMJ without pain was followed by an intermediate phase of abrupt onset, with pain on chewing, biting, or maximal opening, and then by a terminal stage with pain absent. The abrupt onset of the intermediate stage was almost pathognomonic of TMA. Pain typically was located at the TMJ or ear and was increased on loading of the joint. Pain in the TMJ at rest and on motion had a median duration of 5–6 months each. Grating wounds were noted in the intermediate phase in one fourth of the cases. The TMJ pain resolved in all but 3 patients. Most had residual symptoms, chiefly constriction and crepitation. In one third of the

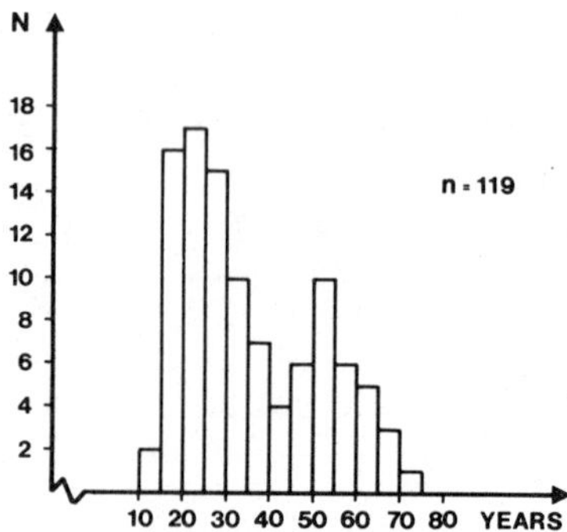

Fig 32.—Age distribution of patients at onset of intermediate stage of TMA: modes, 23 and 51 years; range, 14.5–74.5 years. (Courtesy of Rasmussen, O. C.: Scand. J. Dent. Res. 89:196–203, April 1981.)

Scand. J. Dent. Res. 89:196–203, April 1981.

cases, these features persisted without improving for more than 6 months. Periodic locking in the intermediate stage was less frequent in patients older than age 50 than in younger patients. Younger patients more often had clicking at the onset of the intermediate stage.

The abrupt onset of intermediate-stage TMA appears to represent the actual start of arthropathy. Patient age does not seem to influence the course of TMA significantly. Complete recovery is the most common outcome. Relapses appear to be rare.

Condyloma Acuminatum Involving Oral Mucosa is reported in 2 patients by Richard H. Swan, Raymond K. McDaniel, Bernard B. Dreiman, and William C. Rome. Condyloma acuminatum is a hyperplastic epithelial growth of viral origin. It is commonly present in the anogenital region but rare in the intraoral region. Only 5 documented cases of oral cavity involvement have been reported previously.

The first of the 2 present cases involved a man, aged 18 years, who presented with a growth on the dorsum of the tongue. The growth developed 3 months earlier at the same time as similar lesions developed on the penis. Subsequently, new lesions appeared on the mucosal surface of the upper lip (Fig 33), and new penile lesions also developed. The lesions were excised or cauterized, or treated with podophyllin. The second case was a man, aged 30 years, who presented with multiple papillomatous lesions of the palate and tongue (Fig 34). Both he and his wife had multiple genital lesions.

The virus that causes genital condyloma acuminatum is closely connected with, but not identical to, that which causes common skin

Fig 33.—Two nodular and one cockscomb-shaped lesions on lip. (Courtesy of Swan, R. H., et al.: Oral Surg. 51:503–508, May 1981.)

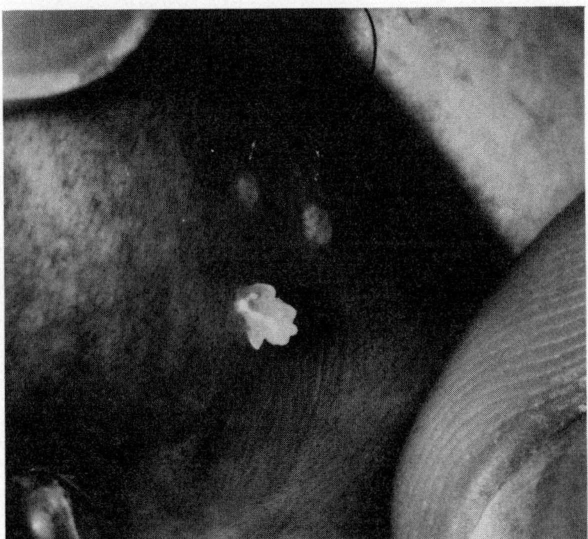

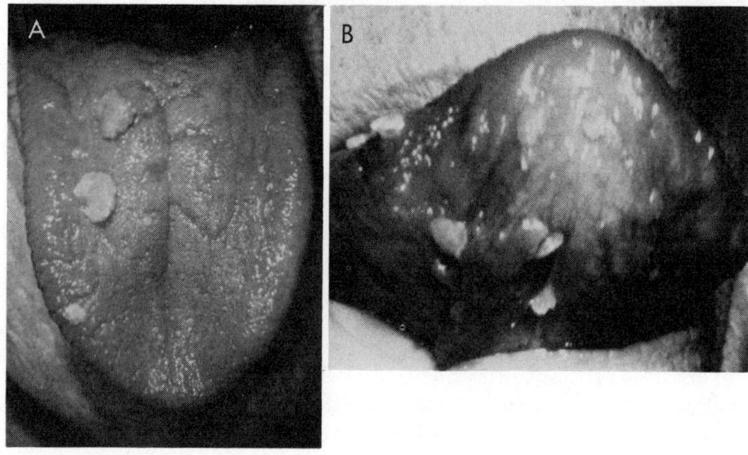

Fig 34.—Lesions on dorsum (**A**) and ventral surface (**B**) of tongue. (Courtesy of Swan, R. H., et al.: Oral Surg. 51:503–508, May 1981.)

warts. Although oral condyloma acuminatum is rare, cases in patients with no history of sexual contact or genital lesions have been reported. It is possible that the causative virus is a variant or mutant strain of the normal genital virus. Generally, small, multiple, white or pink nodules are seen initially, and later they enlarge and may coalesce. The larger lesions can be sessile or pedunculated papillary growths that resemble cauliflowers or cockscombs. Some lesions in 1 of the present cases regressed completely. Spontaneous regression probably is a result of a virus-induced humoral or cellular immune response.

Intraoral lesions of condyloma acuminatum are best eliminated by local excision, electrocautery, or cryosurgery. Podophyllin is not effective against oral growths. The cause of the high recurrence rate is not well understood, although the long incubation period of the virus or reinfection may be partly responsible.

▶ [Although this disease is rare in the oral regions, it should be considered when coalescing pink or white nodules or warty-appearing lesions are observed. The knowledge of coexisting venereal disease is useful in making the diagnosis. After reports of infrequently diagnosed lesions appear in the literature, other cases are often reported. The earlier cases were reported between 1967 and 1969, and it will be interesting to see how many others appear in print.

Marquard and Racey (*J. Oral Surg.* 39:456, 1981) treated a case of condyloma acuminata by repeated application of 15% solution of podophyllin solution in acetone to the oral lesions followed by surgical excision of the residual nodules. Three-year follow-up showed no evidence of recurrence.—H.B.G.R.] ◀

Human Bites to the Face: Management, Review of Literature, and Report of Case are presented by David J. Burton, Joseph G. Chiafair, and Richard G. Davis (Univ. Hosp., Jacksonville, Fla.).

J. Am. Dent. Assoc. 102:192–194, February 1981.

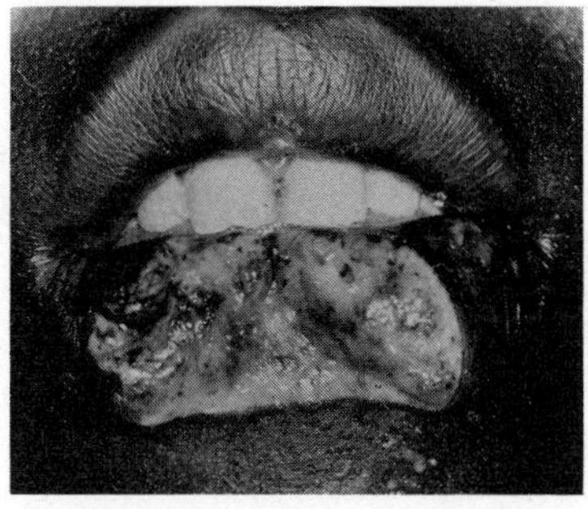

Fig 35.—Frontal view of partial lower lip avulsion caused by human bite. (Courtesy of Burton, D. J., et al.: J. Am. Dent. Assoc. 102:192–194, February 1981. Copyright by the American Dental Association. Reprinted by permission.

Human bite injuries usually are incurred during quarrels, but also may be associated with sexual activity, most often in persons with psychiatric problems. Streptococci are isolated most often, particularly *S. α-hemolyticus.* Secondary infections due to human bites usually are mixed in nature. The injuries are treated by thorough cleansing, irrigation, debridement, and primary closure. Split-thickness grafting of large defects is possible in early injuries that are free from infection. Most workers recommend the use of broad-spectrum empirical antibiotic coverage. Both penicillin G and a penicillinase-resistant penicillin or cephalosporin may be given.

Woman, 20, during an altercation, received a human bite that avulsed about half of the lower lip (Fig 35). Parenteral antibiotics were given, and the wound was covered with betadine soaks. The wound was debrided with

Fig 36.—Procedure for reconstruction of lower lip. **Top left,** midline tissue avulsion. **Top right,** edges of proximal stumps are freshened and developed through-and-through full thickness at white roll line laterally to commissures and are completely undermined and advanced. Midline tissue wedge is then excised with inferior relaxation. **Botton left,** midline closure. **Bottom right,** pedicles closed at midline. (Courtesy of Burton. D. J., et al.: J. Am. Dent. Assoc. 102:192–194, February 1981. Copyright by the American Dental Association. Reprinted by permission.)

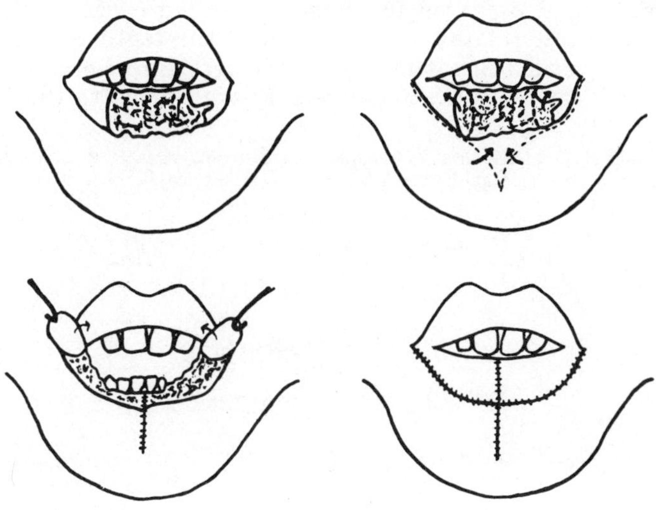

the use of general anesthesia, and flap reconstruction was carried out as shown in Figure 36. The mucosa on the inside of the wound was debrided and trimmed so that the flaps would fit properly. The orbicularis oris muscle was closed as in cleft lip closure, and the V-Y tension-releasing incision at the inferior part of the avulsion was closed from the center outward. Antibiotics were given orally for a week after the operation. There was no evidence of infection. The esthetic outcome was excellent.

Satisfactory functional and esthetic results were obtained in this case without complications by using a technique similar to that used in cleft lip reconstruction. It was not necessary to mobilize the entire commissure of the lips and excise tissue in the alar fold region.

▶ [This is an interesting report of an unusual type of wound in the facial region.— M.L.H.] ◀

Prospective Study of Mandibular Fractures. Randal B. James, Carl Fredrickson, and John N. Kent (Louisiana State Univ., New Orleans) report a 1-year prospective study of 253 patients with 422 mandibular fractures, 230 of whom had follow-up for complications and results of treatment. More than two thirds of the fractures were in patients aged 16 to 30 years. About two thirds of the patients were male. More than half the patients had multiple mandibular fractures. The sites of fractures are shown in Figure 37 and Table 1. Mandibular body fractures were most commonly associated with fractures of the contralateral angle and body. Personal violence was the most common cause of fractures (Table 2).

Closed reduction was performed in 60% of the cases. Dental splints were necessary in 21%. Of 261 teeth directly associated with fractures, 39% were extracted. All patients with compound fractures received antibiotic therapy. Delayed union was seen in 9 patients, nonunion in 3, and malunion in 3. No deaths occurred primarily from mandibular fracture. Nine patients with gunshot wounds that involved the deep neck or floor of the mouth had a tracheostomy.

Infection, which occurred in about 7% of the cases in this series (Table 3), was not related to extraction of the tooth in the fracture line. Most bacteria that caused postoperative infections were sensitive to penicillin. Complications were related more to the sites and

Fig 37.—Areas of fracture location in mandible. (Courtesy of James, R. B., et al.: J. Oral Surg. 39:275–281, April 1981. Copyright by the American Dental Association. Reprinted by permission.)

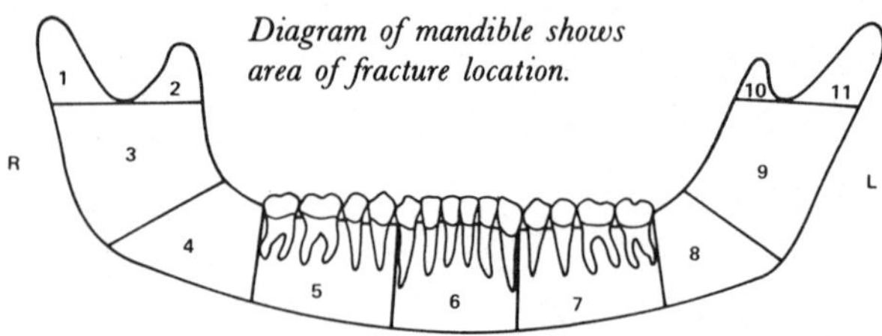

TABLE 1.—FRACTURE DISTRIBUTION ACCORDING TO AREAS IN FIGURE 37

Area	No.	%
1	42	9.5
2	5	1.1
3	17	3.8
4	53	11.9
5	57	12.9
6	63	14.3
7	63	14.3
8	83	18.8
9	8	1.8
10	7	1.6
11	44	10.0
Total	442	100

TABLE 2.—CAUSES OF MANDIBULAR FRACTURES

Causes	No.	%
Interpersonal violence	134	53
Motor vehicular accident	63	25
Other accidents	25	10
Seizure and unclassified	18	7
Gunshot	13	5
Total	253	100

TABLE 3.—POSTOPERATIVE INFECTIONS

Patient no.	Area*	Tooth associated with fracture (mandibular)	Tooth extracted	Surgery†	Infection
24	6	Right lateral incisor	No	OR	Fracture
31	8	Left third molar	Yes	OR	Wound
36	8	Left third molar	Yes	OR	Wound
77	1	None	. . .	CR	Fracture
104	4	Right third molar	Yes	OR	Fracture
113	4	Right third molar	Yes	CR	Fracture
144	8	Left third molar	Yes	OR	Wound
154	6	Right lateral incisor	No	OR	Fracture
170	7	Left second premolar	Yes	OR	Wound
177	5	Right canine	No	CR	Fracture
190	4	Right third molar	No	CR	Fracture
200	4	Right third molar	Yes	OR	Wound
203	4	Right third molar	No	OR	Fracture
208	6	Right central incisor	No	OR	Wound
243	5	Right first premolar	Yes	OR	Wound
252	4	Right second molar	Yes	OR	Wound

*See Figure 37.
†OR, open reduction; CR, closed reduction.

the causes of the fractures than to the specific reduction methods used.

All mandibular fractures should be evaluated individually according to its site, the patient's dentition, medical history, and age, and any associated injuries. The primary goal is to restore masticatory function. A thorough knowledge of occlusion and of the masticatory apparatus is necessary to treat mandibular fractures successfully.

▶ [This study is well worth reviewing by those treating this type of injury. The study is extensive in numbers and it tends to update the treatment rationale for such complex trauma cases.—M.L.H.] ◀

Additional Reading

Darby, W. J.: Why salt? How much? *ASDC J. Dent. Child.* 48:372, 1981.

Driscoll, W. S.: A review of clinical research on the use of prenatal fluoride administration for prevention of dental caries. *ASDC J. Dent. Child.* 48:109, 1981.

Eichenbaum, I. W., et al.: Impact of fluoridation in a private pedodontic practice: Thirty years later. *ASDC J. Dent. Child.* 48:211, 1981.

Gislén, G., et al.: Gingival inflammation in diabetic children related to degree of metabolic control. *Acta Odontol. Scand.* 38:241, 1980.

Katz, S.: A diet counseling program. *J. Am. Dent. Assoc.* 102:840, 1981.

Maw, R. B.: New look at maxillomandibular fixation of mandibular fractures. *J. Oral Surg.* 39:187, 1981.

Rönning, O., and Väliaho, M.-L.: Progress of mandibular condyle lesions in juvenile rheumatoid arthritis. *Proc. Finn. Dent. Soc.* 77:151, 1981.

Simonsen, R. J.: Clinical effectiveness of a colored pit and fissure sealant at 36 months. *J. Am. Dent. Assoc.* 102:323, 1981.

Thylstrup, A.: Is there a biological rationale for prenatal fluoride administration. *ASDC J. Dent. Child.* 48:103, 1981.

Wessberg, G. A., et al.: Transcutaneous electric stimulation as an adjunct in management of myofascial pain-dysfunction syndrome. *J. Prosthet. Dent.* 45:307, 1981.

Wright, J. M., Jr., et al.: Mycosis fungoides with oral manifestations: Report of case and review of literature. *Oral Surg.* 51:24, 1981.

Surgery and Urology

"Definition of 'Minor Surgery': Surgery someone else is having."—
ANONYMOUS

Any surgery is major, especially when it involves an adolescent
who is usually very concerned about his body. The articles and references selected for this section were chosen from several areas of surgery. They should prove useful to the clinician trying to help with the
decision to operate.

The articles and references on reduction mammaplasty are useful
in advising our patients on this procedure. Many times we find that
the adolescent or young adult who chooses this procedure is not fully
aware of the consequences.

The articles on scoliosis offer an update of treatment and the outcome of various procedures. Again, information necessary for advising our patients.

The article on appendicitis by Scher and Coil states that although
mortality from perforation has decreased, the incidence of perforation
has not changed. Perforating appendicitis was more likely to occur in
patients who lived more than 20 miles from the hospital and in patients younger than age 10 years or older than age 60. A large number of perforations occurred in the adolescent population, however.
Those of us who "work up" the acute abdomen, especially in adolescent females, know why this is possible.

From the urologic literature I have included several articles on testicular scanning. Many times the scan can be very useful in deciding
equivocal cases.

Ambulatory Surgery is discussed by Don E. Detmer (Univ. of
Wisconsin). There were early reports that children could be managed
safely on an ambulatory basis, and more recently, well-organized hos-
pital-based and freestanding ambulatory surgical programs for adults
have been developed. In another model of ambulatory surgery, the
patient never occupies a hospital bed in a defined unit but is discharged from the recovery room after surgery with general anesthesia. Some 75 surgical procedures can be done in an ambulatory
care setting. It has been estimated that 20% to 40% of hospital inpatient surgery could be done in an ambulatory setting. If more than
local anesthesia is used, the patient must be examined by a physician
before being discharged. Proof of quality of performance is necessary
to meet requirements of public accountability. Patients treated in an

N. Engl. J. Med. 305:1406–1409, Dec. 3, 1981.

ambulatory setting appear more likely than inpatients to feel that they would choose the same setting again. The patients save time and money and are spared the emotional stress of hospitalization.

Evaluation of the impact of ambulatory surgical care on costs and efficiency is complex. Patient costs are lower if surgery is done on an outpatient rather than an inpatient basis, but it is unclear whether money is ultimately saved at the level of the health care system. Reimbursement for ambulatory surgery varies, although most major insurance carriers reimburse for these services. Many ambulatory surgical units already are independent of hospitals, and outpatient physical therapy and emergency care clinics are expected to compete with hospitals in the future. Demands for cost containment, efficiency, and high-quality services are increasing. The development of ambulatory surgical units is a desirable, achievable, short-range type of objective for the health care system.

▶ [There is a slow but substantial growth in the utilization of ambulatory surgery in the United States. Surgery of the hand especially is mentioned in this article as being appropriate for this. There are other operations that can be done, for example, arthroscopy, both diagnostic and surgical procedures. A break with the tradition of hospitalization for all patients receiving general anesthesia is difficult. It takes incentive and willingness to "experiment" on the part of the orthopedist to utilize ambulatory surgery to a larger degree than in the past. The cost savings are definite and, in many instances, substantial.—M.B.C.] ◀

Reduction Mammaplasty for Moderate Macromastia. Armand D. Versaci (Rhode Island Hosp., Providence) reports experience using a modification of the Ribeiro method to treat moderate macromastia in 23 patients in 1977 to 1979. The nipple-areola site is not chosen until the end of the procedure. The width of the dermal pedicle is limited to one-half the length of the inframammary fold.

TECHNIQUE.—Skin markings are made with the patient standing and the arms at the sides. A thin epidermal graft is removed from the tissue to be used as the dermal pedicle flap (Fig 38). Full-thickness triangles of skin then are removed from either side of the dermal pedicle (Fig 39). The flaps must be separated completely from the breast parenchyma to visualize the boundaries of the glandular tissue. Dissection is carried onto the pectoralis fascia from the medial to the lateral borders of the gland, including an extension into the axilla. Full-thickness incisions are made along the inframammary fold, and the upper pole of the breast is appropriately undermined (Fig 40). Breast resection is then carried out segmentally, and the skin flaps are sutured along the inframammary line. The nipple-areola site then is marked, with an inframammary line-to-areola distance of about 4.5 cm, and the nipple-areola complex is sutured in place after removing a skin button. Suction drainage is used.

An average of 572 gm of tissue was removed from each breast in the 23 patients, who had an average age of 30 years. The longest dermal pedicle was 14 cm. No nipple-areola loss occurred. A conical breast with good support was obtained. Many of the patients were in their late teens or somewhat older and had moderate macromastia.

Ann. Plast. Surg. 6:253–261, April 1981.

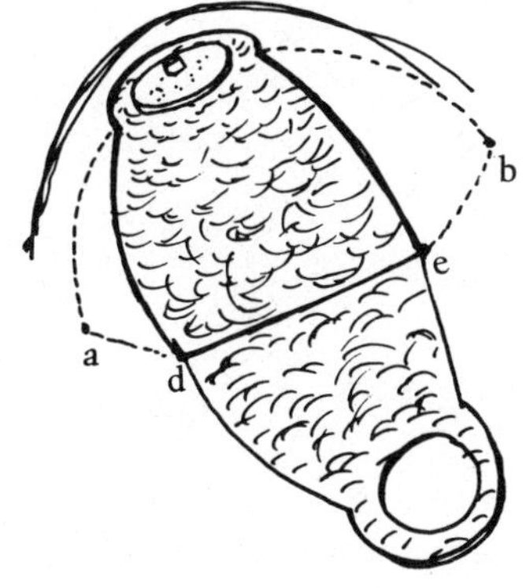

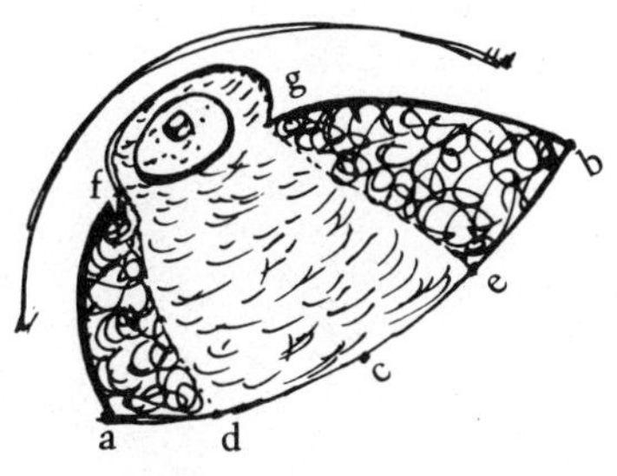

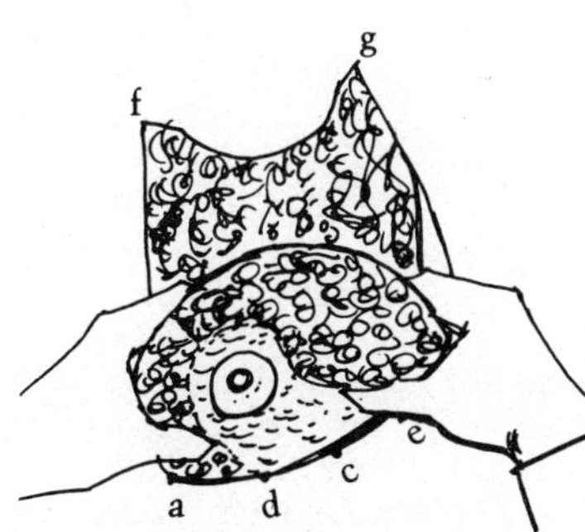

Fig 38 (top left).—First step of operation, the removal of thin epidermal graft from the tissue that will become the dermal pedicle flap.

Fig 39 (above).—Second step, the removal of full-thickness skin triangles from either side of the dermal pedicle.

Fig 40 (left).—Undermining the upper pole of the breast.

(Courtesy of Versaci, A. D.: Ann. Plast. Surg. 6:253–261, April 1981.)

They universally have accepted the limited reductions. Radical reductions were not done in these patients, because the breasts contained more glandular than fatty tissue compared with those of older patients, and the normal aging process can be expected to work toward that end.

▶ [This is a distillation of many other techniques. The article has merit because at some time we all need to vary our reduction. Selection of the new nipple-areolar site at the end of the procedure is highly desirable.—R.O.B.] ◀

Augmentation of the Minimally Ptotic Breast. Mastopexy leads to conspicuous surface scarring, which may be warranted for moderate to severe ptosis or hypertrophy, but not for the small or minimally ptotic breast. Bartels et al. (1976) recently described a periareolar approach to mastopexy, which involves the resection of a doughnut of skin concentrically about the areola, with extension of the inferior part of the incision through the dermis for additional augmentation. Murray W. Seitchik (Hahnemann Med. College, Philadelphia) describes a modification of this approach for augmenting the minimally ptotic breast.

TECHNIQUE.—After the new nipple has been located conventionally in the upright patient, an incision is made through the dermis, and a subdermal

Ann. Plast. Surg. 5:460–463, December 1980.

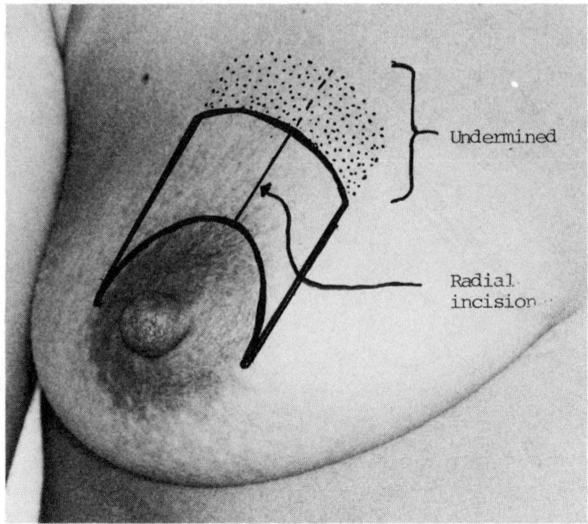

Fig 41.—Undermining beneath the superior skin edge permits a 5-cm radial breast incision. (Courtesy of Seitchik, M. W.: Ann. Plast. Surg. 5:460–463, December 1980.)

plane of dissection is developed beneath the superior skin margin, exposing 5 cm of subdermal tissue just above the areolar border. The breast substance is incised with an electric knife, from the superior areolar border along the entire length of the exposed area (Fig 41), and the incision is deepened to pectoral fascia, where a space is created for the prosthesis. The dense fibers attaching the breast to the pectoral fascia inferiorly are left intact. A 200-cc round implant can be inserted readily. The breast substance is closed with absorbable sutures, and the skin incision is closed in two layers. The disparity in length between the skin and areolar edges is managed by the "halving" suture technique.

This technique elevates the nipple and areola through both augmentation and supra-areolar skin excision. Ready access to the prepectoral space is gained in cases of minimal ptosis. It is not necessary to disturb the richly vascular, dense attachments of the pectoral fascia to the breast at the inferior margin of the muscle. If the supra-areolar skin resection does not exceed 3 cm, hypertrophic scarring should not be excessive, and the areolar shape should not be distorted.

▶ [Here is another procedure for the minimally ptotic breast.—R.O.B.] ◀

Pseudotumor Cerebri: Clinical Profile and Visual Outcome in 63 Patients. James A. Rush (Mayo Clinic) reviewed the findings in 63 patients seen in 1961 to 1978 with pseudotumor cerebri and no associated systemic disease. Follow-up data were available on 16 male and 45 female patients; the average age was 29 years (range, 2 to 67 years). Ten-year follow-up data were available in 75% of cases.

Mayo Clin. Proc. 55:541–546, September 1980.

Thirty-two patients were grossly obese; 5 had recently gained substantial weight. Seven patients had had a recent upper respiratory tract infection. Thrombosis of an intracranial dural sinus was diagnosed in 4 cases. Eight of the 45 female patients had menstrual irregularities at the time of diagnosis.

The median duration of symptoms before diagnosis was 36 days. Headache occurred in 75% of patients; in 6, it was the only presenting symptom. Two thirds of the patients noted disordered visual acuity, 9 as an isolated symptom. Three patients were asymptomatic, papilledema having been found in examination for nonneurologic conditions. Five patients had acuity of 20/30 or worse in at least one eye at the time of diagnosis. Only 4 of 56 patients tested had normal visual fields. Papilledema was mild or moderate in 42 cases. Six patients had evidence of increased intracranial pressure on skull roentgenography.

Six patients recovered spontaneously. Medical treatment sufficed for 48 patients, 43 of whom received corticosteroids alone or with acetazolamide or a diuretic; medical therapy was for 4 months or less in 43 patients. Ten patients required treatment for over a year. Nine patients were operated on; 6 had shunt procedures, 2 had subtemporal decompression, and 1 had decompression of the optic nerve sheath. Seven patients had a final visual acuity of 20/30 or worse, 4 of them unilaterally. Five patients who underwent surgery had a poor visual outcome. Twenty-three patients had recurrent symptoms of pseudotumor cerebri. Four patients had their first or only recurrence more than 4 years after the initial appearance of typical symptoms.

The mechanism of the optic nerve dysfunction producing visual failure in pseudotumor cerebri is not clear. Visual loss did not progress in any patient, but no patient with visual loss had substantial improvement, regardless of the treatment given.

▶ [Mingrino, Scanarini, and d'Avella (*Acta Neurochir. (Wien)* 51:187–193, 1980) consider benign intracranial hypertension probably due to a defect in cerebrospinal fluid resorption. In 8 of the 11 patients with at least a 2-year follow-up, prompt hypotensive effects were noted with intravenous injection of escin, a glycoside similar to saponins, obtained from the horse chestnut. The drug then was given intravenously every 8 hours for 3 days (20 mg), followed by 20–40 mg every 8 hours orally for 20–30 days. One of the 8 patients had a prompt initial benefit, but failed to respond thereafter either to escin or cortisone, and hence had a cerebrospinal fluid shunt. There was a highly suggestive correlation with hyperaldosteronism in 2 patients (elevated plasma renin level but normal blood pressure). Three patients who did not respond to escin did respond to dexamethasone. These may fall in a separate group in which the syndrome is due to disordered membrane transport mechanisms.

Although venous occlusions have been associated with benign intracranial hypertension, at times occlusion produces ventricular dilatation and hydrocephalus. Newman et al. (*J. Pediatr. Surg.* 15:215–218, 1980) report a case in which hyperalimentation (total parenteral nutrition) was used to combat chronic intractable diarrhea in a boy, aged 4 months. First the right internal jugular vein and then the left one had to be sacrificed, with resulting intracranial hypertension and hydrocephalus. When repeated computerized tomography scans showed no improvement, a lumboperitoneal shunt was carried out, with improvement in hydrocephalus and head size. Superior sagittal sinogram showed loci of obstructions in both internal jugular veins, with extensive vertebral venous collateralization.—O.S.] ◀

Juvenile Kyphosis: Histologic and Histochemical Studies. Ernesto Ippolito and Ignacio V. Ponseti (Univ. of Iowa) report the findings in the spine of a boy, aged 16, with juvenile kyphosis, who was killed in an automobile accident. The spinal segment examined was mildly kyphotic. Areas of reduced density and abnormally arranged cartilage cells were seen in the plates of involved vertebrae (Fig 42). Areas with abnormal interterritorial matrix stained strongly with alcian blue in concentrations of up to 1M magnesium chloride. The normal vertebral plate is only weakly alcianophilic with up to 0.4M magnesium chloride. The abnormal areas were only weakly periodic acid-Schiff positive, in contrast to normal areas. Endochondral ossification was altered in some areas of the growth plate, where few capillaries penetrated the cartilage and bone appeared to form directly on the abnormal cartilage. New bone appeared to have remodeled poorly, with large, thick trabeculae. Invaginations of nucleus pulposus into the vertebral body occurred where the cartilage of the adjoining vertebral plate was abnormal.

The vertebral plate of affected vertebrae in juvenile kyphosis has areas that are histologically and histochemically abnormal. Chondrocytes are numerous and often clustered, and the matrix is strongly alcian blue positive, suggesting a high content of proteoglycans or a different structural organization of the matrix. The matrix appears to lack glycoproteins. The findings suggest altered collagen synthesis in areas of the vertebral plate. The vertebral wedging appears to result from stunted ossification due to an abnormal cartilage matrix in the cartilage plate and underlying growth plate and from an increased postural load on the anterior part of the vertebrae. Similar abnor-

Fig 42.—Sagittal section of superior central part of T12 of boy, aged 16, with juvenile kyphosis. In right third of picture, vertebral plate is normal and stains with acid fuchsin. In center and to left, vertebral plate matrix is loose and aniline blue positive. Chondrocytes are clustered, and underlying growth plate is wider. Cason's trichrome; ×27. (Courtesy of Ippolito, E., and Ponseti, I. V.: J. Bone Joint Surg. [Am.] 63-A:175–182, February 1981.)

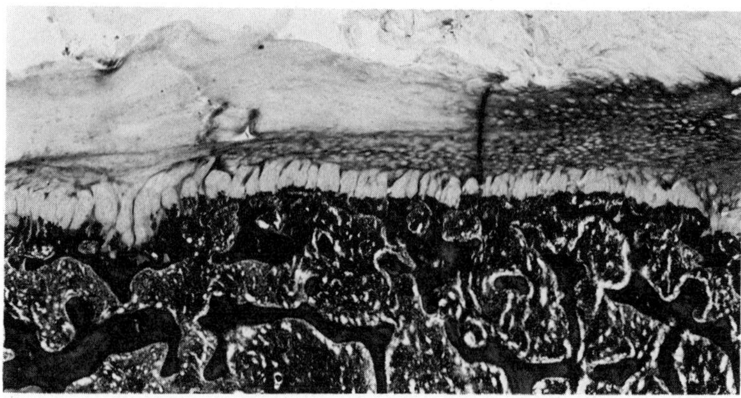

J. Bone Joint Surg. [Am.] 63-A:175–182, February 1981.

malities of growth plate cartilage have been found in slipped capital femoral epiphysis and Legg-Perthes disease, and juvenile kyphosis has been reported to coexist with slipped capital femoral epiphysis. The findings in this study do not support Jaffe's hypothesis of a primary disorder of the intervertebral disk.

▶ [This excellent study confirms that the basic pathology of juvenile kyphosis of the Scheuermann's type is abnormal vertebral and growth plate cartilage. This implies that the clinical diagnosis should rest more on the roentgenographic visualization of stunted ossification of the superior and inferior vertebral body margins than on wedging of the vertebral body, a secondary phenomenon that may occur in many unrelated conditions. The clinical relevance of this study would have been enhanced by showing roentgenograms of the two spines, particularly the abnormal spine to show the degree of spine deformity, irregularity of the vertebral margins, and vertebral body wedging.—H. A. Peterson] ◀

Idiopathic Scoliosis: Long-Term Follow-up and Prognosis in Untreated Patients. Stuart L. Weinstein, Donald C. Zavala, and Ignacio V. Ponseti (Univ. of Iowa) studied recent data on 194 of 219 patients with untreated adolescent scoliosis seen during 1932–1948. The 161 living patients included 136 women and 25 men aged 42 to 70 years (average, 53). The 144 patients who married had an average of 2.8 children. Only 2 women had to have cesarean sections. Of the 161 living patients, 37% had thoracic curves, 25% had lumbar curves, 26% had combined or double major curves, and 12% had thoracolumbar curves. All but 4 of the patients were normally active.

Frequent or daily backache was experienced by 37% of the patients compared with 25% of controls, but it was not disabling. Backache was unrelated to the presence or absence of osteoarthritic changes or to the severity of the curve. The cosmetic deformity of scoliosis was better accepted by the older patients. There was no correlation between the location or degree of the curve and the psychosocial effects. Many idiopathic scoliotic curves continued to increase slowly during adult life, particularly thoracic curves that measured 50–80 degrees. Scoliosis affected pulmonary function only in patients with thoracic curves and did not cause significant limitations in vital capacity and forced expiratory volume in 1 second until the curve approached 100–120 degrees. The pattern in nonsmokers was uniformly characteristic of restrictive lung disease.

The 33 patients who died represented a mortality of 15%, which is similar to the expected rate in the general population matched for age and sex. Scoliosis-related complications caused only 1 of the 33 deaths. Of 5 patients who had spine fusions performed as adults, all 5 had complications from surgery, including rod breakage and pseudarthrosis, and 4 continued to have back pain.

Progressive thoracic curves reaching 50 degrees at skeletal maturity should be fused. Because fusions to L4 and L5 may result in a high incidence of backache 10 years later, and because all patients in this study led normal lives although untreated, fusions of the lumbar

J. Bone Joint Surg. [Am.] 63–A:702–712, June 1981.

component of a double major or lumbar curve are of questionable value. Patients with double major or lumbar curves that are not severe, if skeletally immature, should be treated by bracing techniques because with aging they will not be limited by poor pulmonary function or backache. Patients with thoracolumbar curves who have increasing severity of the curve do not have decreased pulmonary function but they do have a marked degree of cosmetic deformity and increasing, though not disabling, back pain (often associated with a translatory shift of the vertebrae). Thus, surgical treatment of these curves when they reach 50–60 degrees is justified.

▶ [This is a classic study on the natural history of adolescent idiopathic scoliosis, with a follow-up of 194 of 219 patients covering a period from 1932 to 1948. The conclusion of the authors is that scoliosis adds only moderately to the incidence of severe backache in this population group. They also noted that progression of deformity occurred primarily in the thoracic area where curves reached 50 to 80 degrees before skeletal maturity. Some lumbar curves also tended to progress. Therefore, the previous articles by these authors have been substantiated. Much discussion has arisen out of these findings. The practical experience of many orthopedists dealing with adult scoliotics has noted that disabling pain, particularly in the lumbar area, is associated with this degree of scoliosis. However, good comparison studies, as these authors present, are not available. Numerous reconstructive procedures are being performed on adult scoliotics, with reasonably good results with an 85% relief of pain. The morbidity of these procedures is significant, however, and they must be carefully considered before going ahead with surgery.—R. A. Klassen] ◀

The Changing Pattern of Scoliosis Treatment Due to Effective Screening. Gunnar Torell, Anders Nordwall, and Alf Nachemson (Göteborg, Sweden) evaluated the results of a program for the early detection and treatment of scoliosis in a stable Swedish population in 1968–1978. Patients younger than age 20 with idiopathic scoliosis of 20 degrees or more were included in the study. The 725 patients had a mean age at referral of 14 years; 8.7% were male. In the first 5 years, patients with curves of 25–45 degrees were treated in a Milwaukee brace, and those with greater curves were operated on. Subsequently, patients with curves no greater than 40 degrees were managed by bracing; since 1977, the minimum curve considered suitable for brace treatment has tended to be 30 degrees. Since 1976, the Boston brace has been used for progressive curves measuring 25–40 degrees with an apex at T-10 or below. A scoliosis information campaign was begun in 1968, but no strict program for screening was organized.

There was a great increase in referrals and a decrease in the average age of patients referred to the center during the 10-year review period. The average curve also decreased during the study period: the mean curve was 46 degrees in 1968 and 28 degrees in 1978. The average angulation of the ten most severe curves diagnosed each year decreased as well. A total of 59 patients who initially had brace treatment were operated on; most had initial thoracic curves of 40–45 degrees and were seen in the early years of the study. A total of 182 patients were operated on. The proportion declined from 32% to 12%

J. Bone Joint Surg. [Am.] 63–A:337–341, March 1981.

of referred patients, although the indications for surgery were widened in the latter part of the study.

Several years were necessary for the full impact of the information program to be realized. Fewer operations have been necessary. Early detection in combination with early brace treatment of scoliosis appears to reduce the risk of undetected scoliosis deteriorating and is as important as treatment method in obtaining good final results in the population.

▶ [All active scoliosis centers in North America as well as abroad have noted a changing pattern of patient referral, which has resulted in a changing pattern of scoliosis treatment. This article is a definitive study documenting these changes and is the most complete study of its kind to date.—H. A. Peterson] ◀

Hip Pain During Adolescence After Perthes' Disease. Garry D. Grossbard (Royal Natl. Orthopaedic Hosp., London) studied the findings in 12 patients with healed or healing Perthes' disease who experienced pain after a symptom-free period. They were examined clinically and with plain radiography and arthrography. This allowed them to be separated into five groups: osteochondritis dissecans, with and without loose bodies (2 patients each); hinging hip (4); torn acetabular labrum (1); meralgia paresthetica (1); and no diagnosis (2).

Osteochondritis dissecans is an uncommon complication, occurring after the femoral head lesion appears to have healed, but having a variable symptom-free period before becoming clinically manifest. The incidence is highest in male subjects in whom the age of onset of Perthes' disease has been greater than average. The clinical features are generally episodes of stiffness and intermittent pain, which may cause catching or locking of the hip, especially if the osteochondritic fragment is loose.

With overgrowth of the anterolateral aspect of the articular cartilage and crushing of the trabeculae in the bony epiphysis, the unossified portion of the femoral head tends to bulge out from under the lateral portion of the acetabular roof; as a result the leg is adducted, and attempted abduction causes impingement of the femoral head against the superior acetabular rim, which causes the hip to hinge at this point of contact. The resulting pain may be associated with a feeling of the hip "clunking" as it hinges in and out of the acetabulum. This situation is particularly troublesome with an adduction deformity of the hip, when symptoms are produced on attempting to bring the leg into a neutral position.

A torn acetabular labrum may result from an alteration of hip mechanics and shape of the femoral head. After a symptom-free period, development of pain with locking of the hip may be suggestive. This condition occurring after Perthes' disease has not been previously described in the literature.

In meralgia paresthetica, the lateral cutaneous nerve of the thigh either is stretched over a bony protruberance at the site of a prior

J. Bone Joint Surg. [Br.] 63–B:572–574, 1981.

pelvic osteotomy or it is involved in scar tissue within the surgical incision.

The differentiation of these conditions is often difficult clinically. The use of arthrography during general anesthesia has been invaluable in differentiating them and in planning management. In osteochondritis dissecans arthrography is the only method that will determine whether the osteochondritic fragment is loose within the hip. The presence of specific pathologies must be searched for; in this series, simple uncovering of the lateral aspect of the femoral head was not a cause of symptoms.

▶ [Osteonecrotic fragments can develop into osteochondritis dissecans with and without loose bodies. I am surprised that the abnormal shape of the femoral heads after Legg-Calvé-Perthes disease only rarely results in tears of the acetabular labrum. Tearing and erosions of the acetabular labrum are frequent with the "medial type" of coxarthrosis. Cartilaginous osteophytic formation occurs peripherally on the femoral head.—R. H. Fitzgerald, Jr.] ◀

Appendicitis: Factors That Influence Frequency of Perforation. Although mortality from perforating appendicitis has decreased dramatically, the incidence of perforation has not changed over the past 30 years. Kenneth S. Scher and James A. Coil, Jr. (Marshall Univ., Huntington, W. Va.) reviewed the records of 335 consecutive patients treated for acute appendicitis over a 2-year period to determine those factors that may influence the frequency of appendiceal rupture.

There was evidence of perforation in 108 of the 335 patients. Differences regarding race, sex, educational level, family income, health insurance coverage, availability of transportation, and possession of a telephone were not significant between those with and those without perforation. Perforating appendicitis was more likely to occur in patients who lived more than 20 miles from the hospital ($P < .002$) and in patients younger than age 10 years or older than age 60 (table). The mean duration of symptoms before seeking medical attention was 2.5 days in patients with appendiceal rupture and 1.5 days in those without perforation ($P < .001$). Yet, approximately 75% of the patients in each group reported having a "family doctor." The mean number of physician visits before hospital admission was 1.61 in

AGE OF 335 PATIENTS WITH ACUTE APPENDICITIS

Age (years)	No. Cases	No. Perforated	Incidence of Perforation
0-10	60	24	40%
11-20	127	27	21.3%
21-30	69	17	24.6%
31-40	25	6	24%
41-50	21	9	42.9%
51-60	17	10	58.8%
>60	16	15	93.8%

South. Med. J. 73:1561–1563, December 1980.

those with perforation and 1.33 in those without (P <.005). Of the patients with perforating appendicitis, 54.3% had been seen previously by a physician who failed to make the diagnosis.

The results seem to indicate that patient delay in seeking medical attention and failure of the physician to make a correct diagnosis are the principal factors contributing to the frequency of appendiceal rupture.

▶ [Even though the incidence of diagnosis before appendiceal perforation has not changed significantly, the authors point out that treatment has been much improved and mortality reduced. It would be interesting to know the time interval between initial evaluation by a physician and the final diagnosis of perforated appendix in the 54.3% of patients seen prior to the time of final diagnosis. It is rare for an appendix to perforate and within less than 24 hours of symptoms. Seeing and releasing a patient with undifferentiated abdominal pain is a common occurrence in the emergency unit. If a second evaluation is carried out within the next 12 to 15 hours, only a limited number of cases of appendicitis will have proceeded to perforation. Abdominal pain seen earlier in the day "at another institution" deserves special attention and not the attitude of "here comes another hospital shopper."—D.K.W.] ◀

Testicular Scan: Use in Diagnosis and Management of Acute Epididymitis. Jonathan S. Vordermark II, Alfred S. Buck, Stanton R. Brown, and William K. Tuttle III (Madigan Army Med. Center, Tacoma, Wash.) obtained 79 orchiograms in 69 patients with epididymitis seen in 1975–1979. The age range was 12–63 years. Most patients hospitalized with a diagnosis of epididymitis underwent scanning. The supine patient was positioned beneath a gamma camera and, after premedication with potassium perchlorate, 10 mCi of pertechnetate was injected. Children received a dose of 5–10 mCi, based on body weight. Both dynamic and static imaging were carried out.

Scans were consistent with the final clinical diagnosis in 94% of the 69 patients. Four patients had normal scans in the face of clinical epididymitis. Three had "mild" involvement. No patient with a false negative scan had complications. The severity of epididymitis could not be related to the degree of uptake. Scans showed the pathologic features in all 12 patients undergoing exploration on clinical indications.

Testicular scanning has a high false negative rate in patients with mild epididymitis, but it is highly accurate in demonstrating more severe forms of epididymitis. Abscesses at least 1 cm in diameter can be demonstrated by scanning, and testicular hypoperfusion or infraction can be detected. Although very useful in the diagnosis and management of severe epididymitis, the orchiogram is not a substitute for clinical judgment. The orchiogram is the most sensitive method available for the early detection of abscess formation, testicular hypoperfusion, and testicular infarction.

Doppler Ultrasound Versus Testicular Scanning in Evaluation of the Acute Scrotum. There are several causes of an acute scrotum, including torsion of the spermatic cord, which requires im-

JAMA 245:2512–2514, June 26, 1981.
J. Urol. 125:343–346, March 1981.

RESULTS OF RADIOISOTOPIC TESTICULAR SCAN CORRELATED WITH DOPPLER ULTRASONOGRAM AND SURGICAL DIAGNOSIS

	Surgical Diagnosis No. Pts.	Scan Diagnosis		Doppler Diagnosis		
		Correct No. (%)	Incorrect No.	Correct No. (%)	Undetermined No. (%)	Incorrect No.
Torsion	5	5 (100)	0	3 (60)	2 (40)	0
Non-torsion	15	15 (100)	0	11 (73)	4 (27)	0
Totals	20	20 (100)	0	14 (70)	6 (30)	0

mediate surgical treatment. Extreme tenderness precludes adequate examination and makes diagnosis difficult. David D. Rodríguez, Wilmar C. Rodríguez, Jaime J. Rivera, Saul Rodríguez, and Andres Acosta Otero (Puerto Rico School of Medicine, San Juan) compared the diagnostic efficacy of Doppler ultrasound with that of testicular scanning in men aged 35 and younger, seen in a 2-year period with a clinical diagnosis of acute scrotum. Isotope studies were done with pertechnetate.

Forty-seven patients with a mean age of 16 years were evaluated. Torsion of the cord was confirmed operatively in 13 cases. Twenty-one other patients had a surgical diagnosis of epididymitis, and 6 had torsion of the testicular appendages. The Doppler and surgical findings correlated in 62% of the cases of torsion and in 85% of the patients without torsion; the overall diagnostic accuracy was 79%. The Doppler study was misleading in only 1 case, in which torsion of the cord was present. The results of testicular scanning in 20 cases are given in the table. The scan and surgical findings correlated in all cases, and the Doppler and surgical findings correlated in 70% of these cases.

These findings confirm the value of Doppler ultrasonography in evaluating patients with acute scrotum. The study was misleading in only 1 of the present cases. The testicular scan is the most reliable diagnostic method in this setting, especially for eliminating torsion of the cord, but it is more expensive and is a technically elaborate procedure. Where scanning facilities are unavailable, the Doppler study is helpful. If torsion is suspected, immediate exploration is mandatory.

▶ [The differential diagnosis of the acute scrotum usually can be made from the history, physical examination, and urinalysis. Routine use of scanning is unnecessary. In the occasional equivocal case, testicular scanning is very useful. Stage and associates also recently reported (*J. Urol.* 125:334, 1981) a very high rate of accuracy using testicular scanning in patients with an acute scrotum.—S.S.H.] ◀

Testicular Function After Combination Chemotherapy in Childhood for Acute Lymphoblastic Leukemia (ALL). Testicular tubular damage frequently has been observed in boys given combi-

Arch. Dis. Child. 56:275–278, April 1981.

nation chemotherapy for ALL. It has been suggested that vulnerability of the testes to cytotoxic drug damage may vary with pubertal status at the time of treatment. Stephen M. Shalet, Ian M. Hann, Mehroo Lendon, Patricia H. Morris Jones, and Colin G. Beardwell (Manchester, England) assessed testicular function by luteinizing hormone releasing hormone (LH-RH) and human chorionic gonadotropin (hCG) stimulation tests in 44 boys previously or currently receiving chemotherapy for ALL. Twenty-three patients were still on cytotoxic drug therapy at the time of testicular biopsy. Thirty-two boys were prepubertal, 8 were early pubertal, and 4 were late pubertal.

Apart from low basal LH values in prepubertal children, the patients had basal gonadotropin levels and median peak responses to LH-RH similar to those of control children of similar pubertal status. One prepubertal patient had an exaggerated FSH response to LH-RH, and 2 others had exaggerated LH responses. Three of the 8 early pubertal ALL patients had elevated basal serum FSH levels; 1 of them also had an elevated basal LH level. Two of the 4 late pubertal ALL patients had elevated basal serum FSH levels and supranormal FSH responses to LH-RH. One of them also had an exaggerated LH response. The prepubertal and pubertal patients had, as groups, normal testosterone responses to hCG stimulation.

These findings suggest that moderately severe damage to the testicular tubules unassociated with Leydig cell impairment may not be detected in prepubertal boys by current tests of testicular function. The coexistence of abnormal morphological findings and normal function has been partly responsible for the view that the degree of testicular damage in boys given cytotoxic drug therapy may depend on pubertal status at the time of treatment.

▶ [These papers document that boys who are treated for acute lymphoblastic leukemia usually undergo normal puberty and are endocrinologically intact. The following article by Blatt et al. suggests that spermatogenesis may become normal in these boys, but a more detailed biopsy study by the Shalet group (*Lancet* 2:439, 1978) demonstrated definite morphological damage to the testis of boys during and after treatment. It is encouraging that many of these patients will be fertile. Infertile patients who have received chemotherapy should have a complete fertility evaluation and should be followed for several years to determine whether or not spermatogenesis recovers.—S.S.H.] ◀

Covert Bacteriuria in Schoolgirls in Newcastle upon Tyne: A 5-Year Follow-up. Chronic urinary tract infection is a cause of end-stage renal failure and is responsible for one fifth of patients requiring dialysis in Europe. The natural history of covert bacteriuria was investigated by the Newcastle Covert Bacteriuria Research Group (Newcastle upon Tyne, England) in a series of 13,464 girls, aged 4–18 years, who were screened for bacteriuria in 1968–1972. A total of 256 girls (1.9%) were found to have bacteriuria, and 39 of 254 who were examined radiologically (15%) had renal scarring. Of 211 girls followed up, 105 were allocated to chemotherapy for 2 years, prefera-

Arch. Dis. Child. 56:585–592, August 1981.

bly with co-trimoxazole. A daily dose of trimethoprim, 4 mg/kg, up to 160 mg was given for 3 weeks, followed by sulfadimidine, 40–50 mg/kg, up to 2 gm/day. Treatment was stopped after 2 years if it had been effective in the previous 6 months.

About half the girls not given chemotherapy were in remission after 5 years, whereas one fourth of this group had received antibiotics for urinary tract or incidental infection. All but 2 of the girls in the chemotherapy group showed some response. Just over one-third had positive cultures at 5 years, and 10 girls had developed symptoms. Only 2 subjects had persistently positive cultures. Eleven percent of the untreated girls eventually required treatment for symptomatic urinary tract disease. Renal growth was similar in the two groups over the 5-year observation period. Only 1 girl, in the no-therapy group, developed a new renal scar. Most scarred kidneys in patients in an obligatory chemotherapy group exhibited below-average growth, and several patients showed increased renal scarring during follow-up.

It is suggested that, until a reliable nonradiologic method of detecting renal scarring is available, schoolgirls should not be screened for covert bacteriuria.

▶ [Interesting observations in this 5-year study of treated and untreated girls with asymptomatic bacteriuria detected by screening examinations include (1) the infrequency of urinary symptoms among the untreated girls; (2) the absence of renal scarring among the untreated girls; (3) the spontaneous resolution of bacteriuria in approximately 50% of the untreated girls; and (4) the difficulties involved in conducting an epidemiologic study in which it is hoped that a group of patients will not receive antibiotics—Jackson E. Fowler, Jr.] ◀

Urine Culture After Treatment of Uncomplicated Cystitis in Women. A urine culture is often obtained in young women a few days after the end of treatment for a urinary tract infection to determine whether bacteriuria is present and whether antibacterial therapy should be instituted. Occasionally, many follow-up urine cultures are obtained. The need for follow-up cultures may be questioned because of findings that uncomplicated asymptomatic bacteriuria in nonpregnant women does not lead to chronic renal failure or an increased incidence of serious infection. Richard N. Winickoff, Susan I. Wilner, Gail Gall, Thomas Laage, and G. Octo Barnett conducted a retrospective study to determine whether a single follow-up urine culture reduces subsequent episodes of urinary tract infection in women seen in a primary care setting. A total of 141 women with culture-proved symptomatic lower urinary tract infection were studied.

Eighty patients without symptoms had follow-up cultures done within 3 months after initial infection, and 61 did not. The groups were clinically comparable and had similar causes of urinary tract infection. Sulfisoxazole was prescribed for 84% of all initial urinary tract infections. Five patients had resistant organisms. Subsequent urinary tract infection occurred in 15% of the follow-up group and

South. Med. J. 74:165–169, February 1981.

8.2% of the control group. The respective rates of bacteriuria over 1 year were 16.2% and 13.1%. Comparable proportions of the two groups received antibiotics for problems unrelated to urinary tract infection. Only 3.8% of the follow-up culture group had positive cultures, and only 1 of these had a subsequent symptomatic urinary tract infection by the same organism.

Follow-up urinary cultures may not be justified in asymptomatic healthy women treated for uncomplicated urinary tract infection, and the costs of follow-up can be eliminated for many women with sterile urine after a short course of antibiotics.

▶ [In our clinics, women with uncomplicated culture-documented bacteriuria are encouraged to submit a posttreatment urine specimen for culture. No appointment is necessary, a physician need not see the patient, the patient is not charged for a clinic visit, and the cost of the culture is approximately $10. As demonstrated in this study, most asymptomatic patients will have sterile posttreatment cultures. However, we have been impressed that most patients comply with our recommendations and that most patients are reassured when it is proved that their infection has been eradicated.—Jackson E. Fowler, Jr.] ◀

Does Antibacterial Ointment Applied to Urethral Meatus in Women Prevent Recurrent Cystitis? Recurrent urinary tract infection occurs in 5% of females, often even after appropriate antibiotic therapy. The rectal flora is considered the primary reservoir of urinary tract pathogens. H. H. Meyhoff, J. Nordling, P. A. Gammelgaard, and R. Vejlsgaard (Univ. of Copenhagen) undertook a double-blind crossover trial to evaluate the use of an antibacterial ointment in preventing recurrent cystitis when applied to the urethral meatus of women without obstructive uropathy. Twenty-three women who had had at least 2 urinary tract infections treated with antibiotics in the previous 6 months entered the trial, and 17 completed it. The median age was 39 years. About 0.5 ml of 10% povidone-iodine ointment was applied to the urethral meatus each morning and evening and before sexual intercourse. Active ointment and placebo were used for 6-month periods.

The results of urine culture and the number of urinary tract infections did not differ significantly during treatment with active ointment or placebo. The overall incidence of urinary tract infection was reduced from 2 or more to 0.9 per 6 months during the study (both treatments). Side effects were mild. Cultures obtained from the urethral, periurethral, and introital areas during the study yielded results similar to those obtained in pretreatment cultures.

A povidone-iodine ointment, self-applied to the urethral meatus, was of no greater value than placebo in preventing urinary tract infection in women in this study with recurrent nonobstructive cystitis. It is likely that the reduced occurrence of infections was related to improved perineal hygiene. Instruction in perineal hygiene seems preferable to the use of an inert ointment.

▶ [The incidence of bacteriuria during the application of both the antibacterial ointment and the placebo ointment was less than that during the 6-month period prior to

Scand. J. Urol. Nephrol. 15:81–83, 1981.

the study. This probably reflects the natural history of urinary infection in susceptible women that is characterized by clusters of infections over a short time, followed by an infection-free interval of 6–12 months. The need for meaningful controls in the evaluation of any treatment is well demonstrated in this study.—Jackson E. Fowler, Jr.] ◀

Relationship Between Frequency of Sexual Intercourse and Urinary Tract Infections in Young Women. An estimated 10% to 20% of women have a symptomatic urinary tract infection at some time. An association with sexual intercourse has been suggested, but the precise relation between intercourse and the development of infection remains unclear. Arthur B. Elster, Patricia A. Lach, Klaus J. Roghmann and Elizabeth R. McAnarney (Univ. of Utah) examined this relationship in women seen in a 3-month period with symptoms suggestive of acute urinary tract infection and in healthy college-aged women seen in a 1-month period for preventive care. Evaluation was made of 32 students with symptoms of infection and positive cultures for a single organism who had been sexually active in the past 2 weeks and 28 controls. *Escherichia coli* was cultured from the urine in 82% of the study group.

The two groups were similar in age, marital status, age at first coitus, and family history of urinary tract infection or kidney stones. More study women, however, reported that their mothers had had a urinary tract infection. In addition, 70% of the study group had coitus in the past week, and all had been sexually active in the current week. Their average weekly number of coital episodes had increased, whereas that of control subjects had declined. Over 50% of the study group and about 30% of controls had intercourse more often in the current week than in the past week. Genitourinary habits (e.g., perineal wiping and frequency of urination) were comparable in the two groups.

Some healthy young women exhibit an association between an increased frequency of sexual intercourse and the development of symptomatic urinary tract infection. Trauma to the lower genitourinary tract from coitus may alter vaginal adhesiveness and permit vaginal or periurethral bacteria to colonize the urethra and subsequently enter the bladder. However, sexual activity cannot be the only factor predisposing such individuals to urinary tract infection.

▶ [Epidemiologic data indicating that the incidence of bacteriuria in female subjects increases between the ages of 13–20 years and the frequent clinical observation that young women will experience their first episode of bacteriuria shortly after the onset of sexual activity provide convincing circumstantial evidence that intercourse promotes bacteriuria. Nonetheless, the sexual activity of women who are susceptible to urinary infection does not appear to differ from that of women who are resistant to urinary infection. This suggests that other factors, most likely a propensity for colonization of the vaginal introitus by urinary pathogens, predisposes to bacteriuria and that sexual intercourse may increase the possibility of infection in these susceptible women.—Jackson E. Fowler, Jr.] ◀

South. Med. J. 74:704–708, June 1981.

Additional Reading

Ariyan, S.: Reduction mammaplasty with the nipple-areola carried on a single, narrow inferior pedicle. *Ann. Plast. Surg.* 5:167, 1980.

Blatt, J., et al.: Testicular function in boys after chemotherapy for acute lymphoblastic leukemia. *N. Engl. J. Med.* 304:1121, 1981.

Dubousset, A. M., et al.: Autotransfusion with acute hemodilution in the surgical treatment of scoliosis. *Rev. Chir. Orthop.* 67:609, 1981.

Dunnick, N. R., and Javadpour, N.: Value of CT and lymphography: Distinguishing retroperitoneal metastases from nonseminomatous testicular tumors. *AJR* 136:1093, 1981.

Gore, D. R., et al.: Scoliosis screening: Results of a community project. *Pediatrics* 67:196, 1981.

Haderspeck, K., and Schultz, A.: Progression of idiopathic scoliosis: Analysis of muscle actions and body weight influences. *Spine* 6:447, 1981.

Hague, M., et al.: Parental perceptions of enuresis: A collaborative study. *Am. J. Dis. Child.* 135:809, 1981.

Hall, J. E., et al.: Surgical treatment of scoliosis with or without Harrington instrumentation. *J. Bone Joint Surg.* [*Am.*] 63-A:608, 1981.

Hawkins, D. B., et al.: Caustic ingestion: Controversies in management: Review of 214 cases. *Laryngoscope* 90:98, 1980.

Kass, E. J., et al.: Significance of bacilluria in children on long-term intermittent catherization. *J. Urol.* 126:223, 1981.

Kunin, C. M.: Duration of treatment of urinary tract infections. *Am. J. Med.* 71:849, 1981.

Mathes, S. J., et al.: Avoiding the flat breast in reduction mammaplasty. *Plast. Reconstr. Surg.* 66:63, 1980.

Medical Letter on Drugs and Therapeutics: Issue 589—Treatment of urinary tract infections. 23:69, 1981.

Montgomery, S. P., and Erwin, W. E.: Scheuermann's kyphosis: Long-term results of Milwaukee brace treatment. *Spine* 6:5, 1981.

Schultz, A., et al.: Correction of scoliosis by muscle stimulation: Biomechanical analyses. *Spine* 6:468, 1981.

Singer, R., and Krant, S. M.: Intravenous fluorescein for evaluating the dusky nipple-areola during reduction mammaplasty. *Plast. Reconstr. Surg.* 67:534, 1981.

Turck, M.: New concepts in genitourinary tract infections. *J.A.M.A.* 246:2019, 1981.

Sports Medicine

"A healthy mind in a healthy body."—THADDEUS KOSTRUBALA, M.D.,
in *The Joy of Running*

Many health care professionals believe that adolescents and young adults need an exercise program of some type to help them through this period of life. The importance of exercise and a healthy mind and body can not be overemphasized. The field of sports medicine has grown, and exercise programs have forced the clinician to be knowledgeable in different areas of athletic endeavor. The many articles included in this section cover many aspects of sports health care and deserve consideration in our efforts to care for the adolescent athlete.

Sudden Death and Physical Exertion are discussed by Gad Keren and Yehuda Shoenfeld (Tel-Hashomer, Israel). Although physical activity has a number of beneficial effects, it may cause sudden death in both sportsmen and others. Affected sportsmen may have left heart hypertrophy, bradycardia, and disordered intraventricular conduction. Sudden deaths are particularly frequent in sports that require prolonged tolerance, such as marathon running, or an abrupt transition from rest to extreme exertion. Activities associated with extreme vagal stimulation and increased intrathoracic pressure may also be implicated. Diagnoses made in cases of sudden death of sportsmen are listed in the table. Sudden death in inactive persons is chiefly a result of acute myocardial infarction, and it appears that excessive exertion can cause infarction.

Sudden collapse can be attributed to a rise in blood pressure with exercise and a subsequent fall to subnormal levels, especially when

CONDITIONS DIAGNOSED IN SUDDEN DEATH
IN YOUNG PERSONS

Disease	Cases	Ref.
(a) Coronary artery disease	33	7
Acute coronary occlusion	18	6
(b) Coronary malformation	5	15
	2	16
	1	17
(c) Malformation of artery to S-A node	2	18
(d) Tear of aorta	8	7
	1	19
(e) Stenosis of ventricular outlet	3	7
(f) Myocarditis	7	7
	1	20

J. Sports Med. 21:90–93, March 1981.

exertion stops abruptly, and to the Valsalva maneuver or expiratory effort. Bradycardia and extension of the vulnerable period in the ECG compromise the electric stability of the heart and increase the risk of ventricular arrhythmia. Some sudden deaths may be accompanied by chest pain or tachypnea, but heart disease may be unsuspected because of the age of the subjects. Sudden deaths, however, have occurred during or just after physical exertion in sportsmen who underwent thorough examination and were found to be healthy.

▶ [Jokl regards the phenomenon of profound Valsalva or expiratory effort as the principal risk factor affecting the heart during exercise. This phenomenon is most common in wrestlers and weight lifters. It has been noted that intrathoracic pressure may reach 160–220 mm Hg in the course of weight lifting. Excessive internal thoracic pressure can prevent the proper filling of the left ventricle; measurement of blood pressure during such periods may show a systolic pressure as low as 20–25 mm Hg. These two factors in concert—the drop of systolic blood pressure and increase of intrathoracic blood pressure—may be compounded further by the bradycardia of athletes and predispose them to the risk of ventricular arrhythmia. Sports that are associated with sudden, brief, static exertion include wrestling, weight lifting, and tennis.—L.J.K.] ◀

Sudden Death While Playing Professional Football. A recent study of 29 competitive athletes aged 13 to 31 years who died suddenly showed that all but 1 died of cardiovascular conditions, the most common being hypertrophic cardiomyopathy. Three deaths were due to atherosclerotic coronary heart disease. William C. Roberts and Barry J. Maron (Natl. Inst. of Health) report the findings in a professional football player who died suddenly during a game.

The player, who died while walking back to the huddle after running a pass pattern, had developed intense upper abdominal pain 6 weeks earlier, with "aching" in the shoulders, bradycardia, and brief syncope. The pain was nearly absent next day, but fever was present and the serum lactic dehydrogenase value was found to be elevated 2 days after discharge. He was subsequently asymptomatic until death.

Autopsy showed a large transmural healing infarct on the posterolateral wall of the heart, consistent with a duration of 6 weeks. The right, left anterior descending, and left circumflex coronary arteries were diffusely atherosclerotic and severely narrowed by plaques. A small thrombus with underlying plaque hemorrhage was present in the right coronary artery. The liver and spleen were both enlarged.

There was a strong family history of type II hyperlipoproteinemia in this case, and a serum cholesterol measurement of 350 mg/dl had been obtained within a month before death. Extensive hemorrhage into atherosclerotic plaques was observed. This may have been related to contact of the anterior cardiac surface with the sternum in tackling and blocking, with resultant "cracking" of the atherosclerotic plaques. The crack may in turn have led to intraluminal thrombosis. Cracks in plaques might also result from "jarring" without actual contact of heavily atherosclerotic coronary vessels.

▶ [Granted, postmortem examination of this young athlete revealed an unusual anatomical feature, extensive hemorrhage into atherosclerotic plaques about the epicar-

---

Am. Heart J. 102 [Pt. 1]:1061–1063, December 1981.

dial coronary arteries. The authors postulate that trauma caused by the contact of sternum with relatively rigid atherosclerotic vessels was responsible. This may have been the case, but I think the burden of proof is on the person who would contend that this was not a recurrent myocardial infarction in an individual who had sustained documented myocardial infarction in the recent past. The fault, if any, was that at the time of the original abdominal pain associated with diaphoresis and elevated LDH enzyme, a possibly diagnostic cardiogram was not performed, and that he was permitted to resume contact professional football. Coronary artery disease is part of the differential diagnosis of chest or upper abdominal pain, especially if such pain is associated with diaphoresis.—L.J.K.] ◄

Aspirin and Athletics is discussed by Roxanne Caron (Keene State College, Keene, N. H.). Aspirin is one of the most widely used and misused drugs. Team physicians have prescribed it for many painful inflammatory conditions and for the management of pain associated with sprains and strains. The most significant adverse effects of aspirin involve the gastrointestinal (GI) tract and include GI tract bleeding. The GI effects of aspirin can be minimized by using time-release capsules or enteric-coated tablets. Rectal suppositories avoid GI tract symptoms, but absorption is very slow and incomplete. Aspirin increases the prothrombin time, possibly resulting in an increased bleeding time. The central nervous system effects of aspirin include dizziness, headache, and somnolence. Palpitations and tachycardia have been noted. Aspirin may lead to tinnitus, hearing loss, and visual disturbances. Aspirin interacts with various other drugs as well as with alcohol. It interacts with both indomethacin and naproxen. Interactions of aspirin with antibiotics are frequent.

Aspirin overdosage can occur with the administration of presumably "therapeutic" doses, particularly in children, who may exhibit hyperventilation and decreased respiration in the later stages, metabolic acidosis and ketosis, hyper- or hypoglycemia, and twitching. Dehydration and electrolyte imbalance can result from vomiting. Occasionally, internal bleeding occurs. Adults experience lethargy, episodic hyperpnea, tinnitus, and headache in the early stages and, later, loss of hearing, acidosis, hypoglycemia or hyperglycemia, dehydration, and electrolyte imbalance. Some symptoms can be relieved by reducing the dose of aspirin. Sodium bicarbonate hastens the elimination of aspirin. Vitamin K can be given to counteract hypoprothrombinemia. In cases of severe intoxication or hemorrhage, exchange transfusion may be necessary. Sellers et al. suggested the use of activated charcoal in patients with aspirin intoxication. Athletes with aspirin intoxication should be taken immediately to a physician or hospital.

► [Pain is essentially a warning to the body of tissue injury. If the injury is mechanical in nature, as is usually the case in an athlete, there is a need to rest until repair processes are complete. Attempts to override the pain signal by massive doses of aspirin seem an unacceptable form of "doping," with the risks from the drug itself and the incomplete repair process that is ignored.—R.J.S.] ◄

► [Interesting side effects of aspirin not commonly appreciated include augmented sweat loss, increased urinary output, and the inhibition of thirst. In this sense, this

Athletic Training 16:56–58, Spring 1981.

may predispose to hyperthermic problems, especially in such situations as a marathon. Of significance obviously is the rare instance in which aspirin may induce asthma, and the superimposition of salicylate sensitivity expressed as bronchospasm and exercise-induced asthma should be considered. In simple terms, asthmatics probably should not use this agent and exercise. Still to be delineated are reports suggested in the Australian literature that aspirin in high dosage may cause renal damage, including frank necrosis. I am not impressed with Tylenol as a substitute and rather look on that drug as a potential hepatotoxic agent that has had inappropriate pharmacologic promotion by the media.—L.J.K.] ◀

Smoking, Respiratory Symptoms, and Ventilatory Capacity in Young Men: With a Note on Physical Fitness and Acute Respiratory Infections. Previous studies of lung function in young, asymptomatic smokers have given conflicting results. Pekka Kujala (Oulu, Finland) examined the relation between smoking and ventilatory capacity in young servicemen in northern Finland. The 1,076 subjects in the study took 12-minute running tests. Seventeen subjects had evidence or a history of bronchial asthma, and 2 others had undergone lung resection. Nearly two thirds of the subjects smoked, and 9% were ex-smokers. The mean age was 20.1 years.

Smokers had lower values for forced expiratory volume in the first second (FEV_1) and forced expiratory flow than did nonsmokers, but no differences in peak expiratory flow or forced vital capacity were evident. The group difference in FEV_1 was 0.1 L. Function could not be related to the number of cigarettes smoked daily. Smokers had more respiratory symptoms than nonsmokers, including coughing, wheezing, and dyspnea. The incidence of chronic bronchitis was 16% in smokers and 3% in nonsmokers; ex-smokers had an intermediate rate. A history of pneumonia was more frequent in the smoking group. Chronic bronchitis was associated with an increase in other respiratory symptoms, but not with the results of lung function tests or physical work capacity. No significant group difference was found in the number of acute respiratory infections resulting in time off duty. The results of 12-minute runs were poorer in smokers, and correlated negatively with the amount smoked.

Smoking is associated with a reduced ventilatory capacity in young men. The relationship is more evident in tall than in short men. Smoking increases respiratory symptoms, and is associated with impaired physical work capacity.

▶ [The significance of this study is the litany of documented abnormalities observed in young people during a relatively brief interval of time, their military conscription years. The abnormalities identified were not correlated with the number of cigarettes consumed, although prior data would certainly suggest that this has some relevance. If anyone is distressed by the percent (68%) of those recruits who were smoking, it is of further note that this percentage appears to be similar for Norwegian, Swiss, Dutch, American, and Austrian military recruits.—L.J.K.] ◀

Exercise-Induced Asthma: Comparison Between Two Modes of Exercise Stress. Exercise can produce bronchoconstriction in the absence of various exogenous factors. Omri Inbar, Diego X. Alvarez,

Eur. J. Respir. Dis. 62(Suppl.114):7–55, 1981.
Ibid., pp. 160–167, June 1981.

and Harold A. Lyons (SUNY, Downstate Med. Center) compared the effects of an exhaustive effort lasting 50 seconds with those of a 7-minute submaximal effort, which has been documented as causing the most marked bronchoconstriction in asthmatics. Studies were done in 6 male and 4 female asthmatic patients with a mean age of 32.4 years. Two were using prednisone besides bronchodilators. All patients had had extrinsic asthma for at least 2 years. The short treadmill exercise test produced exhaustion within 40 to 50 seconds. The submaximal test produced a heart rate 85% of the age-predicted maximum. The respective mean power outputs were 1,000 and 400 kg per minute.

Minute ventilation, oxygen consumption, carbon dioxide production, and blood pH and lactate concentration were significantly higher during supramaximal exercise. Changes in ventilatory functions are shown in Figure 43. A significant 21% fall in timed forced expiratory volume and a 20% fall in maximal midexpiratory flow (MMEF) occurred with submaximal exercise. The exhaustive challenge led to no significant fall in 1-second forced expiratory volume (FEV_1) but a 26% fall in MMEF occurred. Airway resistance increased about 20% after the submaximal effort, but no significant change followed the brief exercise. Specific conductance decreased 20% after submaximal exercise and about 7% after the short, exhaustive exercise.

Short, exhaustive exercise leads to a marked reduction in MMEF without significant effects on FEV_1 or specific conductance. This type of stress apparently leads to marked obstruction of the small airways without affecting conductance in the large airways. Differences in respiratory heat exchange may be responsible. A short, exhaustive exercise challenge may accurately detect small airways obstruction.

► [It is known that prolonged exercise of seven minutes or longer may bring about large airway constriction and frank asthma. This study shows that exhaustive exercise of less than one minute's duration does not affect conductance in the large airways, but does cause marked obstruction of small airways and clinical asthma nonetheless. The hypothesis remains to be proved that this is a function of heat exchange. It does

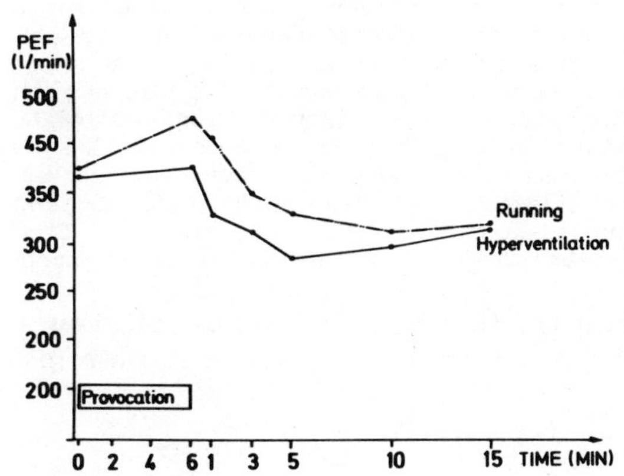

Fig 43.—Changes in 1-second forced expiratory volume (FEV₁), maximal midexpiratory flow rate (MMEFR), and forced vital capacity (FVC) after submaxmal exercise (hatched bars) and short, maximal exercise (solid bars). Means ± SEM are shown. (Courtesy of Inbar, O., et al.: Eur. J. Respir. Dis. 62:160–167, June 1981.)

provide a testing system for inducing small airway obstruction. It may also have therapeutic implications as to whether one is attempting to deal with large or small airway constriction in the asthmatic episode.—L.J.K.] ◄

Effect of Physical Training on Exercise Performance of Children Following Surgical Repair of Congenital Heart Disease. Training programs have been used for patients who had surgery for acquired coronary artery disease, but the use of such programs after the repair of congenital cardiac lesions has received little attention. Barry Goldberg, Raymond R. Fripp, George Lister, Jacob Loke, James A. Nicholas, and Norman S. Talner (Yale Univ. School of Med. and Inst. of Sports Medicine and Athletic Trauma, Lenox Hill Hosp., New York) examined the effects of physical training on exercise performance in 13 male and 13 female patients who underwent surgery for tetralogy of Fallot or ventricular septal defect. A 6-week alternate-day submaximal interval home exercise program was conducted. Work loads were chosen to maintain heart rates of 130–160 beats/minute. The mean age at the time of study was 13.9 years, and at the time of surgery 5.8 years.

Subjects completed an average of 18 of 21 possible training sessions. Maximum work capacity improved 25%. Only 31% of patients performed at less than expected maximal work capacity after training, compared with 65% before training. Significant reductions in oxygen consumption and heart rate were noted at all work levels, indicating improved aerobic efficiency. No significant change in maximum oxygen consumption was observed. Eight patients remained more than 1 SD below Godfrey's norms, and 3 improved to the normal range. Maximum minute ventilation and heart rate were not changed significantly by training.

Many children with congenital heart disease have reduced exercise performance despite excellent hemodynamic results from surgical repair, and a training program can provide the potential for a more normal life style in selected cases. Further studies are needed to determine the program that will provide maximum physiologic improvement while affording safety and promoting compliance.

► [A number of children with repaired tetralogy of Fallot or ventricular septal defect, despite excellent hemodynamic results, continued to have diminished exercise performance values when compared with mean normal values. The finding that those patients with active lifestyles have normal exercise capabilities and that training can improve exercise performance in those with diminished capabilities suggests that the level of cardiovascular conditioning may be a significant factor in postoperative exercise performance. For this reason, postoperative exercise testing is strongly recommended in the medical evaluation of these children. Such testing would have two goals: (1) to permit reliable recommendations of permitted physical activity; (2) to select those who could benefit from rehabilitative intervention in the form of a conditioning program.—L.J.K.] ◄

Exercise-Induced Proteinuria in Children and Adolescents. Physical effort can cause proteinuria in healthy subjects. Both glo-

Pediatrics 68:691–699, November 1981.
Scand. J. Clin. Lab. Invest. 41:583–587, October 1981.

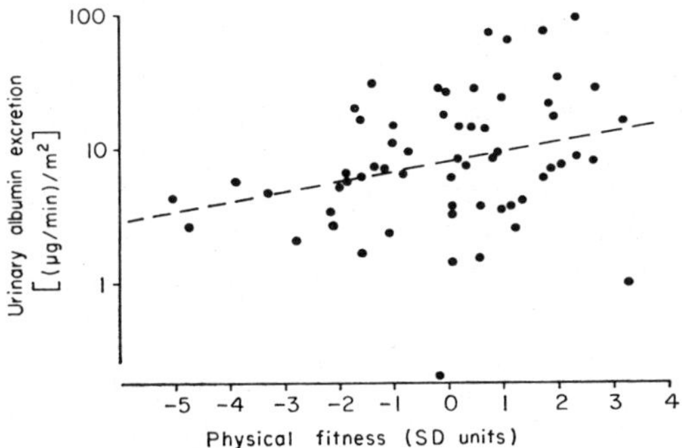

Fig 44.—Correlation between urinary excretion rate of albumin during exercise and physical fitness of subjects; log y = 0.07x + 0.90; r = 0.28; P < .05. (Courtesy of Huttunen, N.-P., et al.: Scand. J. Clin. Lab. Invest. 41:583–587, October 1981.)

merular leakage and impaired tubular reabsorption have been implicated. Niilo-Pekka Huttunen, Marja-Liisa Käär, Marjatta Pietiläinen, Pirkko Vierikko, and Matti Reinilä (Univ. of Oulu) determined urinary albumin and β_2-microglobulin excretion in 60 healthy subjects of both sexes, aged 9–19 years, before and after bicycle exercise. Subjects worked at a rate of 60–70 rpm for 16 minutes at increasing workloads to produce final pulse rates of 170–200 beats per minute.

The mean albumin excretion rate for all subjects increased significantly on exercise, although 19 subjects had decreases. Geometric mean rates of β_2-microglobulin and creatinine excretion were a little higher before than after exercise for the group. No sex differences were apparent in albumin or creatinine excretion, but the boys excreted more β_2-microglobulin both at rest and on exercise. Average urine flows were 1.9 ml per minute per sq m at rest and 1.5 during exercise. Albumin excretion during exercise correlated positively with physical fitness (Fig 44) and with maximal systolic blood pressure, but no correlation was found between albumin excretion and age or urine flow rate.

Physical exercise increases albuminuria in children and adolescents. The increase in albumin excretion appears to be equal in boys and girls and independent of age. Reduced renal blood flow is the most likely explanation for the increased albumin excretion associated with exercise.

▶ [The increase of urinary albumin excretion during exercise without concomitant increase in β_2-microglobulin excretion indicates a glomerular leaking type of proteinuria during physical stress in this study group of children and adolescents. This can be thought of as a consequence of reduced renal capillary blood flow during exercise stress.—L.J.K.] ◀

Immunologic Responses to Training in Conditioned Runners. The long-term effect of intense daily physical exercise on the immune

Clin. Sci. 60:225–228, February 1981.

system and host defense status of athletes is unknown. P. G. Hanson and D. K. Flaherty (Univ. of Wisconsin) investigated the immunologic response to training in 6 well-conditioned male runners. Total leukocyte count, subpopulations of leukocytes, and immunoglobulin and complement levels were measured 15 minutes before and 10 minutes and 24 hours after a continuous 8-mile training run (estimated work intensity, 72% of $\dot{V}_{O_2}$ maximum).

All parameters were within the normal range before the start of the run. At 10 minutes after completion of the run, a statistically nonsignificant increase in total leukocytes was observed, which included variable increases in mature neutrophils, T lymphocytes (E rosettes), B lymphocytes (EAC rosettes), and mononuclear EQ-IgG rosettes (table). With the Chang liver cell assay, a significant increase was observed in the antibody-dependent cytotoxic activity of K lymphocytes ($P < .05$). At 24 hours postexercise, all cellular populations had returned to the normal, preexercise range. However, the cytotoxic activity of K lymphocytes remained significantly elevated ($P < .05$). Immunoglobulin and complement levels were not significantly changed at 10 minutes or 24 hours.

Chronic exercise training does not appear to have an adverse effect on circulating cellular or humoral immune components in healthy, well-conditioned adults. In addition, the increase in K lymphocytes may provide added host defense capacity during and after periods of physical stress.

IMMUNE RESPONSES TO EXERCISE

Response	Rest	Postexercise	
		+10 min	+24 h
Component leucocytes (mm^{-3})			
Total leucocytes	5373 ± 1995	7166 ± 2569	4996 ± 1889
Neutrophils	3046 ± 1385	3930 ± 854	2667 ± 788
Bands	62 ± 111	10 ± 24	64 ± 59
Eosinophils	118 ± 46	105 ± 138	71 ± 99
Basophils	11 ± 27	35 ± 45	23 ± 28
T-Lymphocytes	1361 ± 554	1690 ± 1047	1390 ± 609
B-Lymphocytes	446 ± 236	557 ± 565	434 ± 217
EA-IgG rosettes	228 ± 318	658 ± 978	254 ± 193
Antibody dependent cytotoxic activity (%)			
K-Lymphocytes	67 ± 10	79 ± 14*	83 ± 12*
Mononuclear cells	35 ± 9	41 ± 11	41 ± 10
Immunoglobulins (i.u.)			
IgG	148 ± 29	151 ± 32	146 ± 28
IgA	128 ± 48	131 ± 43	122 ± 48
IgM	134 ± 69	180 ± 52	173 ± 32
IgE	296 ± 381	315 ± 326	224 ± 272
Complement (mg/100 ml)			
C$_3$	83 ± 10	92 ± 14	96 ± 13
C$_4$	27 ± 7	28 ± 6	28 ± 7

*$P < .05$ compared with the resting value (Student's paired t test).

▶ [There has been surprisingly little study of the influence of physical activity on an individual's susceptibility to infections. It is recognized that exercise may cause localization of some viral infections in active tissues (anterior poliomyelitis, acute viral myocarditis). One recent study noted that six-year-old children were absent from school more frequently if they were enrolled in an activity program, but older students (aged 7–11 years) behaved much the same way as a control group (Shepard, R.J., *Physical Activity and Growth,* London, Croom Helm, 1982). In theory, the stress of prolonged running would be expected to alter immune responses. Hanson and Flaherty found no change, but it may be that an effect would have been detected with more severe effort; the 8-mile run at 72% of maximum oxygen intake may be compared with a 26-mile marathon event at 82% of maximum oxygen intake by some of our "postcoronary" patients.—R.J.S.] ◀

Immune Function in Marathon Runners. Many runners claim reduced susceptibility to respiratory infections. Apart from denial of pain or a "runner's high," augmentation of host immunity is a possibility. Richard L. Green, Sandra S. Kaplan, Bruce S. Rabin, Carl L. Stanitski, and Ursula Zdziarski (Univ. of Pittsburgh) examined the immunologic status of 20 male marathon runners, 6 of whom had completed marathon races in the past month. Two were studied within 3 days of completing a marathon, and 3 had blood samples taken within an hour of a 10-mile run. Mean immunoglobulin values were within normal limits. Half the runners had slightly low total lymphocyte counts. Leukocyte phagocytosis and killing were consistently normal. Nine subjects reported that resistance to respiratory infections had increased and 1 that it had declined, but these findings could not be correlated with significant changes in measures of immune function.

Long-distance running has no effect on immune function. No consistent augmentation of immune function was demonstrated in this study, but the rigorous demands of a marathon training schedule appear not to affect immune variables adversely.

▶ [The normal immunologic integrity or immunity depends upon certain intact variables in the host; these include the capacity of the white blood cells to phagocytize and kill invading organisms; the presence of humoral antibody that is capable of defending against bacteria and viruses; the presence of lymphocytes that defend via cellular immune mechanisms against viruses, fungi, and bacteria; and lastly, the presence of complement in an adequate amount for immune adherence and phagocytosis. Normal leukocyte phagocytosis and killing, and normal quantitative immunoglobulin levels were shown in the 20 marathon runners. Quantitative immunoglobulin concentrations were not any greater or less in the world-class runners and were indistinguishable from those of runners in a slower, low-mileage group. One hypothesis is that, in a marathon or any extreme exertion, a poorly trained person is certainly capable of weakened host defenses. This is analogous to the stressed rat and has anecdotal support in human subjects in the literature. Impaired immune defenses are likely to be present in the stressed individual at high altitude, and this is an area that still must be documented with precision.—L.J.K.] ◀

Renal Function Abnormalities Induced by Marathon Running. Castenfors reported changes compatible with renal ischemia after short periods of cycling, and isolated cases of acute renal failure requiring dialysis have followed exercise. James A. Neviackas and

Ann. Allergy 47:73–75, August 1981.
South. Med. J. 74:1457–1460, December 1981.

John H. Bauer (Univ. of Missouri, Columbia) assessed renal functional changes induced by marathon racing in 4 normal men, aged 26–48 years, who completed either 1 or 2 marathon runs of 26.2 miles. All were experienced marathon racers who trained an average of 60–100 miles a week. They were allowed to deplete and load carbohydrates as they wished. All decreased their mileage in the week before the races.

The runners did not have muscle cramps during or after the warm- or cold-weather marathons. The average weight loss during the warm-weather races was 7.7 lb. Serum electrolyte levels were unchanged. The creatine phosphokinase level was increased after the race, but was normal after 1 week. Numerous urinary red blood cells, granular casts, renal tubular epithelial cells, and heavy proteinuria were observed in initial postrace specimens, but all subjects had normal findings subsequently. The warm-weather runners had positive urinary myoglobin tests after the race but normal findings at 1 week. The inulin clearance was 50% of baseline after warm-weather races. The para-aminohippurate (PAH) clearance was slightly below normal in 2 of 3 runners. The postrace filtration fraction ranged from 11.5% to 14.5%; it was normal at 1 week. One runner had a slightly abnormal creatinine clearance after the race. Values at 1 week were clearly depressed in 2 runners. The fractional excretion of creatinine increased after the race in all 3 runners, and decreased to below unity at 1 week. Cold-weather runners had no decrease in inulin or PAH clearances. One of 3 runners had a further depression of creatinine clearance 1 week after the race. All runners had an abnormal fractional excretion of creatinine after the race, with normal findings at 1 week.

These asymptomatic runners exhibited renal functional alterations after a marathon run. There was no evidence of prolonged ischemia. Runners should be warned that warm-weather marathon racing may precipitate significant renal functional abnormalities.

▶ [There has been much debate concerning the significance of proteinuria and other changes in renal function that accompany vigorous exertion. The present report shows that when healthy competitors cover a marathon distance in warm weather, sustaining fairly severe dehydration, the creatinine excretion is still abnormal one week later. At this stage, inulin clearance has been restored to its baseline value, and it thus remains controversial whether the reduced excretion of creatinine reflects a continuing abnormality of renal function; possibly, it is due rather to replenishment of muscle creatine stores lost during the bout of sustained exertion.

Nevertheless, the present report is of value in showing the acute depression of inulin clearance, and in establishing that changes are more severe when the same subjects run a marathon distance in warm, rather than cold weather.—R.J.S.] ◀

Jogging and Diabetes Mellitus. David R. Jones and Kenneth A. Johnson (Mayo Clinic) encountered a woman aged 20 who had had diabetes for several years, complicated by proliferative retinopathy and peripheral neuropathy despite reasonably good control with insulin. She experienced mild calcaneal pain in both feet while jogging.

Foot Ankle 1:362–364, May 1981.

Her x-ray films showed an infraction of the inferior calcaneal margin of the left foot and a displacement of the calcaneal apophysis of the right foot. Increased technetium uptake was seen in both calcanei. Both feet healed with the use of short-leg walking casts for 3 months, and the patient then was given total plantar contact shoes. Another insulin-dependent diabetic woman, aged 21, complained of bilateral calcaneal pain during long-distance jogging, which had persisted months after running was stopped. A technetium scan showed increased uptake in both calcaneal regions and in the navicular region of the left foot. Pain resolved when weight-bearing was reduced.

Diabetes previously has been related to stress fracture of the calcaneus. Neuropathic bone changes are not uncommon in patients with diabetes. Neuropathy may permit repeated stresses to accumulate without a normal pain response; jogging stresses may also be applied in an unusual manner. Vascular disease may be a factor in stress fractures in diabetics. Reduced bone mass has been described. Diabetics who jog should be cautioned about the risks involved. If pain develops but roentgenograms are negative, a stress fracture should be considered. The technetium bone scan is useful both for diagnosis and for monitoring bone healing during treatment.

▶ [The relationship of diabetes mellitus to stress fracture of calcaneus has been reported previously by Coventry in the *Journal of Bone and Joint Surgery* in 1979 and by Daffner in *Skeletal Radiology,* 1978. It is postulated that in multisystem disease such as diabetes, an associated peripheral neuropathy, vascular disease, or primary bone disease could cause the fracture. Neuropathic bone changes are not uncommon in patients with diabetes mellitus and may be the presenting feature leading to the diagnosis. The hypothesis further contends that the neuropathy may permit repetitive stresses, as well as the supplemental stress of jogging, without triggering the normal pain response. It is harder to implicate the vascular disease of diabetes. Reduced bone mass also has been described in patients with diabetes mellitus. The fracture risk appears to be for leg and ankle alone. Persistent pain in an impact type area in a diabetic or nondiabetic, even if initial roentgenograms are negative, warrants a technetium bone scan as the definitive diagnostic test.—L.J.K.] ◀

Fractures and Refractures in Intercollegiate Athletes: An 11-Year Experience. James A. Whiteside, Samuel B. Fleagle, and Alexander Kalenak (Pennsylvania State Univ., University Park) discuss the incidence of fractures and refractures occurring among intercollegiate athletes participating in 18 sports at Pennsylvania State University during an 11-year period from the fall of 1968 through the spring of 1979.

During the study period, 231 fractures occurred at 17 different injury sites in 185 male and 34 female intercollegiate athletes. The greatest number of fractures occurred in men's (M) football, followed by basketball (M), wrestling (M), soccer (M), women's (W) gymnastics, lacrosse (M), and lacrosse (W), and the greatest percentage of fractures in specific squad populations occurred in football (M), followed by basketball (M), gymnastics (W), volleyball (W), lacrosse (W), and soccer (M). The fracture rate was 3.05% for the specific squad popu-

Am. J. Sports Med. 9:369–377, Nov.–Dec. 1981.

lation of men and 1.98% for women. Overall, the fracture rate was 2.46% for the athletic population. Of the 231 fractures, 119 (52%) occurred in football, at a rate of approximately 11 per year. Although most of these fractures occurred in practices, the fracture incidence was 1 (12.5%) per 8 games and only 1 (7%) per 14 practices. More fractures occurred in winning than in losing seasons. The most common fracture sites were the finger, hand, face, foot, nose, and leg, regardless of sport or gender.

Of 28 fractures of the fifth metatarsal, 50% occurred in football. The most common fracture site overall was the proximal shaft, followed by the widest portion of the base and the proximal base. Except in 3 cases where refractures occurred, a noncasting, nonoperative, aggressive rehabilitation program was successful.

Of the 15 refractures, 14 occurred in collision or contact sports and involved the hand and finger, tibia, fifth metatarsal, clavicle, and rib. The mean interval between fracture and refracture was about 26 weeks (range, 8.3–44.4 weeks). Essentially, the refractures assumed the same fracture line as the initial break, and the same mechanical forces caused both fractures.

▶ [Attempting to tabulate and "analyze" a variety of different fractures occurring among a variety of different intercollegiate teams can be likened to counting the vegetables in an Irish stew. If that is your thing, fine. However, from the standpoint of data analysis it can serve no useful purpose. A second error is noted in the authors' failure to appreciate the different healing patterns of the variety of fractures that occur in the fifth metatarsal. Also, their designation of the "Jone's type" fracture occurring at the base, rather than in the proximal shaft distal to the tuberosity, is not correct. The attempt to demonstrate a relationship between the incidence of fractures and the relative success or failure of Penn State's football team is not statistically valid.—J.S.T.] ◀

High School Sports Injuries. Robert A. Shively, William A. Grana, and Dennis Ellis compared the injury rates in boys and girls participating in 8 predominantly noncontact interscholastic sports in 79 Oklahoma high schools during the 1978–1979 school year. The sports were track, cross-country running, swimming, tennis, volleyball, soccer, basketball, and baseball/softball.

There were 165 injuries in 6,478 boys and 132 injuries in 4,807 girls, for an injury rate of 25.4 and 27.4 injuries per 1,000 participants, respectively. Major injuries were significantly more common in girls than in boys ($P < .05$). One girl basketball player died, apparently as a result of cardiac arrest. Both groups had a similar pattern of injury by anatomical area, although the girls had a significantly higher incidence of knee injuries than boys ($P < .01$). Sprains and strains were the most frequently reported injury, and there was no marked difference between the sexes in any specific type of injury. The most frequently sprained area was the ankle, and the girls had a significantly greater frequency of major ankle injuries ($P < .05$). The girls lost more time as a result of their injuries than did the boys, even though the severity of their injuries was similar. Twenty-one

Physician Sportsmed. 9:47–50, August 1981.

boys and 27 girls were lost for the season, and 11 boys and 12 girls underwent surgery for treatment of their injuries. More injuries occurred in practice than in competition in both boys (95 injuries) and girls (90 injuries). Slightly more injuries were sustained during the second half of the season than the first half.

Although the overall injury rates did not differ significantly between boys and girls, the girls lost more time as a result of injury. This may be because there is less emphasis on year-round conditioning programs for girls, and girls may have less motivation to return rapidly to competition because there is less peer pressure to do so. More information is needed to determine whether the trends toward more ankle sprains and more major knee injuries in girls are real.

▶ [The authors should be complimented on their methodology in conducting this epidemiologic study on Oklahoma secondary school sports injuries. Their findings support the published work of Garrick et al. (*Pediatrics* 61:465–469, March 1978; and *JAMA* 239:2245–2248, May 26, 1978) on Seattle high school athletes. The significantly greater number of knee injuries and major ankle injuries experienced by female athletes is discussed in terms of anatomical differences between boys and girls as well as the decreased emphasis on year-round conditioning programs associated with female athletics.—J.S.T.] ◀

Weight Training-Related Injuries in the High School Athlete. Skilled high school coaches are competent in training specific performance capacities of their athletes, but they may not be aware of the disabilities resulting from overtraining. Thomas A. Brady, Bernard R. Cahill, and Leslie M. Bodnar retrospectively reviewed the records of 80 junior and senior high school athletes who sustained weight training-related injuries between August 1976 and August 1980.

It was difficult to determine the exact cause of injury in 37 of the 80 patients, because history also revealed a program of running excessive mileage or running repetitive laps in the gymnasium. Of the remaining 43 athletes with injuries caused almost exclusively by a weight training program, 29 experienced lumbosacral pain. These 4 girls and 25 boys had an average age of 15.8 years. A history of using the Leaper as part of a weight training program was cited by 17 of the 29 patients. In 6 patients the lumbosacral syndrome developed as a result of combining Leaper workouts with Universal Gym workouts. Dead weight lifting accounted for 4 of the lumbosacral injuries and workouts on the Universal Gym alone accounted for the remaining 2. Surgical treatment was required in 4 of these patients; 3 others were hospitalized, but treated conservatively. Home treatment with a hospital bed and pelvic traction was required by 20 patients.

Avulsion of the anterior superior iliac spine was the second most frequent injury, occurring in 6 of the 43 patients. Complete avulsion occurred in 2 of these patients while they performed hyperextension back exercises on the Universal Gym. Partial separation of the anterior superior iliac spine occurred in 2 athletes while performing on the Leaper and in another 2 while performing dead weight lifting.

Am. J. Sports Med. 10:1–5, Jan.-Feb. 1982.

None required surgery. Four athletes sustained meniscal laceration, 2 while performing leg curls and 2 while performing dead weight lifting. All of these patients underwent surgery for a torn meniscus. Acute cervical sprain occurred in 4 athletes while working out on the Leaper, and all responded to conservative treatment.

This review demonstrates the importance of taking an adequate history regarding the weight training program used by the injured athlete. Most weight training-related injuries are insidious, having a gradual onset. Weight training programs should be supervised to allow safe increases in the use of sophisticated weight training routines within specific limits.

▶ [This article attempts to demonstrate a relationship between weight training and injuries sustained by young athletes while participating in a weight training program. The results do not support this: 50% of the injuries reported could not be linked to weight lifting. The authors do, however, point out the need for knowledgeable, direct supervision with attention to training technique as means of preventing most of the injuries that occur as a result of this activity.—J.S.T.] ◀

Cost of High School Soccer Injuries. Soccer is the most widely played sport in the world and today is increasing in popularity in the United States. James W. Pritchett (Phoenix, Ariz.) obtained data on the cost of high school soccer injuries from the largest single insurer of secondary school students in 6 Western states for the 1976 and 1977 seasons. Claims were reported for 4.1% of 10,634 players. The average claim cost was $127. Minor injuries (e.g., sprains, strains, contusions, and abrasions) constituted about 75% of all injuries and about 50% of all costs. Lower extremity injuries accounted for more than 50% of all injuries and costs. Knee injuries accounted for 11.7% of all injuries and 28% of all medical costs paid by the insurance companies.

Injuries are 20% as frequent in soccer as in football. It is expected that medical expenses for soccer players will be less than 16% of those for an equal number of football players. Knee injuries and internal derangements of the knee are about equally frequent in injured soccer and football players. Lower limb injuries are more frequent in soccer players, but all other body regions are injured less frequently. The proportion of injuries costing more than $285 is about equally frequent in the 2 sports.

▶ [The conclusions drawn from the data as presented, is somewhat misleading regarding "equal frequency" of knee injuries and internal derangements of the knee among football and soccer players. All injuries, including knee injuries, occur five times more frequently in football; i.e., the incidence of knee injuries in a population of soccer players is one fifth that of a comparable population of football players. What is similar is the distribution of knee injuries (11%) in both groups, not the frequency or incidence.—J.S.T.] ◀

Injuries in Interscholastic Wrestling are reviewed by Ralph Requa and James G. Garrick. The injuries associated with participation in 19 interscholastic sports during a 2-year period were investigated.

Am. J. Sports Med. 9:64–66, Jan.–Feb. 1981.
Physician Sportsmed. 9:44–51, April 1981.

Certified trainers were placed in 4 schools to document male and female interscholastic sports injuries. Both practices and matches were monitored. An injury was defined as a condition which caused the participant to be removed from practice or competition, or to miss a subsequent practice or event. In wrestling the term injury has a broader definition and can include time-out periods.

The 234 wrestlers sustained 176 injuries, for a rate of 75.2 injuries/ 100 participants/season. Of the sports investigated, only football had a higher injury rate (81.1 injuries/100 participants). The likelihood of sustaining a more severe injury was somewhat higher in wrestling than in football. The number of strains and sprains was similar and accounted for almost 75% of the wrestling injuries. The upper extremities were involved in 29% of injuries, the lower extremities in 33%, and the spine and trunk in 34%. The most common injuries were paraspinous strains, knee sprains, and sprains and strains of the upper extremities, especially the shoulder. There was 1 shoulder dislocation-subluxation, and the shoulder was involved in 3% of sprains and 14% of strains. Knee sprain is often associated with football, but was much more common in wrestling. There were no significant brain or spinal cord injuries in this study.

More than 1 in 5 injuries represented a reinjury, although in the shoulder, knee, elbow, and ankle about 1 in 3 was a reinjury. About one third of ankle sprains were reinjuries, but the initial injury did not necessarily occur in wrestling.

Although they involve only 15% of the wrestler's activity at most, competitive events accounted for a high proportion of injuries. When activity time is expressed in minutes at risk, matches constitute only 1% of wrestling time.

Injuries can also be related to the position of the wrestler at the time of occurrence. One third occurred with the wrestler in the neutral position. In injuries which occurred when 1 wrestler had the advantage, 85% were to the one having the disadvantage. Wrestling has been criticized for promoting extreme, possibly hazardous, weight reduction practices, but no overt injury problems related to these practices were seen in this study.

The individual risk of injury in wrestling is at least equal to that in tackle football.

▶ [Having described an injury rate of 75.2 injuries per 100 participants per season, the authors conclude that ". . . medical or paramedical coverage should be present at all competitive events." It appears that such data would better serve as the impetus for implementation of preventive measures by identifying etiologic factors.—J.S.T.] ◀

Injuries in Interscholastic Track and Field. High-school track and field is one of the most popular interscholastic activities among both sexes. It encompasses diverse activities and provides opportunities for people with varying skills to participate. Previous studies of injuries often lack precise diagnostic information. Use of an oversimplified injury classification system hinders any attempt to create le-

Physician Sportsmed. 9:42–49, March 1981.

gitimate injury prevention programs. Superficial investigations also lack control information about the population at risk and probably underrate injuries that have subtle transitory symptoms or cause marginal decrements in performance. R. K. Requa (Goldwater Found., Sun City, Ariz.), and J. G. Garrick (Center for Sports Med., San Francisco) discuss the results of a study conducted over a 2-year period in 4 high schools. Each school had trained personnel to identify, classify, and follow all sports injuries. An injury was defined as a traumatic medical condition resulting from athletic participation that necessitated the athlete's removal from practice or a competitive event, or resulted in the missing of a subsequent practice or event.

During the study, 308 boys and 208 girls participated and had 101 and 73 injuries, respectively. Injuries were sustained during practice in two thirds of cases in all sports and in three fourths of cases in track and field. For girls, 89% of injuries occurred during practice, compared with 64% of injuries in boys. The severity of injuries was slightly lower than in the all-sport average. Track and field had a high proportion of injuries resulting in more than 5 days of lost time; 40% of girls' injuries and 30% of boys' injuries fell into this category, and 19% of girls' and 14% of boys' injuries resulted in a loss of more than 10 days.

Musculotendinous injuries constituted the largest category. Inflammations occurred more often than in most other sports, but sprains were less common, as were contusions, lacerations, and fractures. The lower extremities are used extensively in all track and field events, and 85% of the injuries in this series involved the lower extremities. The thigh was the most common site of injury, followed by the leg and knee. Thigh strains, primarily those involving the hamstrings, were common and constituted 55% and 52% of the strains and 28% and 21% of all injuries for boys and girls respectively. Shinsplints, muscle and tendon injuries of the leg, and various inflammatory knee problems made up most of the injuries to these areas. Ankle injuries were rare.

More than 70% of track injuries in girls occurred in events of distances of 440 yards or less, compared with 36% in boys. Almost 40% of the boys' track event injuries occurred in the hurdles category, but girls had few injuries in hurdles. There is no apparent explanation for this difference in injury pattern, which cannot be explained by the variety of events alone. More than 10% of injuries to both sexes occurred during warm-up exercises.

▶ [It is difficult to understand how the authors disparage the use of oversimplified injury classification systems and then proceed to define injury in this study as ". . . a traumatic medical condition resulting from athletic participation that necessitates removal from practice or a competitive event and/or resulted in the missing a subsequent practice or competitive event." Also, they fail to identify the specific populations studied.—J.S.T.] ◀

Physiologic Alterations in Young Swimmers During 3 Years of Intensive Training. Previous studies of child athletes have failed

J. Sports Med. 21:179–185, June 1981.

to show whether they achieve superior function through training, or possess it before the start of training. Christian W. Zauner and Norma Y. Benson (Univ. of Florida, Gainesville) attempted to determine whether further training of highly successful young competitive swimmers would result in improvement in already above-average function. Seven female and 8 male age-group swimmers age 9–19 years participated in the study. Both groups jointly held more than 60 Florida AAU and Junior Olympic titles, all acquired during the 3-year study period. The athletes trained in the summer in twice daily sessions of 6,000–10,000 meters each, and in the winter at least 6 times a week with long yardage and weight training.

The mean maximal oxygen uptake, adjusted for size, increased significantly from year to year during the study. The physical work capacity also increased significantly from year to year when adjusted for size. Both measurements were consistently greater in the male athletes. Body surface area and forced vital capacity both increased significantly over time. Mean forced vital capacity became significantly greater than predicted in the second year of the study and remained so in the third year.

Young elite athletes exhibit progressive increases in maximal oxygen uptake and physical work capacity with continued training. Training during growth appears to be important if full potential is to be achieved. Forced vital capacity may be increased beyond that expected through prolonged intensive training in childhood. In future studies, volume-pressure curves should be recorded during training in childhood.

▶ [Considering the duration of prior intensive training, the significant increases in the size-compensated maximal oxygen uptake, in physical working capacity, and in forced vital capacity are impressive. The shortcoming of the study is the lack of a control group, and that the values for forced vital capacity, impressive as they are, are reported without size compensation.—L.J.K.] ◀

Analysis of Roller Skating Injuries. Between 1974 and 1980, the number of roller skating injuries in the United States increased annually from 50,000 to 176,000; 7 deaths were reported (table). Richard D. Ferkel, Larry L. Mai, Karlis C. Ullis, and Gerald A. M. Finerman (UCLA Center for the Health Sciences) retrospectively reviewed the records and x-ray films of 186 patients treated for roller skating-related injuries between July and December 1979.

Of the 186 patients, 44% were male and 56% were female, average age 25.3 years (range, 7–58). Injuries totaled 202, and of these 130 were fractures and 72 involved soft tissues. The upper extremity was injured in 72% of patients and the lower extremity in 26%. Most injuries involved the wrist (47%), elbow (14%), and ankle (10%). Fractures accounted for 74% of the wrist injuries, 86% involving the distal radius. Radial head fractures accounted for 65% of the elbow injuries. Most upper extremity injuries, including those of the wrist, forearm,

Am. J. Sports Med. 10:24–30, Jan.–Feb. 1982.

COMPARATIVE STUDIES OF ROLLER SKATING INJURIES

	National	Ferkel	Carmody and Scott	Schwarzman
Number of patients	176,194	186	150	100
Average age	19.3	25.3	27.5	28.1
Sex ratio (M/F)	0.39	0.79	0.66	0.59
Injury ratio (F/S)*	0.52	1.78	1.86	1.86
Regions most frequently injured	1. Distal radius + ulna 2. Radius	1. Distal radius + ulna 2. Radial head	1. Distal radius + ulna 2. Radius	1. Distal radius + ulna 2. Radial head
Deaths associated with roller skating	7	0	1	0

*F/S = percentage of fractures or dislocations/percentage of soft tissue injuries.

and elbow, were associated with reflex hyperextension of the wrist and elbow.

Lower extremity injuries tended to be more severe and required surgery more often. Of the 20 ankle injuries, 80% were fractures, 85% of which required surgery. Thus, 46% of all surgical cases involved ankle fractures. Examination of the x-ray films showed that all ankle fractures were either pronation-external rotation or rupination-external rotation injuries. Posterior malleolus fracture occurred in 75% of the incidents.

Inexperienced skaters were involved in 77% of all accidents, although injuries in experienced skaters required surgery twice as often. Female skaters were injured more frequently, but operation was required 3 times more often in males. More than 90% of the skaters did not wear protective equipment. Skaters who seldom participated in sports had a greater likelihood of being injured earlier than skaters who had a high level of sports activity. "Loss of balance" was the most frequent explanation for the injury (61%); "irregular riding surfaces" accounted for 26%, and "collisions" contributed to 11%. Supination-external rotation ankle injuries appeared to be associated with high-top rather than low-top skates.

The results indicate that the occurrence of roller skating injuries is influenced by skating experience, surface texture, skate type, and whether protective equipment is worn. Differences between data from the National Electronic Injury Surveillance System and local studies suggest that the latter may be biased by the types of injuries seen and by the nature of the injury surveillance.

▶ [This retrospective report on UCLA's experience with roller skating-related injuries is very timely in light of the increase in number of participants in this activity, and dramatic increase in injuries.

One important point is worth repeating: 90% of the injured wore no protective gear. Of the seven deaths in skating since 1973, one was due to a pulmonary embolus, two were due to myocardial infarction, and four resulted from head injury. The importance of protecting the head cannot be overemphasized.—J.S.T.] ◀

Roller Skaters—More and More Frequent in the Emergency Ambulance: A First Analysis of Injuries From This Fashionable Sport is reported by G. Pfaff and A. Meinel (Univ. of Heidelberg). The many technical improvements of roller skates increased the speed and the risks of this popular sport. Five years ago, when the first medical analyses of skateboard accidents were made, only brief reports were available concerning roller skating injuries. The American National Electronic Injury Surveillance System (NEISS) reported 95,103 injured roller skaters in 1979, a number that has more than doubled since 1974. At the Surgical University Hospital in Heidelberg, 78 patients were seen with injuries that followed roller skating accidents during the first 6 months of 1980. This marks a 7-fold increase compared with 1978 figures.

A total of 119 roller skating injuries were evaluated. There was a

Chirurg. 52:178–181, March 1981.

wide span of ages, with the youngest patient being 5 years of age and the oldest 38 years old. Accidents occured most frequently in the age group between 10 and 14 years. Most of the injured persons were female skaters. More than half the injuries were fractures, about one fourth contusions, and the rest were dislocations, wounds, and luxations. Most frequently observed were injuries of the upper extremity (67.7%). This predominance is even more impressive among the group of fractures, about 90%, with 80% occurring in the forearm and wrist. The authors attribute this pattern of distribution to the fact that roller skaters tend to protect themselves with their forearms when falling. Unlike the skateboard rider, the roller skater is fastened to the skate and cannot jump off when threatened by a sudden fall.

Most patients were treated on an ambulatory basis; about 9% needed hospitalization from 2 to 15 days. Protective clothing prevents soft tissue lesions, but roller skating, like any other sport, has to be learned.

Skateboarding Fractures. Richard W. Hawkins and E. Dennis Lyne (Henry Ford Hosp., Detroit) retrospectively analyzed the clinical records of 49 patients with 50 fractures sustained while skateboarding and evaluated the results of a follow-up questionnaire. The follow-up period ranged from 3 to 24 months.

The patients were aged 2–40 years, average 14 years. Of the 50 fractures, 38 occurred in the upper extremity, with fracture of the distal radius occurring in approximately 50%; there was no predilection for the dominant hand. Six of the 12 fractures in the lower extremity were in the ankle. There were no compound fractures. Three fractures required surgical treatment. Of the 37 patients who returned the questionnaire, 25 reported full recovery from their fracture. Fourteen had been skateboarding for less than 6 months at the time of injury; 5 patients were injured during their first time on a skateboard. Loss of balance was the most frequently cited mechanism of injury (35%), followed by striking an irregularity in the riding surface (32%). Four (11%) patients reported equipment failure to be a factor in the injury, although this appeared to be the result of maintenance failure rather than design failure. At the time of injury, 24 patients were wearing tennis shoes, 12 were wearing no protective clothing, 7 wore a helmet, 7 wore knee or elbow pads, and 5 wore the full complement of protective equipment.

▶ [In their introduction, the authors cite a 1977 Consumers Product Safety Commission report regarding skateboard injuries. However, the more recent 1980 report shows skateboard injuries were down to one fifth of their 1977 peak and that roller skating injuries far exceeded the high seen in skateboarding (Ferkel, R.D. et al.: *Am. J. Sports Med.* 10:24–30, 1982). There are many similarities in the epidemiology and the injury prevention recommendations of these two activities.—J.S.T.] ◀

Urban Cowboy Syndrome is described by Stephen B. Seager, Leonora Jui-Aenlle, and Nelson Faux (Phoenix, Ariz.). Since its origin at a Houston bar and its publicity in a hit movie, mechanical bull

Am. J. Sports Med. 9:99–102, Mar.–Apr. 1981.
Ann. Emerg. Med. 10:252–253, May 1981.

riding has become a very popular pastime. All 20 patients discussed here presented with 3 findings in common: orthopedic problems, either fractures, contusions, or sprains; no previous bull-riding experience; and consumption of a significant amount of alcohol.

Of the 20 patients, 13 were men and 7 women. The women were aged 22–50 years, and the men were aged 19–49 years. Only 1 had any previous bull-riding experience. The most common injuries were joint sprains of the wrist, elbow, ankle, or knee. Fractures of the rib, wrist, thumb, or lumbar vertebrae were seen in 6 patients. Contusions alone were seen in 3 persons, and a laceration was the chief complaint in 1.

The injuries from mechanical bulls can be divided into 3 categories. The bucking of the bull produces 3 directions of force. There is an up-and-down "bucking" action, as well as a side-to-side rotation and a front-to-back undulation meant to simulate the transfer of the animal's weight from front to hind legs. There is a control to monitor the speed. Some form of padding covers the floor surrounding the bull. One hand is placed in a grip attached to the front end of the bull.

Most injuries occur to those who are thrown off the bull, from contact with the floor. In this group, 8 persons were injured in this manner. Another group sustained injuries from tangling with the bull while falling. Hand injuries were common in this group. The third group hit the bull with parts of the body as they were thrown off. Four patients were injured without actually being thrown off; 2 sustained sprains and 2 suffered fairly severe compression fractures of lumbar vertebrae.

Patrons of mechanical bull devices should be aware that serious injuries can occur. However, given the popularity of this form of entertainment, it is likely that these injuries will continue to be seen until the fad runs its course.

▶ [Along with turf-toe and joggers' nipple, the urban cowboy syndrome can hardly be considered one of the important sports medicine syndromes. However, since a case of quadriplegia has been associated with the riding of a mechanical bull, the matter should be taken seriously. It should be noted that none of the twenty patients injured in this series had previous bull-riding experience, and they had consumed a significant amount of alcohol.—J.S.T.] ◀

Neck Pain, Headache, and Loss of Equilibrium After Athletic Injury in a 15-Year-Old Boy. Although considered to be a congenital lesion, developmental os odontoideum has been reported in 9 patients. Radiographically, this lesion appears as a small corticated ossicle in close continuity with the anterior arch of the atlas, which is separated from the base of the odontoid by a variable distance. This leaves the atlantoaxial joint susceptible to structural instability. Donald L. Roback (St. Luke Hosp., Pasadena, Calif.) reports a case of os odontoideum that occurred in a boy after athletic injury.

Boy, 15, experienced diffuse neck pain, severe headache, and loss of equilibrium 2 days after a flexion injury of the neck that was sustained when he

JAMA 245:963–964, Mar. 6, 1981.

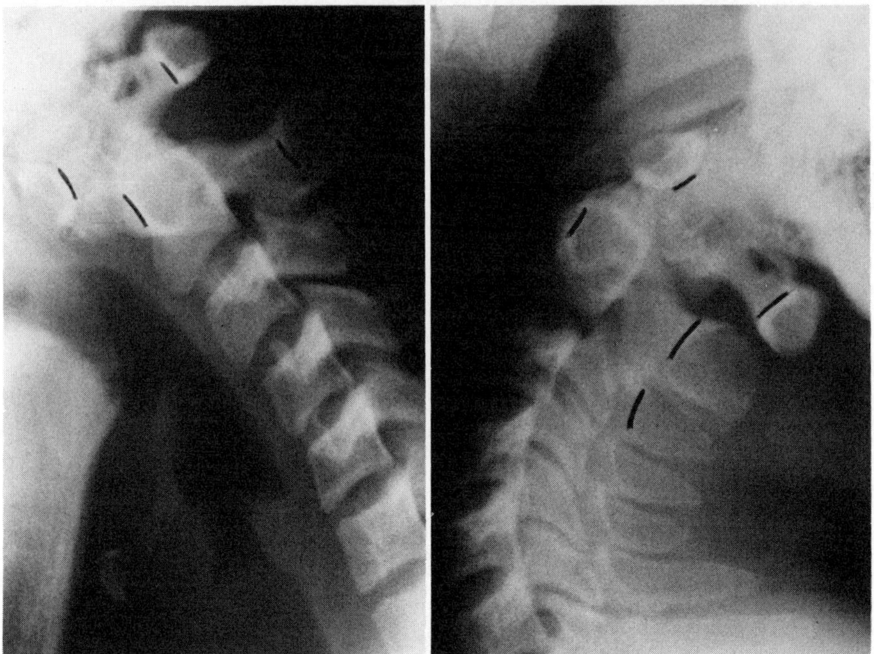

Fig 45.—Anterior and posterior dislocation at the atlantoaxial joint in boy, 15, with os odontoideum that followed trauma. (Courtesy of Roback, D. L.: JAMA 245:963–964, Mar. 6, 1981.)

was struck from behind while playing football. The patient had no history of neurologic illness and denied experiencing radicular pain, blurring vision, double vision, weakness, numbness, or difficulties with speech or memory. Physical examination revealed moderate tenderness over the posterior spine in the C2–C3 region, and paraspinal muscle spasm was present over the upper cervical region. Otherwise, neurologic findings were normal. Voluntary flexion and extension views demonstrated a 1-cm anterior and posterior dislocation at the atlantoaxial joint (Fig 45). After the patient was stabilized in a neck brace, he underwent a posterior cervical fusion that was tolerated well. The postoperative course was uneventful.

It is recommended that when os odontoideum is suspected, the examination include tomography and, if possible, voluntary flexion and extension views to determine if excess motion is present. Os odontoideum should not be regarded as an incidental finding after trauma but as a potential cause of severe neurologic dysfunction.

▶ [As the author has noted, "The accepted management of unstable or symptomatic os odontoideum is generally agreed on as posterior fusion. Controversy exists as to the management of stable os odontoideum."—J.S.T.] ◀

Conservative Treatment of Tennis Elbow is discussed by Robert P. Nirschl and Janet Sobel (Virginia Sports Medicine Inst.). Confu-

---

Physician Sportsmed. 9:43–54, June 1981.

sion about the pathology and treatment of tennis elbow is common. It is a form of tendinitis that may be lateral, medial, or posterior. The authors refer to the pathologic tendon changes in tennis elbow as "fibroangiomatous hyperplasia," which is also present in other forms of tendinitis. The key element in healing is the change of the immature fibroangiomatous hyperplasia to the mature form. The best chance for healing occurs after the initial injury.

The basic treatment of tennis elbow includes relief of pain and inflammation, promotion of healing, exercises to strengthen the arm, correction of the stress that originally caused the problem, and surgery if conservative treatment fails.

Ice and rest are important in reducing pain and inflammation. Total immobilization is not recommended, but activities that cause pain must be eliminated. If symptoms occur only with the backhand stroke, the patient need not stop playing tennis completely. Anti-inflammatory medications are helpful but must be tailored to the patient's needs. Cortisone injections should be used sparingly because multiple intratendinous injections result in tendon atrophy or dissolution. The cortisone is not injected directly into the tendon.

The criteria for healing include absence of pain without medication, full return of flexibility, and full return of strength and endurance. The process depends on the natural healing capacity of the patient. High-voltage galvanic stimulation has been used for its analgesic effect and to stimulate healing.

Progressive controlled exercise is also important. Exercise is difficult to monitor, but monitoring strength is a more objective measurement. Grip testing with a hand dynamometer is useful for recreational athletes and Cybex testing for competitive athletes. Exercise should be daily and monitored periodically. Healing is indicated by return to normal strength, endurance, and flexibility and by control of inflammation.

Once the patient has recovered, it is important to eliminate the overload forces that initially caused the injury. This can be accomplished by using a counterforce brace, modifying the player's technique, and modifying the equipment.

Conservative treatment was successful in 92% of the patients treated by the senior author. Those for whom surgery was necessary had the following clinical characteristics: technique that emphasized excessive forearm use, chronic pain in the other arm and shoulders, intense pain during activity and at night, short-term response to cortisone, lack of tissue resistance to cortisone injection, aggravation of symptoms by high-voltage galvanic stimulation, and no relief with counterforce bracing. Surgery improved symptoms in 97% of these patients.

▶ [This article is a basic primer dealing with the pathology, treatment, and prevention of this common problem. However, the authors have failed to elaborate on the appropriate exercise regimen which is so important in the management of tennis elbow.—J.S.T.] ◀

Stress Fractures Through the Distal Femoral Epiphysis in Athletes: A Previously Unreported Entity. Richard W. Godshall, Carl A. Hansen, and David C. Rising (Sellersville, Penn.) report 2 cases of this previously undescribed condition. Both patients were male; 1 was black and 1 was white.

CASE 1.—Youth, 15, had vague pain in the left knee area centered mostly in the area of the distal femur. In the past 2 months he had undertaken an extensive physical fitness program involving long periods of running. About 1 month after training began, he started to have pain, particularly while running, which subsided shortly thereafter. There was no injury, swelling, or giving way. Despite pain, he continued his fitness program, but the pain gradually became so severe that he could no longer run. The only physical finding was circumferential pain on deep palpation over the distal femur. Widening and loss of the normal architecture of the distal femoral epiphyseal line was seen radiologically. He was instructed to use crutches for 4 weeks and was kept from running and jumping for 12 weeks. The fracture healed without long-term complications.

CASE 2.—Youth, 14, had had intermittent pain in the right knee for several months, mainly after running. He played junior high school basketball also. Initially, the symptoms subsided after the event. Later, they lasted 6–12 hours beyond the game. Palpation elicited slight pain over the lateral aspect of the distal femoral epiphysis. Roentgenographic findings are shown in Figure 46. He was placed on crutches for 3 weeks and physical activity was limited for 3 months. Follow-up films showed complete healing.

Stress fractures of the distal femoral epiphysis should be considered in differential diagnosis of knee pain after activity in young athletes.

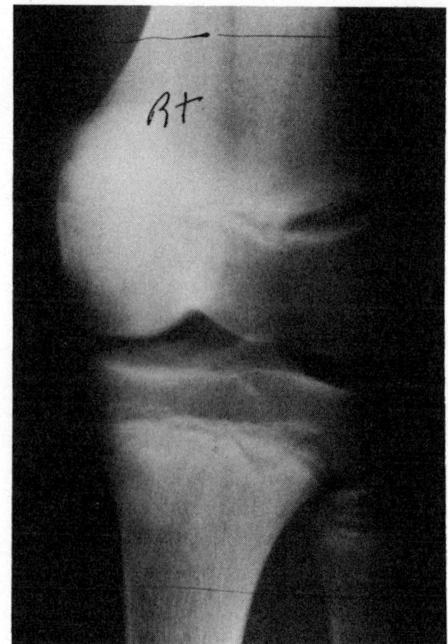

Fig 46.—Stress fracture of distal femoral epiphyseal line. (Courtesy of Godshall, R. W., et al.: Am. J. Sports Med. 9:114–116, Mar.–Apr. 1981.)

Am. J. Sports Med. 9:114–116, Mar.–Apr. 1981.

► [Observations presented in this article would have been enhanced by radionuclide bone scans, tomograms, and a more erudite roentgenographic interpretation of the films. The authors' conclusion that "failure to recognize this condition could lead to dire consequences" deserves further elaboration.—J.S.T.] ◄

Functional Versus Organic Knee Pain in Adolescents: A Pilot Study. Various investigators have found psychologic factors to be of significance in certain groups of adult orthopedic patients, particularly those with low back pain. However, little is known about the role of psychologic factors in children and adolescents with orthopedic complaints. Gregory K. Fritz, Eugene E. Bleck, and Irene Susan Dahl (Children's Hosp. at Stanford, Palo Alto) conducted a pilot study of 28 consecutive adolescents whose primary complaint was knee pain. The patients completed the Junior-Senior High School Personality Questionnaire (HSPQ), and information on other variables was obtained before the first orthopedic visit. Follow-up evaluation was carried out 6–8 months after the first visit.

The 19 girls and 9 boys ranged in age from 12 to 16 years, mean 14. Although many of the patients participated in athletic activities, no visit was prompted by an acute, sports-related injury. Based on a review of the case material and the orthopedic diagnosis, the patients were divided into 3 groups. Group I included 17 patients (61% of the total); this group had symptoms, physical signs, roentgenographic changes, and arthroscopic or surgical findings consistent with orthopedic damage. The 6 group II patients (21% of the total) had an ambiguous or insufficient organic etiology to account for the degree of disability present; arthroscopic findings were limited to poor patellar tracking or mild patellar chondromalacia. The 5 group III patients (18% of the total) did not have any discernible organic disease after extensive evaluation. In addition, each of the group III patients had at least 2 of the following clinical features: history of the symptom varying considerably in the telling; reports of pain dramatically out of proportion to the findings on examination; pain described with vague or diffuse adjectives; and marked evidence of emotional difficulties. These patients were considered to have functional knee pain. Of the 14 HSPQ scales, only scale 2 (group dependency vs. self-sufficiency) significantly differentiated the groups ($P < .05$). Overall, 84% of the patients with an average or greater tendency to be socially group dependent were in group I. Each of the group III patients had a score on Scale J indicative of a high degree of internal restraint. Groups II and III patients had had knee pain for 6 or more months ($P < .05$). The percentage of those who had undergone previously unsuccessful treatment for knee pain increased from 41% in group I to 50% in group II to 100% in group III. Forty-seven percent of the girls, but only 22% of the boys were in group II or III. The ability to tolerate pain and adhere to exercise regimens tended to be more common in group I patients.

The HSPQ appears to have little practical value for the clinician

Am. J. Sports Med. 9:247–249, July–Aug. 1981.

attempting to assess the functional component of a complaint in an adolescent. Further studies involving larger populations of highly athletic adolescents are needed to understand and differentiate orthopedic pathology and psychopathology.

Surgical Procedure for Osgood-Schlatter Lesion. The Osgood-Schlatter lesion (OSL), caused by traumatic separation of part of the cartilaginous apophysis of the proximal tibial epiphysis by stresses occurring at the insertion of the patellar tendon, usually heals spontaneously; however, the prolonged reduction in physical activity necessary in affected young persons may cause them considerable frustration and emotional disruption. These patients often are intent on sports or strenuous activities such as ballet. Andrew G. King and G. Blundell-Jones evaluated the simple procedure advocated by Dunkerly in 66 of 78 patients operated on between 1967 and 1978, who had 77 knees treated. Symptoms were present for a mean of 13.3 months before surgery.

The procedure is illustrated in Figure 47. After the fragment is dissected from tendinous attachments, the split tendon is united with a single suture. The separated fragment should be removed in 1 piece with minimal trauma. The patient is allowed to bear weight when he can perform a good quadriceps contraction. Patients with unilateral involvement returned to full athletic activity after a mean of 3.8 months and bilaterally affected patients after 6 months. Sixteen patients had a lump at the operative site. Nine had some discomfort on kneeling, and 3 had a scar or numbness. The only disabling symptom was locking of the knee in 1 patient; this was found to be due to a coexisting meniscal tear. There were no relapses.

Many active young persons with the OSL can avoid prolonged withdrawal from athletic and strenuous social activities and repeated periods of immobilization by undergoing this operation. The procedure appears to relieve pain and permits an early return to full activity without relapse. The operation is considered for severely affected young persons who are intent on sports activities and in patients whose symptoms recur after prolonged conservative management.

▶ [The Osgood-Schlatter lesion (OSL) can be categorized into three separate forms distinguished by the appearance of a lateral roentgenogram of the knee. A roentgenogram of grade I OSL appears normal, particularly the appearance of the tibial tubercle apophysis. Actually, this form represents an insertional patellar tendinitis. Grade II OSL appears as an irregular, sclerotic proximal tibial apophysis and probably represents a form of osteochondrosis at the site of the insertion of the patellar tendon. Grade III OSL is characterized by the presence of an intertendinous ossicle that is easily recognized on roentgenograms.

The surgical procedure described in this article is effective for dealing with the grade III OSL. In those youngsters with marked symptomatology who have not responded to conservative management, extirpation of the intertendinous ossicle affords total relief of pain.

It is questionable that 30% of youngsters with OSL require surgery (Migal, M. A., et al.: *J. Bone Joint Surg.* [Am] 62–A:732–739, 1980). Although the authors state OSL, ". . . is caused by traumatic separation of a portion of the cartilaginous apophysis

Am. J. Sports Med. 9:250–253, July–Aug. 1981.

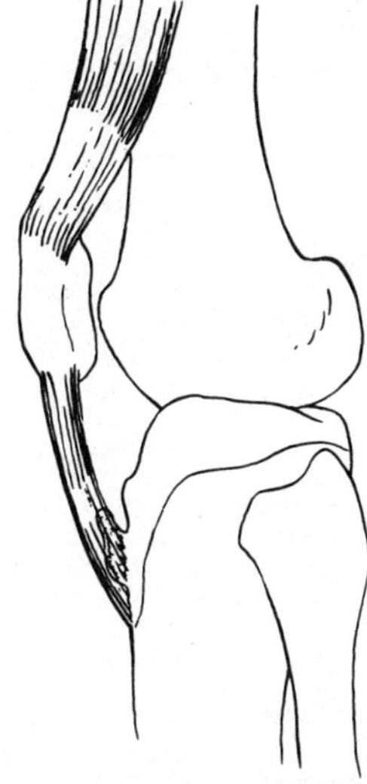

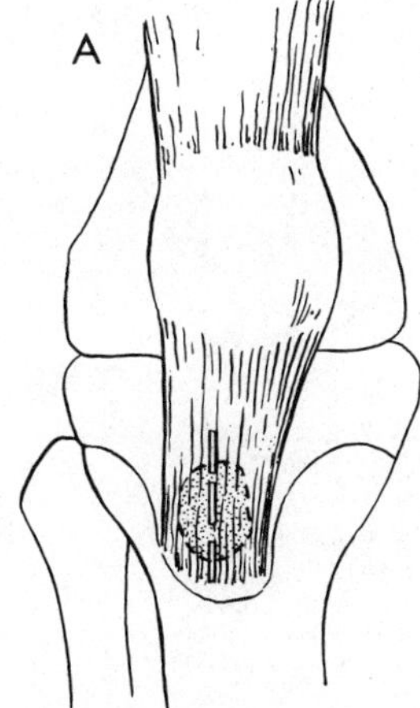

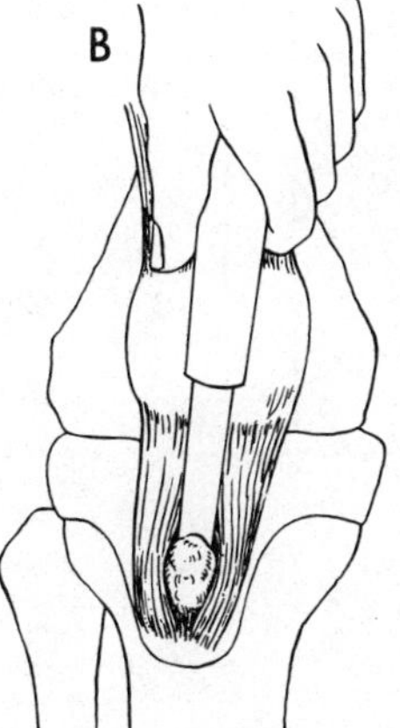

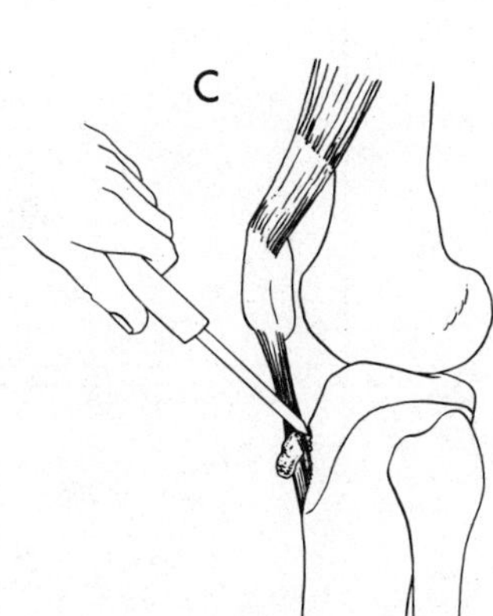

Fig 47 (left).—Soft tissue defect seen proximal to right patella; **below,** ossicle is removed by splitting tendon and excising only attachment of ossicle to underlying apophysis.

(Courtesy of King, A. G., and Blundell-Jones, G.: Am. J. Sports Med. 9:250–253, July–Aug. 1981.)

of the proximal tibial epiphysis" and OSL ". . . usually heals spontaneously," no documentation of either statement is provided.

As stated, in those youngsters with a symptomatic intertendinous ossicle, the procedure is quite effective. Essentially, with surgery, the youngster trades pain and a lump for a scar and a lump.—J.S.T.] ◄

Problems in Diagnosis and Treatment of Ankle Injuries. Frederick W. Reckling, Gerald R. McNamara, and Arthur A. DeSmet (Univ. of Kansas) reviewed the records of 371 patients treated for ankle fractures between 1965 and 1979. Evaluation was made of findings in 92 patients with 93 fractures after an average follow-up of 11 months. The classification system used is illustrated in the chart. A fifth type of injury, the pronation-dorsiflexion or pilon fracture, in-

J. Trauma 21:943–950, November 1981.

CLASSIFICATION OF ANKLE INJURIES*

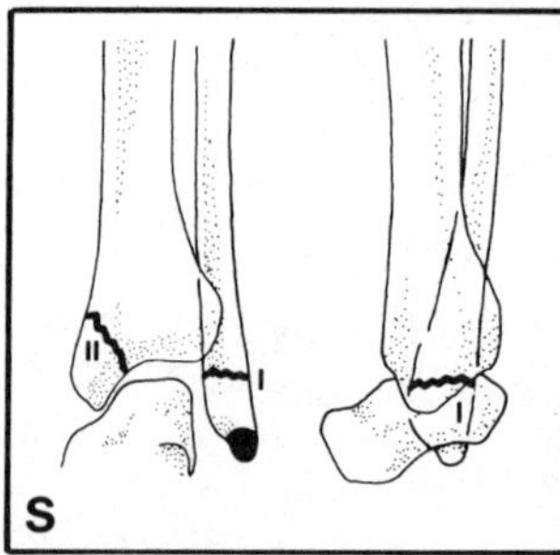

SUPINATION FRACTURE (S)

STAGE I. *transverse fracture of lateral malleolus*
II. vertical fracture of medial malleolus

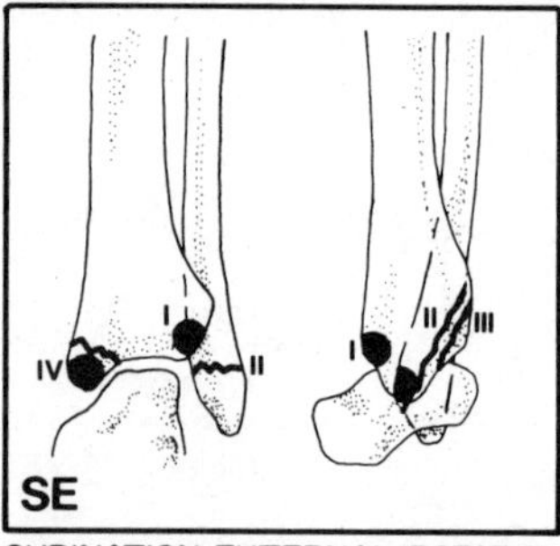

SUPINATION-EXTERNAL-ROTATION FRACTURE (SE)

STAGE I. avulsion of anterior tibio-fibular ligament
II. *oblique fracture of lateral malleolus*
III. fracture of posterior tibial margin
IV. fracture of medial malleolus

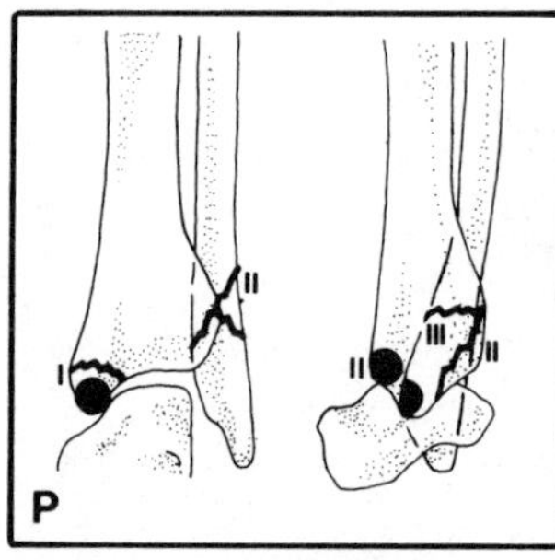

PRONATION FRACTURE (P)

STAGE I. fracture of medial malleolus
II. avulsion of anterior and posterior tibio-fibular ligaments and fracture of posterior tibial margin
III. *bending fracture of lateral malleolus*

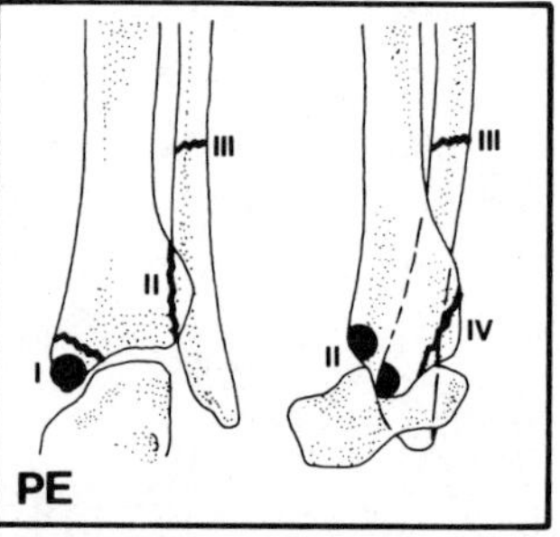

PRONATION-EXTERNAL-ROTATION FRACTURE (PE)

STAGE I. fracture of medial malleolus
II. rupture of all syndesmotic ligaments
III. *fracture of fibular shaft*
IV. fracture of posterior tibial margin

*Laüge-Hansen classification as modified by Burwell and Charnley.

cludes less common injuries, e.g., anterior marginal fractures and certain injuries of the lower third of the tibial shaft involving the ankle.

The 1 stage I supination injury was managed by closed reduction, and 1 stage II fracture was treated by screw fixation of the medial malleolus and plate fixation of the fibular fracture; the outcome was good in both patients. Treatment of 2 stage III pronation fractures by anatomic reduction and fixation of the fibula with a semitubular plate and repair of the ruptured deltoid ligament gave good results. Most stage II supination-external rotation injuries were managed by closed reduction and a short leg plaster dressing; 7 of 8 such patients had good results. Twenty-nine of 33 stage IV supination-external rotation injuries were treated by open reduction and internal fixation or ligamentous repair. All 15 patients having screw fixation or tension band wiring of the medial malleolus and plate fixation of the fibular fracture had a good result. Three of 5 patients having plate fixation of the fibula and repair of the deltoid ligament had good results, as did 3 of 4 having screw fixation of the medial malleolus only. Screw fixation of the medial malleolus and plate fixation of the fibula gave good results in patients with stage III pronation-external rotation lesions. All 6 pronation-dorsiflexion lesions were treated by open methods. Twenty-three Dupuytren's fractures were encountered in this series. Twelve of 15 patients had good results when treated by accurate anatomic reduction of the fibular fracture, application of a semitubular plate, insertion of a fibulotibial transfixion screw through the plate, and repair of the deltoid ligament or internal fixation of the medial malleolar fracture.

In difficult ankle injuries, more anatomic reduction generally gives better results regardless of the method of repair. A fibulotibial transfixion screw is necessary when severe diastasis of the tibiofibular syndesmosis is present, but it cannot substitute for accurate reduction of the fibula at its anatomical length. Pilon fractures are best managed by open reduction with restoration of the articular surface and internal fixation with supplemental bone grafting.

▶ [This article makes two important points. First, "The extent of involvement of the articular surface of the tibia as seen on the original postinjury roentgenogram correlated closely with the extent of subsequent ankle arthrosis." Also, "The second most important prognostic feature was recognition or failure to recognize rupture of the distal tibiofibular syndesmosis, its reduction, and maintenance of reduction until complete healing had occurred."—J.S.T.] ◀

Osteoid Osteoma of the Ankle in an Athlete. Evaluation of pain of the lower extremity in the young athlete can be difficult, especially if the pain is periarticular. If the patient is a male athlete between 10 and 20 years of age and thigh or leg pain occurs predominantly at night, osteoid osteoma should be considered. David F. Apple, Jr., and Edward C. Loughlin, Jr. (Emory Univ.) describe a case of osteoid osteoma of the ankle in a basketball player.

Boy, 14, a basketball player, presented with pain in the anterolateral aspect of the left ankle. The pain was not related to any specific traumatic event, only to the rigors of daily practice. Motion was not limited, and there was no swelling or crepitus, though there was tenderness at the joint line between the tibia and fibula. Roentgenograms were normal, and a diagnosis of chronic capsular sprain was made. The patient continued to play despite the pain. About 6 months later, he complained of continuing anterolateral pain that was made more intense by pressure on the ball of the foot. Tenderness was noted over the anterior ankle, which increased with extreme dorsiflexion. Roentgenograms revealed a radiolucent area in the anterior distal tibia (Fig 48). The patient revealed that he had experienced pain at night, which was relieved by aspirin. A diagnosis of osteoid osteoma was considered.

Am. J. Sports Med. 9:254–255, July–Aug. 198

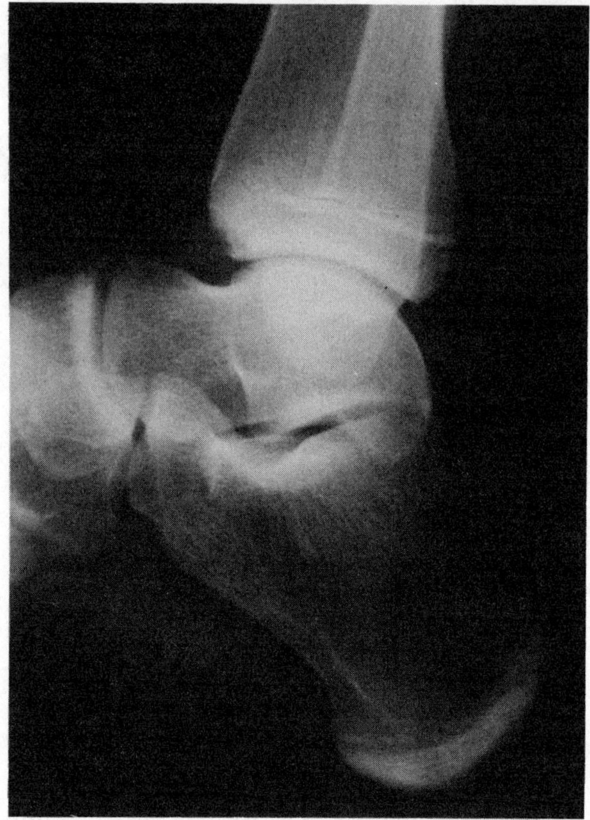

Fig 48.—Radiolucent area on anterior tibia within the joint in boy, 14, with osteoid osteoma. (Courtesy of Apple, D. F., Jr., and Loughlin, E. C., Jr.: Am. J. Sports Med. 9:254–255, July–Aug. 1981.)

Tomography revealed a lesion consistent with osteoid osteoma. Surgery was deferred until aspirin was no longer effective. A bloc excision was performed, and the patient now attends college and plays intramural basketball without complaint.

The growing frequency of joint injuries in athletes increases the possibility of misdiagnosis. It is suggested that tomography and scintigraphy may lead to an earlier diagnosis of an intra-articular osteoid osteoma.

▶ [Noteworthy is the failure of the authors to present histologic substantiation of the clinical diagnosis.—J.S.T.] ◀

Additional Reading

Alpert, B. S., et al.: Hemodynamic and ECG responses to exercise in children with sickle cell anemia. *Am. J. Dis. Child.* 135:362, 1981.

Balfour-Lyon, L., et al.: Relationship of exercise-induced asthma to clinical asthma in childhood. *Arch. Dis. Child.* 56:450, 1981.

Berson, B. L., et al.: Epidemiologic study of squash injuries. *Am. J. Sports Med.* 9:103, 1981.

Bohlmann, J. T.: Injuries in competitive cycling. *Physician Sportsmed.* 9:117, 1981.

Bundgaard, A., et al.: Importance of ventilation in exercise-induced asthma. *Allergy* 36:385, 1981.

Canale, S. T., et al.: A chronicle of injuries of an American intercollegiate football team. *Am. J. Sports Med.* 9:384, 1981.

Clement, D. B., et al.: Survey of overuse running injuries. *Physician Sportsmed.* 9:47, 1981.

D'Alessio, D. J., et al.: Study of the proportions of swimmers among well controls and children with enterovirus-like illness shedding or not shedding an enterovirus. *Am. J. Epidemiol.* 113:533, 1981.

Dressendorfer, R. H., et al.: Development of pseudoanemia in marathon runners during a 20-day road race. *J.A.M.A.* 246:1215, 1981.

Dujardin, C., et al.: Treatment of severe fractures of the lower end of the radius by Ledoux's bipolar pin method. *Ann. Orthop. Ouest.* 13:71, 1981.

Gangitano, R., et al.: Volleyball injuries: Clinical and statistical findings. *Ital. J. Sports Traumatol.* 3:31, 1981.

Goldberg, B., et al.: Preparticipation sports assessment: An objective evaluation. *Pediatrics* 66:736, 1980.

Grana, W. A., and Rashkin, A.: Pitcher's elbow in adolescents. *Am. J. Sports Med.* 8:333, 1980.

Hang, Y.-S.: Tardy ulnar neuritis in Little League baseball player. *Am. J. Sports Med.* 9:244, 1981.

Hixson, E. G.: Injury patterns in cross-country skiing. *Physician Sportsmed.* 9:45, 1981.

Jaffin, B.: An epidemiologic study of ski injuries: Vail, Colorado. *Mt. Sinai J. Med. (N.Y.)* 48:353, 1981.

Koiwai, E. K.: Fatalities associated with judo. *Physician Sportsmed.* 9:61, 1981.

Lewis, J., et al.: Exercise-induced urticaria, angioedema, and anaphylactoid episodes. *J. Allergy Clin. Immunol.* 68:432, 1981.

Mackie, J. W., and Webster, J. A.: Deep vein thrombosis in marathon runners. *Physician Sportsmed.* 9:91, 1981.

Malpass, C. A., Jr., et al.: Waterslide injuries. *Ann. Emerg. Med.* 10:360, 1981.

Marcus, N. A., et al.: Hot air ballooning injuries. *Am. J. Sports Med.* 9:318, 1981.

Pavlov, H., et al.: Nonunion of olecranon epiphysis: Two cases in adolescent baseball pitchers. *AJR* 136:819, 1981.

Routson, G. W., and Gingras, M.: Surgical treatment of tennis elbow. *Orthopedics* 4:769, 1981.

Weiler-Ravell, D., and Godfrey, S.: Do exercise- and antigen-induced asthma utilize the same pathways? Antigen provocation in patients rendered refractory to exercise-induced asthma. *J. Allergy Clin. Immunol.* 67:391, 1981.

Williams, A. F.: When motor vehicles hit joggers: Analysis of 60 cases. *Public Health Rep.* 96:448, 1981.

Miscellaneous

A lumper lumps, a splitter splits, and some things fall between.

The nice thing about having a miscellaneous section is that any articles that don't quite fit elsewhere are guaranteed a home. In general this section covers topics which may not be specific for adolescents and young adults but are very important in delivering health care. For example, the articles on prostaglandins, interferons, and drug fever cover all ages, but information acquired from them is applicable to this age group.

The Prostaglandins. Peter M. Olley and Flavio Coceani (Hosp. for Sick Children, Toronto) discuss the prostaglandins (PGs), 20-carbon unsaturated fatty acids whose structure comprises a cyclopentane ring with two aliphatic side chains. Each PG if designated by a letter dependent on its cyclopentane substituents and a subscript numeral indicating the number of carbon-to-carbon double bonds in the side chains. The thromboxanes differ from the PGs in having an oxane ring structure.

Prostaglandins are biosynthesized from dihomo-γ-linolenic acid (eicosatrienoic acid, results in the "1" series of PGs) and arachidonic acid (eicosatetranoic acid, precursor of the "2" series), which are both derived from the essential dietary fatty acid, linoleic acid; the "3" series of PGs is biosynthesized from eicosapentanoic acid. Prostaglandins have been found in all mammalian tissues studied; they are not stored preformed but are synthesized and released as required. Arachidonic acid is split from cell membrane phospholipids by phospholipase A_2, and once released may be transformed via one of three pathways (Fig 49). The finding that leukotriene C is identical to slow-reacting substance A raises the possibility that pathways 2 and 3 may equal or exceed in importance the cyclooxygenase pathway; the term "PG system" may not be appropriate to indicate the entire group of active substances derived from arachidonic acid, and the alternative term "eicosanoids" has been proposed. Conversion of arachidonic acid to the endoperoxides by cyclooxygenase is inhibited by nonsteroidal anti-inflammatory drugs, e.g., aspirin and indomethacin; lipoxygenase pathways are not blocked. Imidazole and benzydamine hydrochloride interfere with thromboxane synthesis. Steroids and quinacrine hydrochloride also interfere with PG formation.

It is highly probable that arachidonic acid metabolites are involved in the pathogenesis of inflammation, pain, and fever. Patency of the

Am. J. Dis. Child. 134:688–696, July 1980.

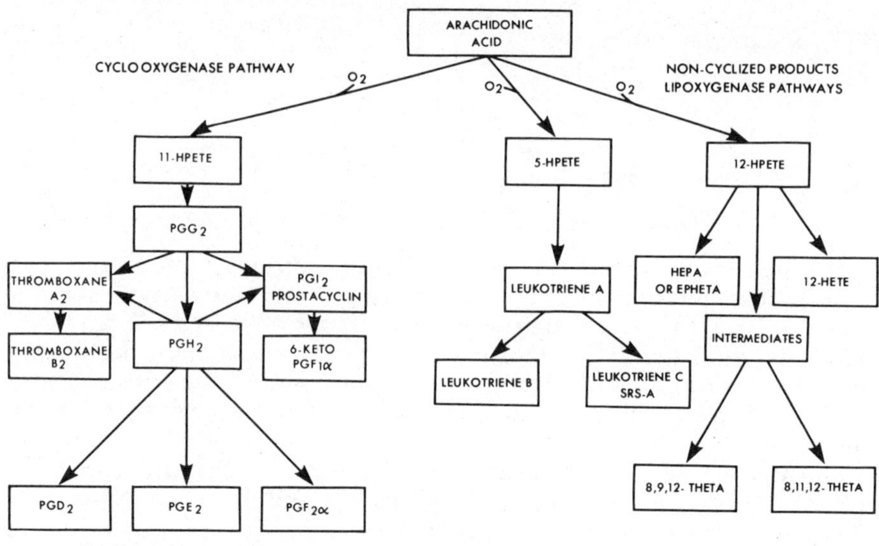

Fig 49.—Transformation of arachidonic acid by three pathways, *PG*, prostaglandin; *11-HPETE*, 11-hydroperoxy-5,8,12,14-eicosatetranoic acid; *5-HPETE*, 5-hydroperoxy-6,8,11,14-eicosatetranoic acid; *12-HPETE*, 12-hydroperoxy-5,8,10,14-eicosatetranoic acid; *12-HETE*, 12-hydroxy-5,8,10,14-eicosatetranoic acid; *HEPA*, 10-hydroxy-11,12-epoxy-5,8,14-eicosatrienoic acid; *8,9,12-THETA*, 8,9,12-trihydroxy-5,10,14-eicosatrienoic acid; *8,11,12-THETA*, 8,11,12-trihydroxy-5,9,14-eicosatrienoic acid; *SRS-A*, slow-reacting substance A. (Courtesy of Olley, P. M., and Coceani, F.: Am. J. Dis. Child. 134:688–696, July 1980; copyright 1980, American Medical Association.)

fetal ductus arteriosus is regarded as sustained by continuous intramural production of PG. Prostaglandins can act locally on pulmonary vascular smooth muscle; their action is influenced by the level of oxygenation or baseline vascular tone. The effects of PGs on pulmonary vessels are paralleled by their effects on bronchomotor tone. Exogenous PGs contract the human uterus by direct action on myometrial cells. Thromboxane A_2, which has a strongly proaggregatory action on platelets, is also a potent arterial vasoconstrictor. Prostaglandin I_2 has a strong antiaggregatory action on platelets and is a powerful vasodilator. Aspirin irreversibly inactivates platelet cyclooxygenase by acetylation of active sites, thereby preventing thrombane A_2 formation; dipyridamole potentiates the action of PGI_2 on platelets by inhibition of phosphodiesterase. Increased production of $PGF_{2\alpha}$ (a pulmonary vasoconstrictor and bronchoconstrictor) from linoleic acid occurs in children with cystic fibrosis. Also, increased PG synthesis has been found in children with diabetes mellitus and may be related to vascular complications. Overproduction of E-type PGs has been proposed to explain the pathogenesis of Bartter's syndrome.

▶ [These ubiquitous substances play important roles in such fundamental defenses as pain, inflammation, and fever. The elucidation of their structure and metabolic pathways is an achievement of the first rank. The therapeutic potential of various prostaglandins (PG) and their homologues is great, although only in its beginning phases of application. Prostaglandin E_2 has been used effectively for inducing labor, whereas other PGs have been used for inducing abortion (*Prostaglandins* 18:162, 1979). Prostaglandin synthetase inhibitors, such as indomethacin have been used to prevent premature labor. Indomethacin and other inhibitors of PG synthesis (excepting aspirin) are useful for treating dysmenorrhea (*Science* 205:175, 1979). When patency of the ductus arteriosus is needed to sustain circulation in patients with multiple congenital cardiac defects, PGE has been useful. On the other hand, when the ductus arteriosus fails to close normally, indomethacin has been used successfully in lieu of surgery (*N. Engl. J. Med.* 295:530, 1976). The vasodilating effects of PG have been used for treating chronic ischemic foot ulcers and painful ulcerations associated with Raynaud's disease. Prostaglandin E compounds are bronchodilating and possibly may be useful for treating bronchial asthma. Hypertensive patients have responded to infusions of PGE or PGA_1 with reduction of arterial pressure to normal levels without compromise of renal blood flow or of sodium or potassium excretion (*Ann. Intern. Med.* 74:703, 1981). Prostaglandin E compounds are thought to protect the gastric mucosa, by increasing secretion of gastric mucus and bicarbonate and decreasing secretion of gastric acid (*Adv. Prostaglandin Thromboxane Res.* 2:529, 1976). Thus, these compounds may be useful not only for treating spontaneously occurring acid-peptic disease, but also that induced by chronic treatment with large doses of anti-inflammatory drugs. The anti-inflammatory action of many compounds is now known to be related to the ability to inhibit PG synthesis. We shall be hearing a great deal more about these most important substances.—L.E.H.] ◄

Clinical Status of Interferons: Will Their Promise Be Kept?

William E. Stewart II (Meml. Sloan-Kettering Cancer Center) discusses the clinical status of interferon, the "hottest" medical topic since antibiotics. Interferon is a natural cell product, nontoxic, yet possessing strong antiviral activity.

The present definition of an interferon (a somewhat arbitrary one) is any cellular protein that can induce nonspecific virus resistance in cells by mechanisms involving cellular RNA synthesis. The first rough classification of interferons included three species: leukocyte, fibroblast, and immune or type 2. These three species are at present called "alpha," "beta," and "gamma." All interferon molecules thus far characterized are of almost identical length—either 165 or 166 amino acid residues. Interferons can be made almost anywhere in the body (after injection of a virus into the organism). In an oversimplification, the alpha interferons seem to be produced primarily by the B lymphocytes, the gammas by the T lymphocytes, and the betas by the body's solid tissues.

Potential clinical applications of interferon include its use as a virus inhibitor and cell stimulator (to produce the cell's own interferon). Interferon, depending on the dose, also can induce and block synthesis of various cellular products, both proteins and nonproteins. The virus-inhibitory effects of interferon are transient. A second clinical application of interferon is in cancer therapy, but caution is needed in this case because available clinical evidence is sparse. When interferon has been used clinically to treat tumor, patients have shown evidence of one or more of the characteristic antitumor activities of interferon. A third major clinical area in which interferon can be expected to be valuable is in immunosuppression. In high doses, inter-

Hosp. Pract. 16:97–105, May 1981.

feron can suppress certain immune reactions and thereby prolong graft survival in experimental animals. There is also evidence that interferon may prove useful in promoting wound healing and as an analgesic.

The side effects of interferon include a fever response (probably due to impurities), suppression of bone marrow, and loss of hair. A potential problem with this type of treatment deals with the peculiarities of manufactured versus native interferon. The native interferons appear to differ from the manufactured product in a few amino acids, but these differences are not yet known to be biologically significant.

It is concluded that, even if interferon fulfills only half of its present clinical promise, its development will mark a major advance in medicine.

▶ [The increased availability of interferons due to their manufacture by recombinant DNA techniques will soon make possible the numerous clinical trials that will provide the ultimate assessment of their value in clinical medicine. A good summary has been published of the clinical trials on interferons until relatively recently (*Br. Med. J.* 1:1558, 1980). Virtually all studies up to that time used interferons as a prophylaxis against viral disease, as a treatment for established acute viral illness, or as a treatment for chronic virus infection. Many years will pass before interferons become available for treating common colds.—L.E.H.] ◀

Drug Fever is discussed by Benjamin A. Lipsky and Jan V. Hirschmann (Univ. of Washington). Adverse drug reactions occur in about 10% of hospitalized patients and 2.5% of outpatients receiving drugs. Fever is the sole or most prominent clinical feature in about 3% to 5% of these reactions (table). Elevated temperature from administration occurs during or shortly after a drug is given. Certain drugs like bleomycin and amphotericin B regularly induce fever in a large proportion of recipients by unknown mechanisms apparently unrelated to exogenous pyrogens. Occasionally the pharmacologic ef-

TYPES OF DRUG FEVER

Administration related
    Exogenous pyrogens of microorganisms
    "Pyrogenic effects"
    Injection-induced inflammation
Pharmacologic action
    Therapeutic reaction
    Tissue injury
Direct alteration of thermoregulation
    CNS stimulation
    Peripheral effects
        Increased metabolic rate
        Peripheral vasoconstriction
        Decreased sweating
Idiosyncratic susceptibility from a hereditable
    biochemical defect
Hypersensitivity
    Fever with other reactions
    Fever alone

JAMA 245:851–854, Feb. 27, 1981.

fect itself induces fever; an example is pyrexia after antibiotic therapy for spirochetal diseases. Other drugs directly alter the normal thermoregulatory mechanisms, either centrally as with amphetamines and cocaine derivatives or peripherally to increase the metabolic rate or impair heat dissipation. The most common mechanism of drug fever is probably immunologic.

Fever from drug allergy typically appears after 7 to 10 days of treatment. Fever from drug hypersensitivity appears to be more common with atopy and severe infection and in systemic lupus erythematosus. Patients often appear to be well and frequently lack tachycardia, but the range of reactions is wide. Fever from drug allergy resolves rapidly when administration of the responsible agent is stopped. Drugs cause 1% to 2% of cases of prolonged fever of unknown origin in both adults and children.

Failure to consider or exclude drug fever may lead to unnecessary diagnostic procedures and inappropriate therapy. Resolution of fever after withdrawal of a drug is strongly suggestive, but the only definitive evidence is its recurrence on reexposure to the agent. If hypersensitivity fever is suspected in patients receiving multiple drugs, the best approach is to discontinue all inessential medications and then rechallenge with each drug if the fever abates. If several essential drugs are being given, they may be stopped one at a time at 2- to 3-day intervals and a chemically unrelated substitute prescribed if possible. If a drug causing fever must be continued, corticosteroid therapy usually suppresses the fever and any accompanying manifestations. Attempts at desensitization have been largely unsuccessful.

▶ [Some frequently used drugs that commonly may cause drug fever include antihistamines, barbiturates, penicillins, methyldopa, phenytoin sodium, procainamide, quinidine sulfate, salicylates, and sulfonamides. Fever after administration of vaccines is also common.—L.E.H.] ◀

Adverse Drug Reactions Advisory Committee: Report for 1979. This committee has reported to the Australian Minister of Health on 2,686 cases of suspected adverse drug reactions during 1979. Age and sex of these patients are shown in Figure 50. A total of 701 separate drugs were listed as "suspected," an average of 1.12 drugs for each patient. Eleven drugs—trimethoprim with sulfamethoxazole, sodium diatrizoate, amoxycillin, propranolol, naproxen, ampicillin, methyldopa, labetalol, indomethacin, allopurinol, and cimetidine—accounted for 23.7% of the severe reactions. In 48 fatalities reported, it was suspected that concurrent drug therapy may have contributed to the outcome. Twenty-five episodes of possible drug interaction were reported.

With the β-adrenoreceptor blocking drugs, no pattern of adverse effects could be detected. With psychotropic drugs, the rapid tranquilization technique involving frequent administration of large doses of drug appeared to affect 2 patients who suddenly and unexpectedly

---

Med. J. Aust. 2:569–571, Nov. 15, 1980.

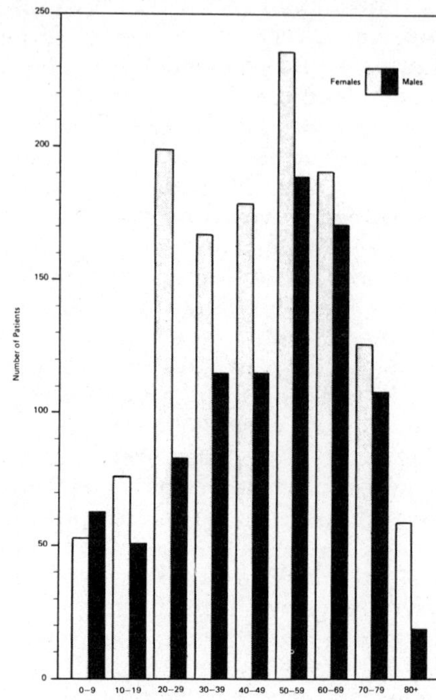

Fig 50.—Age and sex distribution of 2,198 patients who experienced a suspected adverse drug reaction (excluding 488 patients whose age and/or sex was not specified). (Courtesy of Adverse Drug Reactions Advisory Committee: Med. J. Aust.: 2:569–571, Nov. 15, 1980.)

experienced cardiopulmonary arrest while receiving haloperidol orally and parenterally. With nonsteroidal anti-inflammatory drugs, reports continue to be filed on life-threatening and occasionally fatal haematologic disorders associated with use of these drugs. Two normotensive drug addicts receiving clonidine to control opiate withdrawal symptoms suffered from faint-headedness and drowsiness while taking the clonidine. With regard to over-the-counter drugs, the committee received six reports that a pediculocide shampoo had caused severe corneal irritation when it accidentally entered the eyes. The committee also received five reports of skin reactions associated with topical use of benzoyl peroxide preparations for acne treatment, and it continues to receive reports of unanticipated hypertensive episodes associated with high doses of phenylpropanolamine (an appetite suppressant).

The Adverse Drug Reactions Advisory Committee believes that an adequate feedback of information to all health professionals is essential to its work in promoting drug safety.

▶ [A similar report is available from New Zealand (*N.Z. Med. J.* 93:194–198, 1981). Both articles emphasize the difficulty in ascertaining the event that causes attention and the drug or drugs being taken by the patient. Only slightly more than 25% of the Australian reports were considered to be certain or probable drug reactions.— L.E.H.] ◀

Transdermal Scopolamine in Prevention of Motion Sickness at Sea. N. M. Price, L. G. Schmitt, J. McGuire, J. E. Shaw, and G. Trobough (Stanford Univ.) note that use of scopolamine to prevent motion sickness is well established. They therefore examined the efficacy and side effects of scopolamine delivered by a transdermal therapeutic system (TTS) that, when placed in the postauricular area, provides controlled dosage of the drug to the systemic circulation (Fig 51).

The incidence of nausea and vomiting during use of transdermal scopolamine, oral dimenhydrinate (Dramamine), or placebo was compared in 4 double-blind clinical trials at sea. Healthy men and women, aged 16–55 years, with a history of motion sickness were randomly assigned to treatment groups. Subjects who requested it received supplemental medication during motion (200 μg of scopolamine hydrobromide intramuscularly).

Compared with placebo, transdermal scopolamine provided protection ($P = .0001$) against motion sickness. In study 2, because so few placebo users became sick, the protection provided by TTS or dimenhydrinate was not significant. In study 3, dimenhydrinate did not provide significant protection during the roughest seas. In study 4, when TTS was taken 16 hours prior to motion, it afforded the greatest protection (no one became sick.) When TTS was applied 4 hours before motion, there was some protection ($P = .04$) against motion sickness. Use of transdermal scopolamine resulted in some side effects before motion, including dry mouth, drowsiness, and blurred vision.

When administered by TTS, scopolamine protected against motion sickness at sea and induced few side effects associated with conventional dosage forms of the drug. The overall efficacy of transdermal

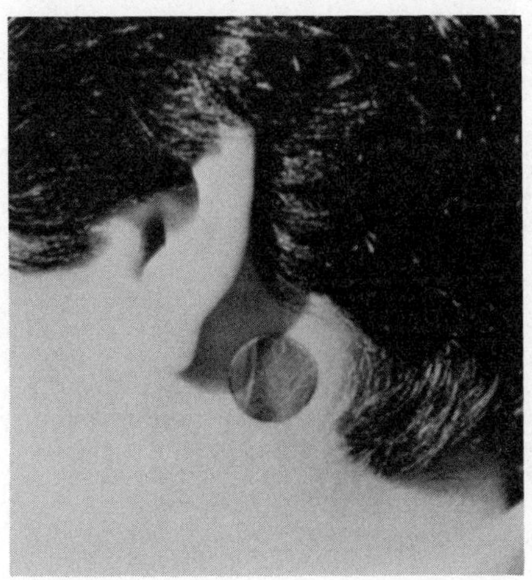

Fig 51.—Transdermal therapeutic system (TTS) in place behind the ear. (Courtesy of Price, N. M., et al.: Clin. Pharmacol. Ther. 29:414–419, March 1981.)

Clin. Pharmacol. Ther. 29:414–419, March 1981.

scopolamine in these studies reached a level of $P = .0001$ and oral dimenhydrinate a level of $P = .05$.

▶ [Scopolamine has long been recognized as the most effective preventive for motion sickness. Unfortunately, when the drug is administered systemically, side effects may be severe. It would seem, therefore, to be an ideal candidate for a specialized drug delivery system. The transdermal approach described above preserved the efficacy of the drug in preventing motion sickness, but was associated with many fewer systemic effects. Sustained low doses of drugs may be the way to go with many compounds which, while efficacious, exact too great a toll in side effects.—L.E.H.] ◀

Natural History of Childhood Asthma to Adult Life. Alfred J. Martin, Louise A. McLennan, Louis I. Landau, and Peter D. Phelan (Melbourne) studied physiologically and clinically a randomly selected group of 331 asthmatics who had started to wheeze in childhood and a control group of 77 children. They were studied prospectively from age 7 to age 21 years.

Most subjects improved during adolescence and about 55% of those whose wheezing had started before age 7 years and stopped before adolescence remained wheeze free. Forty-five percent of subjects who had apparently ceased to wheeze at age 14 years had minor recurrences of wheezing between ages 14 and 21 years. Fewer than 20% of those with persistent symptoms in childhood had become totally wheeze free during adolescence, although there was amelioration in symptoms. Girls did less well during adolescence than boys, so that there was no longer an increased preponderance of boys with increasing severity of asthma. Normal growth was achieved by subjects with all grades of asthma, despite persistence of symptoms in many. At age 21 years, patients often had features of airway obstruction during an interval phase, especially those who had more persistent symptoms.

Although the prognosis for wheezing that starts in childhood may not be as good at age 21 years as it appears at age 14 years, about half of children who start wheezing before age 7 years will be wheeze free in early adult life. Most of those with continuing symptoms are less troubled at age 21 than they were at age 14 years. As a group, children with asthma can be expected to achieve normal stature by age 21 years, even though asthma has persisted in some. Clinical and physiologic signs of airway obstruction can be found in an interval phase, especially in those with persistent wheezing during childhood and adolescence.

▶ [Pediatricians can use information such as this when attempting to arrive at some answers for parents' questions about how their children will do down the line with their asthma. There have been several studies on the same topic in recent years. The reason for this most probably reflects the fact that we are getting differing opinions as to who will and who will not do well with asthma. The British seem to be light-years ahead of us in studying this problem. The British National Child Development Study looked at a longitudinal survey of all children in England, Scotland, and Wales who were born during 1 week in March 1958 (Peckham et al.: *J. Epidemiol. Commu-*

Br. Med. J. 280:1397–1400, June 14, 1980.

nity Health 32:79, 1978). Three percent of the children had unequivocal asthma during the first 7 years of life. Of this group, 43% were still wheezing by age 11 and 7% had "wheezy bronchitis." Another 4% of children who had had no history of asthma before age 7 developed it between ages 7 and 11. In another British study, Blair (*Arch. Dis. Child.* 52:613, 1977) looked at children born between 1948 and 1952 and followed for an additional 20 years. He found that half of the group was symptom free, 21% suffered from attacks every few months, and 27% remained well only to relapse eventually. The average age of relapse in this study was 18 years. The sum impression of all these data, although the numbers differ a bit, seems to indicate that children who wheeze stand a reasonable chance of continuing to wheeze and will constitute a group of patients the internists will have to deal with. In an absolutely excellent review of this area, Kuzemko (*J. Pediatr.* 97:886, 1980) arrived at a series of conclusions related to factors affecting the prognosis of childhood asthma. I think they are well worth mentioning. He suggested that a favorable prognosis was associated with prolonged breast-feeding, allergen avoidance in early infancy, persistently negative allergy skin tests, absence of another atopic condition, and a negative family history of atopy. Unfavorable prognoses were related to artificial feeding, severe symptoms at presentation, presence of another atopic condition, history of atopy in a first-degree relative, and nasal polyps. There have been quite a few other suspected unfavorable prognostic factors. These remain questionable but include male or female sex, early age of onset, early diagnosis, poor medical care, multiple positive skin tests, removal of the tonsils, and excessive requirement for corticosteroids.—J.A.S.] ◄

Evaluation of Neck Masses. Although isolated neck masses are not commonly seen in family practice, it is important that the physician appreciate the potential complexity of this problem. Ernest A. Weymuller, Jr. (Univ. of Washington, Seattle) presents general principles to assist the physician in organizing a logical approach to the evaluation and treatment of neck masses.

Initial evaluation should attempt to differentiate between neck masses caused by acute, subacute, or chronic infection, anatomical derangement, benign tumor, or frank malignancy (table). Neck masses in children 15 years of age or younger tend to be infectious lymphadenitis or benign congenital neoplasms. From 15 to 35 years of age, the probability of lymphoma increases, although infection and benign lesions predominate. After 35 years of age, there is an increased probability of metastatic carcinoma. More than 50% of all neck masses are the result of primary thyroid disease. Excluding benign thyroid disease, 80% of adult lateral neck masses are malignant. If the mass is carcinoma of a lymph node, the probability that the primary tumor is a squamous cell carcinoma of the upper airway is 85%. In children, the most common malignant neck masses are lymphoma (54%), sarcoma (20%), and other rare tumors (26%). Regional symptoms (ears, nose, throat) related to neck masses include pain, dysphagia, hoarseness, and unilateral hearing loss, while systemic symptoms include weight loss, fever, chills, malaise, and diaphoresis. A complete history appropriate for the evaluation of neck masses would include duration, pain and tenderness, change in size, and prior history.

Most neck masses fall into the group of infectious nodes, lipomas, furuncles, and thyroid enlargement. If a mass does not respond to

J. Fam. Pract. 11:1099–1106, December 1980.

NECK MASSES BY ANATOMICAL UNIT INVOLVED AND GENERAL NATURE OF PRESENTATION

Anatomic Unit	Acute Infection and Inflammation	Subacute and Chronic Infection and Inflammation	Anatomic Derangement and Benign Tumor	Malignancy
Skin and Subcutaneous Tissues	Furuncle	Comedone	Lipoma Sebaceous cyst Dermoid cyst Thyroglossal duct cyst Branchial cleft cyst	Basal cell Squamous cell Melanoma Cutaneous metastases Teratoma
Vasculature and Deep Neck Spaces	Lateral pharyngeal space infection Carotid sheath infection Ludwig angina	Arteritis	Tortuous vessels Aneurysm Arterio-venous fistula Carotid body tumor Angiomatous tumors Paraganliomas	Hemangiopericytoma
Lymph Nodes and Lymphatics	**Bacterial** Streptococcus Staphylococcus Brucella Tularemia Diphtheria Syphilis (1° and 2°) Pasteurella **Viral** Herpes zoster Coxsackie Cytomegalovirus Measles Rubella Mumps Trachoma	**Mycobacterial** Tuberculosis Atypical **Parasites** Toxoplasmosis Leishmania **Bacterial** Leprosy Actinomycosis **Fungal** Histoplasmosis Coccidiomycosis Sporotrichosis Blastomycosis **Miscellaneous** Cat scratch Sarcoidosis Drug induced Serum sickness	Benign reactive lymphadenopathy Cystic hygroma Hamartoma	Lymphoma Metastatic carcinoma
Thyroid	Thyroiditis (viral, bacterial)	Thyroiditis (Hashimoto's radiation)	Goiter Adenoma Follicular cyst	Carcinoma Lymphoma
Parathyroid			Adenoma Cysts	Carcinoma
Larynx-Pharynx	Laryngopyocele Acute laryngeal dislocation (cricothyroid joint)	Relapsing polychondritis Gout	Laryngocele Chondroma Post traumatic asymmetry	Carcinoma
Neuro-Muscular	Masseteric hypertrophy	Myositis ossificans	Traumatic hematoma	Sarcoma

simple treatment or the initial diagnostic effort is uncertain, the patient should be referred to a competent head and neck surgeon for thorough evaluation.

Prognosis in Postural (Orthostatic) Proteinuria: 40- to 50-Year Follow-up of 6 Patients After Diagnosis by Thomas Addis. The excellent prognosis generally associated with postural proteinuria has recently come into question. David A. Rytand and Stephen Spreiter reevaluated 6 cases diagnosed by Addis 42 to 50 years ago.

N. Engl. J. Med. 305:618–621, Sept. 10, 1981.

The patients were among 54 in whom Addis had diagnosed "orthostatic albuminuria." Three patients had died of nonrenal causes without renal disease having been detected. The other 3 are alive after 42 to 45 years without proteinuria and with apparently normal renal function, although 1 initially had some severe disease with decreased renal function. Three of the 5 men had had transient urinary tract infections in the past decade.

This experience indicates that long-term survival can be expected in patients with postural proteinuria. Abnormal urinary protein was absent at late follow-up in these 6 patients. No glomerulopathy was found on microscopic study in 1 patient. The importance of urographic abnormalities in subjects with postural proteinuria remains to be established, but they probably are not important with regard to survival or persistence of proteinuria.

▶ [It is nice to have this long-term follow-up, spanning almost half a century, to reassure us about the benign nature of proteinuria, i.e., urinary protein present only in the upright position. Dr. R. R. Robinson recently confirmed this in a 20-year follow-up of military trainees in whom "fixed and reproducible" orthostatic proteinuria had been detected (*Kidney Int.* 18:395–406, 1980). The mechanism of orthostatic proteinuria probably involves a disproportionate decrease in renal plasma flow as compared to glomerular filtration rate, as a result of efferent arteriolar constriction in the upright posture. In consequence, filtration fraction rises, and the concentration of plasma albumin in glomerular capillaries is increased.—F.H.E.] ◀

Additional Reading

Chandra, R. K., et al.: Penicillin allergy: Anti-pencillin IgE antibodies and immediate hypersensitivity skin reactions employing major and minor determinants of penicillin. *Arch. Dis. Child.* 55:857, 1980.

Chipps, B. E., et al.: Diagnosis and treatment of anaphylactic reactions to Hymenoptera stings in children. *J. Pediatr.* 97:177, 1980.

Goldman, P.: Metronidazole: Proven benefits and potential risks. *Johns Hopkins Med. J.* 147:1, 1980.

Golla, J. A., et al.: An immunologic assessment of patients with anorexia nervosa. *Am. J. Clin. Nutr.* 34:2756, 1981.

Goodall, R. J. R., et al.: Relationship between asthma and gastroesophageal reflux. *Thorax* 36:116, 1981.

Greenberger, J. S., et al.: Results of treatment of 127 patients with systemic histiocytosis (Letterer-Siwe syndrome, Schüller-Christian syndrome, and multifocal eosinophilic granuloma). *Medicine (Baltimore)* 60:311, 1981.

Homcy, C. J., et al.: Ischemic heart disease in systemic lupus erythematosus in the young patient: Report of six cases. *Am. J. Cardiol.* 49:478, 1982.

Hosea, S. W., et al.: Imparied immune response of splenectomized patients to polyvalent pneumococcal vaccine. *Lancet* 1:804, 1981.

Imbach, P., et al.: High-dose intravenous gammaglobulin therapy of refractory, in particular idiopathic, thrombocytopenia in childhood. *Helv. Paediatr. Acta* 46:81, 1981.

Irwin, R. S., et al.: Chronic persistent cough in the adult: Spectrum and frequency of causes and successful outcome of specific therapy. *Am. Rev. Respir. Dis.* 123:413, 1981.

Kirsner, J. B.: Irritable bowel syndrome: Clinical review and ethical considerations. *Arch. Intern. Med.* 141:635, 1981.

Korman, M. G., et al.: Influence of smoking on healing rate of duodenal ulcer in response to cimetidine or high-dose antacid. *Gastroenterology* 80:1451, 1981.

Merrett, T. G., et al.: Screening for IgE-mediated allergy. *Allergy* 35:491, 1980.

Oster, J. R., et al.: Laxative abuse syndrome. *Am. J. Gastroenterol.* 74:451, 1980.

Pastides, H.: Iron deficiency anemia among three groups of adolescents and young adults. *Yale J. Biol. Med.* 54:265, 1981.

Rossing, T. H., et al.: Emergency therapy of asthma: Comparison of acute effects of parenteral and inhaled sympathomimetics and infused aminophylline. *Am. Rev. Respir. Dis.* 122:365, 1980.

Schwartz, A. L., et al.: Management of acute asthma in childhood: A randomized evaluation of β-adrenergic agents. *Am. J. Dis. Child.* 134:474, 1980.

Shore, A., and Ansell, B. M.: Juvenile psoriatic arthritis: An analysis of 60 cases. *J. Pediatr.* 100:529, 1982.

Strohl, K. P., et al.: Progesterone administration and progressive sleep apneas. *J.A.M.A.* 245:1230, 1981.

Subject Index

W

X

Z